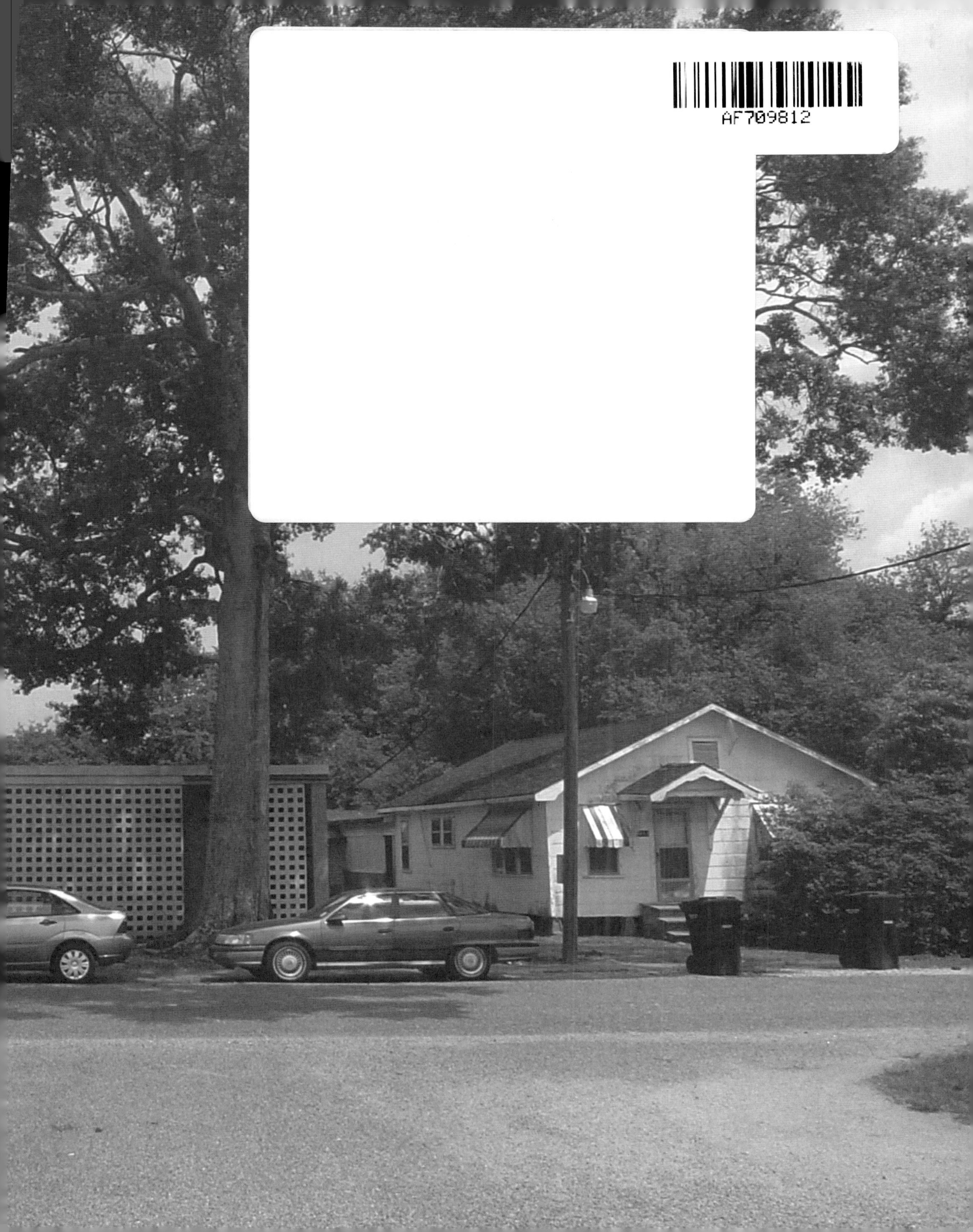

Compassion in Architecture

Compassion In Architecture

Evidence-based Design for Health in Louisiana

Stephen Verderber

Center for Louisiana Studies
Lafayette, LA
2005

Stephen Verderber is a Professor of Architecture in the School of Architecture and Adjunct Professor in the Department of Health Systems Management, at Tulane University. He is a registered architect and a founding principal of R-2ARCH, Los Angeles and New Orleans. Verderber earned a doctorate from the University of Michigan, has published widely in international journals on the subject of architecure and health, and has received numerous national awards. He is the first author of *Healthcare Architecture in an Era of Radical Transformation* (2000) and in 2005 was the recipient of the National Distinguished Professor Medal from the Association of Collegiate Schools of Architecture.

Front cover: (top) Ouachita Parish Health Unit, West Monroe; (bottom, left to right) Lafayette Parish Health Unit in Lafayette, Avoyelles Parish Health Unit (Bunkie) proposal, Jefferson Parish Health Unit in Metairie.

Back cover: (top) Beauregard Parish Health Unit in DeRidder; (bottom, left to right) Calcasieu Parish Courthouse in Lake Charles, Richland Parish Health Unit (Rayville) proposal, 1940s Mobile TB Screening Unit.

Front endsheets: Vermilion Parish Health Clinic, Abbeville, La., 1952.

Back endsheets: Lafayette Parish Health Clinic, Lafayette, La., 2002.

Center for Louisiana Studies
University of Louisiana at Lafayette
P.O. Box 40831
Lafayette, LA 70504-0831

Printed in the United States of America

ISBN: 1-887366-63-6
Library of Congress Control Number: 2005931503

Printed on acid-free paper.

http://cls.louisiana.edu

CONTENTS

August 29, 2005

In requiem

In memory of all Louisianians and Gulf Coast residents

who perished in the wrath of merciless Hurricane Katrina and her aftermath

Acknowledgments

Louisiana is a fascinating place to live and work. My experience in collaborating with people throughout the state made it possible to develop the ideas and sense of purpose embedded in this book. It is my hope that this spirit of cooperation and sustained support is at least in some small way imparted to you, the reader. Without question, this book would not have been possible without the support of the Louisiana Office of Public Health. Many thanks are owed to those dedicated individuals who work so hard, through this agency, on behalf of the people of Louisiana. I overheard a conversation some time ago between two nurses in a rural town. One nurse said, "You know, public health-care is the type of thing most people don't know they need until they actually need it." To this the other nurse replied, "I suppose, in a way, we are doing our jobs at the highest level at those times when we are most invisible to the general public." Public health services are essential to the well being of a community. The Office of Public Health provides immunizations, nutritional education for expectant and young mothers, family planning, STD screening and treatment, HIV/AIDS screening, fresh water monitoring, food and sanitation permit inspections, licensing and oversight, anti-bioterrorism rapid response programs, vital records services, treatment for chronic diseases, school-based health centers, health statistics, smoking cessation and anti-obesity health education.

In September 1990, I knew little of the inner workings of the Louisiana Office of Public Health. Assistant secretary Joel Nitzkin, Deputy Assistant Secretary Joseph Kimbrell, and Eric Baumgartner were instrumental in supporting the belief that architecture was a missing component in furthering the goals and efficacy of the agency relative to its mission. The assistant secretaries who have followed Dr. Nitzkin, to date, have been Larry Hebert, Dr. Baumgartner, Jimmy Guidry, Madeline McAndrews, and Sharon Howard. Each has supported the goal of upgrading Louisiana's public health architectural infrastructure by supporting the redevelopment of its network of public health community care facilities. Thanks to Claude Carbo, for his wisdom, wit, and introduction to the political fine points of working collaboratively with the parish police juries across the state. His "learn by doing" crash course in the political landscape in Louisiana, as it relates to public healthcare, was invaluable. Joan Bostick was instrumental in getting the program off and running. She most ably accompanied the team into the field from 1990-94. Sylvia McKee served as program liaison and field guide from 1994-96, followed by Kay Harned (1996-2002), Darlene Smith (2002-2005), and Barbara Woodard (2005-). These talented individuals have been extremely important to the success of this initiative. Nothing of consequence would have occurred without them.

Thanks to the region administrators, without whom access to the various parishes would have been next to impossible. This group consists of Joan Smith, Avis Grey, Jamie Roques, Jimmy Gum, David Thomas, Fred Duplechin, Paul Landry, Larry Richard, Tina Stefanski, H. Dohn Alexander, B.J. Foch, Jerre Perry, John Naponick, the late Billy Goins, Bille Strickland, and Steve McAdams. Various region and central office medical, nursing, and environmental health coordinators and their support staff have also been instrumental, including Shelley Coates Jones, Jerrell Mathison, Gary Peck, M.D., Bobby Savoie, Henry Bradford, Craig Peters, Larry Fox, Doris Brown, and Antoinette Lewis.

Many thanks to the dedicated professionals housed within the health units across the nine OPH regions. Their assistance and collaborative support has been essential because that is where "the rubber meets the road" with regard to architectural intervention. Space does not allow for me to thank all these persons individually. The clerks, nurses, and sanitarians employed in the various parishes are dedicated healthcare professionals. Just keep doing what you do each day, for you are the end-user occupants. The public appreciates what you do. Also, thanks to the many patients who took the time to complete surveys and post-occupancy interviews, and to the local elected officials in the parishes and statewide elected officials—you also have a difficult job. Public healthcare in Louisiana deserves your support.

A community health center is a civic building. Buildings are expensive, and the public expects a viable return on the investment of their tax dollars. A debt of gratitude is due to the many architects, contractors, and others who have applied the compendium of planning and design guidelines in their work on behalf of the Office of Public Health. Thanks to the Center for Louisiana Studies at the University of Louisiana at Lafayette, for their support in producing this book, and especially Carl A. Brasseaux, director of the center, James Wilson, the center's assistant director, and Jennifer Cooper, production director. My partner in R-2ARCH, Ben J. Refuerzohas provided of support and insight. Many, many thanks to the talented students in the Tulane School of Architecture and the young practitioners who have worked on this project since 1990. This group includes John G. Davis, David Riebe, Francisco J. Arens, Maria Ximena Blacut, Daniel Gero, Barbara Carter, Ott Gira, Chris Roth, Todd Welch, Ava Brucato, Aaron Selinger, Romy Diaz, Erin Rensink and most recently, Kevin Frank, Julia Ford, Claudia Foronda, Victoria Yee, and Jessica Gramcko. In addition, a number of Jessica Gramcko's photographs appear in the book, as does the architectural design work of Julia Ford and Claudia Foronda. Further thanks to Reed Kroloff, Dean of the Tulane University School of Architecture, and to David J. Fine, former chair of the Department of Health Systems Management at Tulane University, for their research support.

Special thanks to my two children, Alexander and Elyssa Leigh, and my wife, Kindy, and my parents, for their unwavering support. You have been patient, especially during my many sojourns crisscrossing the state, logging over 125,000 miles on the odometer along the way. And incidentally, the appetizing food in Louisiana is probably America's best. Many thanks to all the local restaurant owners who keep Louisiana's unique culinary traditions alive, provocative, and vibrant—*laissez le bon ton roulé!* This archi-cidental tourist has learned much. It is hoped that individuals and organizations near and far will in some way benefit from this book as a means to improve the everyday life of their community through architecture.

Stephen Verderber
New Orleans
August 2005

Chapter 1

Introduction

This narrative is about places—healthplaces—where individuals and families suffer from health disparities. An alternative way of making buildings is needed in order to improve these persons' quality of life. It has been said that America has become a nation whose citizens, like fish, taking no notice of the water surrounding them, pay no heed to their milieu, being neither aware of nor cognizant of the places where they live out their lives. This is a sad commentary on contemporary America, for it signifies a moral devaluation of human experience and the traditional importance of the built environment in shaping our lives. The ramifications are innumerable and continue to disproportionately affect the powerless and the marginalized. By extension, the very definition of community is being called into question in an age of instant gratification, as we immerse ourselves in a burgeoning sea of digital media. This transformative technology is increasing in sophistication to the point where real-time human experience has become unable to match its virtual counterpart.

Besides the profound influence of digital media saturation, special interests, and complex, at times conflicting, alliances perpetuate health inequalities, and these disparities manifest in the architectural environment. Taken together, these trends point to the validity of an area of research that gained considerable momentum in the late twentieth century.[1] In this field of scholarship, an effective case for studying the ordinary everyday setting in American life has been put forth. Previously neglected topics have been studied. This broad bandwidth of scholarly work ranges from the origins of post-World War II suburbia, the impact of the automobile in American history, to the ubiquity and pervasiveness of roadside vernacular architecture, to the adverse effects of globalization on rural America in the past decade. Paul Groth defines the field of cultural landscape studies as:

> The term *landscape* means more than a pleasing view of scenery. Landscape denotes the interaction of people and place: a social group and its spaces, particularly the spaces to which the group belongs and from which its members derive some part of their shared identity and meaning. All human intervention with nature can be considered as cultural landscape: the high-style cathedral or office tower, as well

> as the depression-era Hooterville hut, a farmer's barbed-wire fence, or a kitchen garden. Cultural landscape studies focus most on the history of how people have used everyday space— buildings, rooms, streets, fields, yards—to establish their identity . . . the conviction . . . is that better knowledge of ordinary environments can foster deeper understanding of American people and American culture and can lessen the environmental dangers caused by people who cannot see and interpret their surroundings.[2]

Architecture is but one ingredient within a polymorphic cultural landscape. A portrait of a given building or building type across multiple site contexts may be delineated through systematic documentation and assessment in the field. The people who inhabit places within an architectural landscape possess a wealth of verbal, visual, and spatial knowledge culled through individual experience. This knowledge manifests in a mix of archival and synchronous information. These latter types of data are obtained through surveys, interviews, visual documentation, and research methods borrowed from the social sciences. Multifaceted assemblages of data have been the heart and soul of the most fascinating work in this field to date. As such, the level of critical discourse on this topic has evolved and increased in sophistication in recent years. Cultural geographers, literary theorists, biologists, art historians, historians, social theorists, anthropologists, landscape architects, and architects have all made worthwhile contributions.[3]

Jay Appleton, a cultural geographer, extends Groth's reasoning in that this interdisciplinary field is not focused on any particular discovery, theory, breakthrough, or philosophical position, such as a cure for diabetes. It is, however, an interdisciplinary assemblage of individuals who have traditionally been connected only remotely to one another. Systematic critical inquiry in the realm of the everyday built environment is considered peripheral—whether in architecture, geography, or sociology.[4] Architecture, as a profession and academic discipline, has been no exception. The architecture of the everyday milieu, especially that of underrepresented minorities in American society, continues to receive comparatively little meaningful scholarly or professional attention.

Louisiana, with a population of 4.3 million, is a unique cultural landscape with a colorful and conflicted history. Its history is deeply rooted in Europe, the Maritime Provinces of Canada, the islands of the Caribbean, and West Africa.

The state's geography has been and continues to be a powerful determinant in the lives of its residents. In South Louisiana, roadside burial sites are common amid the state's ubiquitous wetlands and roadside settings. Any relatively dry land available will do, as the caskets must be buried above a shallow subsurface water table line (Fig. 1.1). Louisiana is bordered on the west by the Sabine River, which separates the state from Texas. Arkansas sits to the north. Much of Louisiana's north–south border with Mississippi is cut by the formidable currents of the Mississippi River as it meanders its way southward to the Gulf of Mexico. The state's southeastern region stretches eastward to Pearl River. Were it not for the continuous intervention of the U.S. Army Corps of Engineers, the Mississippi River would have altered its course several generations ago. An abrupt redirection of the river, if this should occur, would profoundly dislocate the residents of the southernmost third of the state. As it is, a complex system of manmade levees boldly hems the mighty Mississippi into its precariously balanced course.

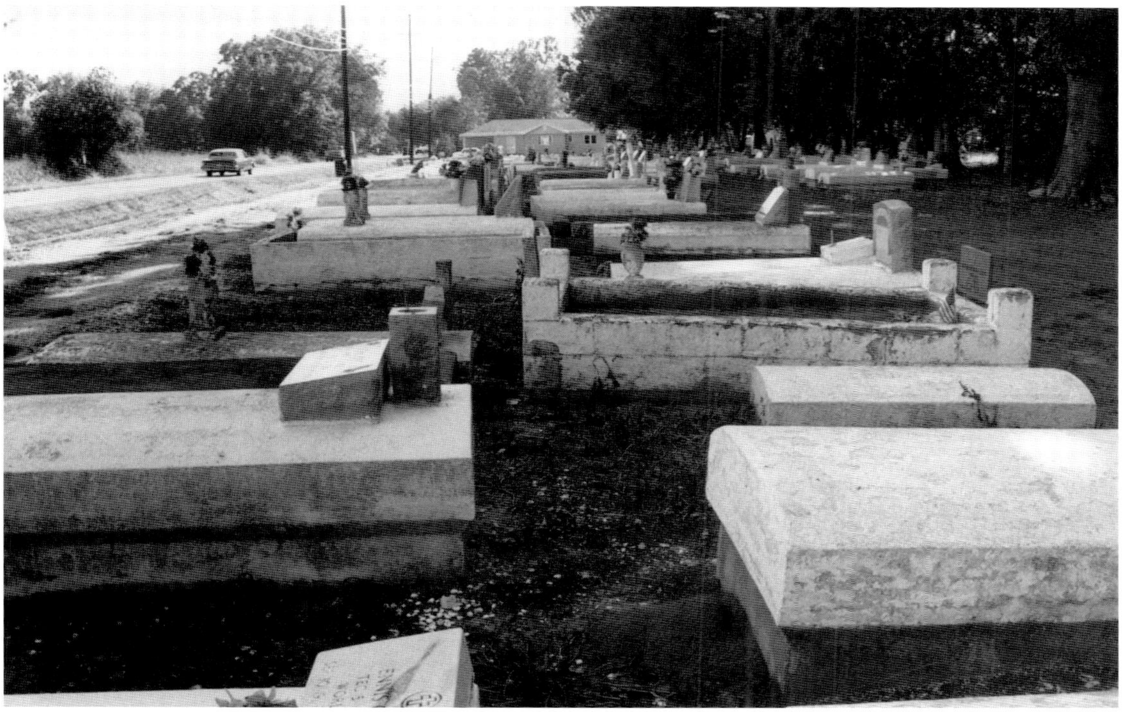

Fig. 1.1

The ubiquity of the relationship between water and the reality of everyday life sets the stage for a fascinating, if rather tenuous, balance between the forces of nature and human civilization. The threat of flooding associated with the potential catastrophic damage caused by hurricanes is constant, as these violent storms can sweep in from the Gulf of Mexico on short notice. This, combined with the deleterious effects of decades of oil and gas exploration, and the resulting land subsidence, has resulted in significant erosion along Louisiana's gulf coast. A parcel of land along the Louisiana coast roughly the size of Manhattan is lost each year to the forces of coastal erosion. This is a very serious matter for communities near the coast. Beyond matters of the physical environment, the lingering effects of generations of institutionalized racism in the South continue to warrant programs to alleviate racial discrimination. Despite these and other challenges in everyday life, Louisianans are justly proud of their physical environment and its inhabitants' unique cultural heritage.

Sometimes, a single serendipitous event can alter the course of a professional life. In the fall of 1990, this author received a phone message that read: "Please return call." When I called back the next morning, the voice on the other end began by saying "I was given your number from a friend in the School of Public Health . . . it was suggested I contact you to see if you can help us." This agency, the Louisiana Office of Public Health, had a stack of dusty surveys lying around for five years in a box thrown into a forgotten corner of a bleak office in a state office building in New Orleans. The caller, it turned out, was searching for some old memos on an unrelated topic, and unknowingly stumbled upon the forlorn surveys that had never even been read. These surveys were an inventory of all facilities in its network. Five years earlier, staff housed in the agency's parish-based care settings had dutifully filled them out, one survey per program site. But by 1990 no one seemed to know why they had ever been distributed in the first place or if anything had come of them. In 1990, by happenstance, the agency's recently appointed director, Joel Nitzkin, became curious when learning his central administration lacked any overview of its inventory of facilities, either individually or collectively. As a result of his puzzlement when he learned of the ill-fated 1985 surveys, he instructed an assistant to determine if the survey data remained relevant.

Meanwhile, Nitzkin made numerous excursions into the field and quickly learned firsthand the deplorable conditions of most of the health units. He was further puzzled as to the investment value of devoting energies to planning new community health programs and strengthening existing programs without any coordinated effort to improve the architectural infrastructure and facility management aspects of the facilities. Any significant improvement in the agency's public health programs, he reasoned, would require a thorough rethinking. The agency was burdened with an inventory of functionally obsolete buildings. The U.S. Public Health Service, with assistance from the Rockefeller Foundation, built dozens of Hill-Burton box clinics in the aftermath of the devastating Flood of 1927—with many still in use as of 1990.[5] This building evolved as a distinct type. Modernist architects in the American South applied the International style to the design of the parish health unit—the term unit borrowed from military deployment contexts. To be awarded a commission to design a parish health unit was a source of prestige, particularly in tough economic times.[6] With the network of facilities having since fallen into serious need of replacement and repair, the challenge ahead required an open mind and the suspension, as has often been said, of "one's system of disbelief."[8]

Architecture, Health, and Evidence-based Design

Architecture—the art and science of making a building—is essentially an act of optimism. Unfortunately, the profession of architecture continues to operate from a deficient knowledge base. Its disciplinary core of professional practice is particularly sparse in comparison to the health science professions from the standpoint of making use of research findings. Design decisions are too frequently based on prior quasi-educated assumptions, intuition, complacency, or an attitude of "that's just the way we've done it before." In general, as a result, it has been an uphill struggle to develop an adequate foundation of empirical data on how buildings actually influence human health and well being.[9] However, more and more practitioners in architecture for healthcare, and their clients, are just now beginning to appreciate the positive outcomes attainable from blending evidence-based research into their modus operandi. A fledging field, dubbed design therapeutics by this author, has begun to influence the planning and design of hospitals, care settings for the aged pediatric facilities, outpatient care clinics, and other healthcare building types. Only relatively recently have public health providers and health professionals, including the federal Centers for Disease Control and Prevention (CDC), and professional journals in the field of public health, made the explicit connection between the value of investing in high quality architecture, urban planning, and the role of the built environment with respect to the control and eventual abatement of chronic diseases, including heart disease and obesity. It is now an accepted fact that counter-therapeutic physical settings contribute to deleterious health outcomes in humans.[10]

The evidence-based design movement in architecture for health predated yet parallels the evidence-based medicine movement in the United States although the term "evidence-based" is borrowed to a large extent. It denotes assessment, systematic assessment. The reasoning goes something like this: If it is routine procedure for an attorney to conduct a post-trial case review, or for a physician to predict the effects of a given drug in a patient, why should an architect not be held accountable to being able to predict that the design one "prescribes" will work? In order to do this, he or she must revisit one's completed buildings to learn firsthand how things turned out. But this is seldom done systematically. In architecture, the movement over the last fifteen years to assess in order to predict outcomes has more frequently been referred to as research-based design. [11] Evidence-based research and design (EBR&D) for healthcare may therefore be defined as the systematic study of the functional needs, goals and aspirations of the occupants who live, work, and receive care in healthcare settings, with the objective of improving their well being and health status through therapeutically resonant architectural design. One underlying assumption stands out: the need is great for a substantiated, reliable knowledge base for practitioners. This application, the translation process, applies as much in architecture and its related design professions as it does in the health science

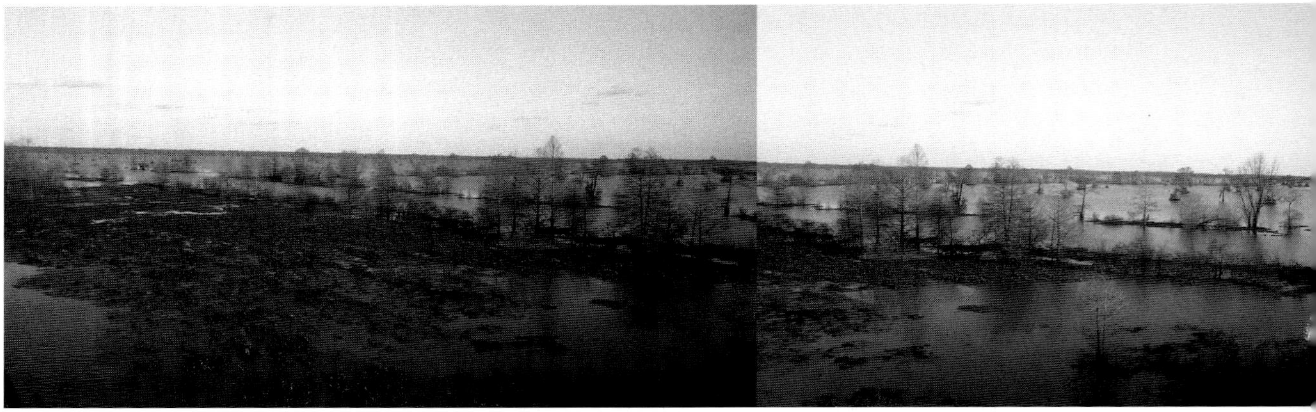

Fig. 1.2 a

professions. It is a subject that is attracting increasing international attention at this time.

With this said, telltale signs surround us in our everyday world that architects and urban planners are experiencing diminishing influence. Drive down nearly any suburban commercial strip or through any recent subdivision—sprawl has become the norm rather than the exception.[12] For the architect, the intertwined effects of myth and taste, coupled with the responsibility of providing a service to ensure "public health, safety, and welfare" has become problematic. The client unwittingly assumes the architect antecedently works in full knowledge before construction in terms of how the resultant building will actually perform in everyday use. Critics counter that architects therefore have little interest in engaging in such activities as EBR&D because this takes needed time and money away from far more pressing things, especially if the results of any such investigation are to be considered non-proprietary and thus available to anyone, including one's competitors, and especially if the findings are not to the architect's liking.

Many disciplines are required to work harmoniously in order to create a successful work of architecture. Unfortunately, in a professional landscape subdivided into myriad disciplines, sub-disciplines, and areas of consulting expertise, each domain develops in time its own "turf," intellectual traditions, and myths to protect itself from encroachment. For the architect it is no different: these behaviors function to retain control, as a defense mechanism against any outsider profession or specialist deemed by the architect as a competitor. One consequence of this syndrome is an unwillingness to collaborate in an open, unfettered, transparent manner. Collaborations tainted by fear and uncertainty are rarely productive. Useful interdisciplinary, evidence-based knowledge in

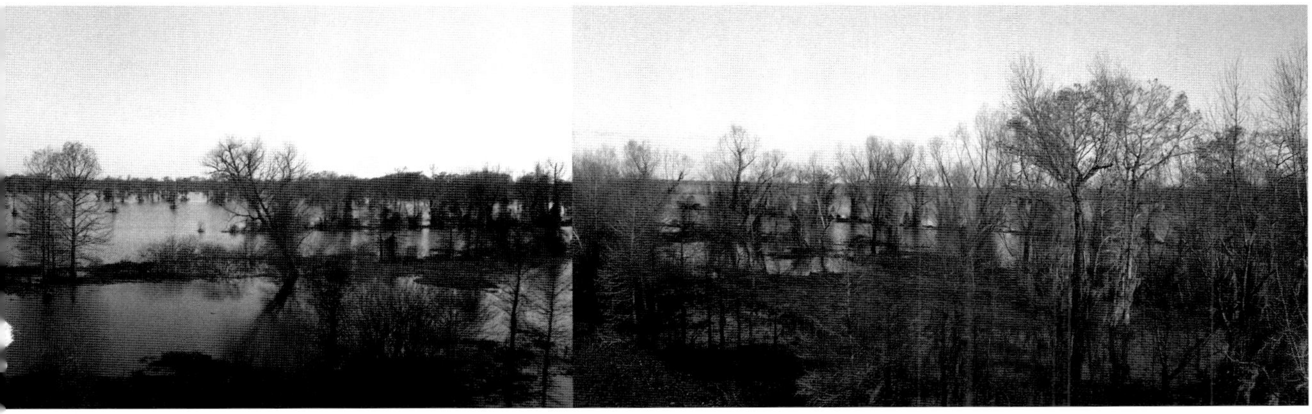

Fig. 1.2 b

day-to-day professional practice consists of research apriori (prior to, and during, design) as well as apostiori (after construction and occupancy). This broadened perspective can yield useful aesthetic and functional information from empirically validated findings.[13]

Many years ago the British architect and educator Peter Stringer called for a redefined architectural discipline premised on a solid foundation of factual knowledge.[14] This would counter the didactic relationship between architects and political power, and would, in turn, result in a far more accountable holistic paradigm, which would subsequently increase the architect's value to society. Stringer's view consisted of a synthesis of two worlds, which, by and large, function in different spheres—one, an architectural discipline, and another, an architectural profession.[15] This book is about extending beyond the traditional limits of architectural research and practice. Research and practice need not remain disconnected. More specifically, this book is about how the fields of medicine, nursing, environmental health, epidemiology, health nutrition, architecture, engineering, interior design, landscape architecture, community health, and local government are linked.[16]

A fifteen-year (and running) effort has centered on intrapreneurship—a protocol for innovatively working within and on the behalf of a government bureaucracy to achieve tangible change.[17] The community-based programs provided by the Louisiana Office of Public Health consist of family planning, immunizations, treatment for communicable diseases such as HIV/AIDS and related sexually transmitted diseases, school-based clinics, and tuberculosis, child and maternal health, and health education on such issues as domestic violence, tobacco cessation, and obesity eradication. In addition, the range of environmental health programs provided by the agency consist of water and food monitoring programs based on enforcement of the state sanitary code, and the enforcement of regulations mandated by the Louisiana Department of Environmental Quality (DEQ), as well as local jurisdictional sanitary and sewage permitting programs. The nutritional health program remained wholly dependent on the federally funded Women/Infant/Children (WIC) program. In the 1987-88 fiscal year this federal program alone provided Louisiana with $87 million in externally based funding. The WIC program provides prenatal and early childhood nutritional education and the issuance of food stamps for the purchase of milk, formula, and certain pre-approved foods. The vital records program maintained by the Louisiana Office of Public Health (OPH) is the sole state repository for all birth, death, divorce, and marriage records. The vital record offices in each region issue all vital record permits and all permanent records dating from the state's inception in the early nineteenth century. These archives are housed in central repositories in New Orleans and Baton Rouge, and offices are operated in parish health units throughout the agency's nine geographical regions. In all, four types of programs are housed at each parish health unit—clinical services, environmental health services, nutritional health services, and vital records services.

The total OPH budget for the 1990-91 fiscal year was $156.6 million. During the same period, federal funding support amounted to $89.6 million, of which, $74.5 million was the state's share of the federal WIC program. By the 2003-04 fiscal year the agency's budget had increased to $299.3 million, and WIC program funding during the 2004-05 fiscal year totaled $135 million. Despite this, the agency weathered a succession of hiring and expenditure freezes during the 1990s, and all OPH programs, as well as the WIC program, experienced cutbacks of one sort or another: the number of nurses alone shrunk by nearly 400, and some clinics were closed. As mentioned, by 2000 the total number of program sites (clinics and support facilities such as the nine administrative offices and the seven region labs) had been reduced nearly 25 percent through a combination of closures and consolidations.

Louisiana, paradoxically, is a poor state despite an abundance of physical and human resources. The southern portion of Louisiana is scenic by virtually any definition, as evidenced by this view of the Atchafalaya Basin wetlands (Fig. 1.2a-b). Although blessed with one of the nation's most captivating cultural and physical landscapes (Figs. 1.3 and 1.4),[18] the Pelican State is mired in poverty. Between 1990 and 2000, Louisiana was the nation's second poorest state in terms of per

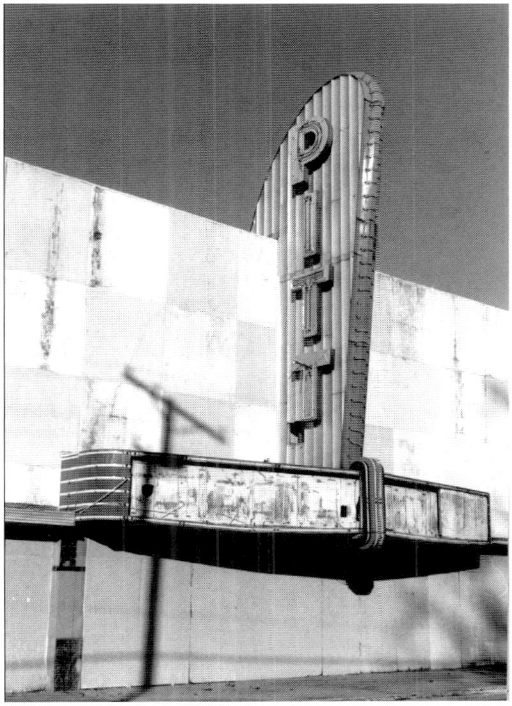

Fig. 1.3

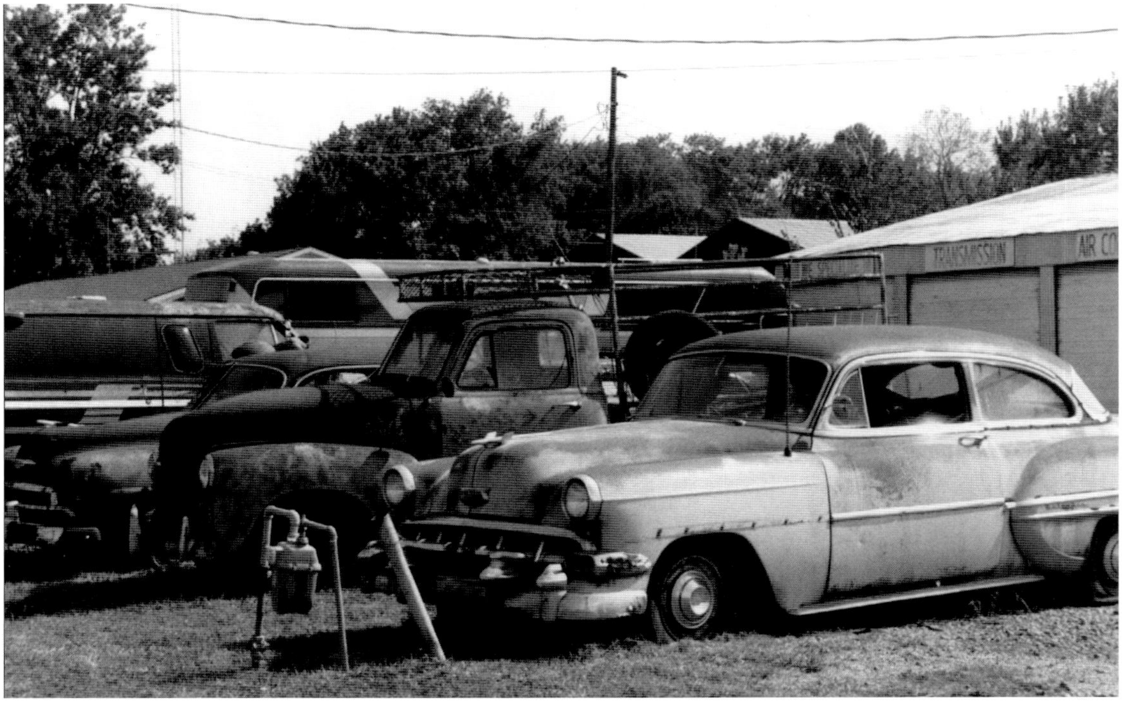

Fig. 1.4

capita income (behind New Mexico) and, indeed, the region lagged behind many developing nations in this category. In 2002, 37 percent of all Louisiana children below the age of five lived in poverty and 12.1 percent of the state's families received food stamps (as compared to the national average of 6.9 percent). It is thus hardly surprising that Louisiana's public health "report card" is poor in comparison with those of other states.[19] Louisiana's rates of cancer, cardiovascular, and diabetes-related deaths, and the state's infant mortality rate, remained significantly higher than that of the nation as a whole. A 1996 national report concluded that Louisiana was the unhealthiest state in the nation. This ranking was based on residents' high rate of smoking, obesity, violent crime, low high school graduation rate, high employment rate, low access to primary healthcare, high rate of worker disability claims, high rate of heart disease and diabetes, high rate of mortality across all segments of the population, and high rate of premature infant deaths. A similar study published in 2004 reaffirmed this ranking.[20] Making matters worse, competing political special interests clashed between the public and private sector care providers and their corresponding healthcare bureaucracies.[21] The backbone of the public health system for the uninsured poor and working poor remains nine Charity Hospitals operated by DHH and sixty-seven parish-owned, but state-run, health units.[22] The vast majority of patients are provided care at no little or no cost. Fees for services are based on a sliding scale according to one's ability to pay. Reimbursement is provided through the aforementioned combination of state and federal funds.

In 1990, 66 percent of all OPH facilities were found to have been in operation in their present building for thirty years or longer. Most of these buildings had long since passed the end of their useful lives. Obsolescence had become the rule rather than the exception in this healthcare milieu (Fig. 1.5). Despite this, the staff heroically strove to make the best of their bad situation. Often, this resulted in exam rooms with buckets strategically arranged on the floor to catch water seeping through the roof; major leaks sometimes flooded the exam rooms and shut down entire clinics (Fig. 1.6). Patients sat in hallways because there were no seats in the cramped waiting room; records in some places were stored in open view in the hallway, unlocked and unsecured (Fig. 1.7). Patients on crowded clinic days waited outside in the wind and rain, and boxes of medical records and supplies were strewed about in a seemingly random manner, often in direct violation of the State Fire Code, even in mechanical equipment rooms (Fig. 1.8). Such were the sights routinely encountered at that time. Many nurses and other clinic and clerical

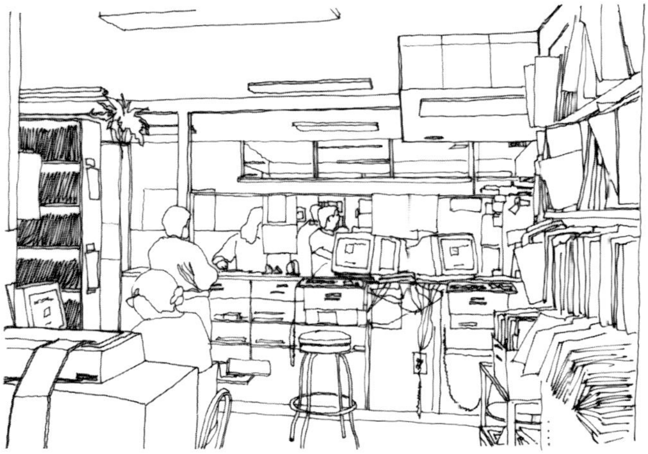

Fig. 1.5

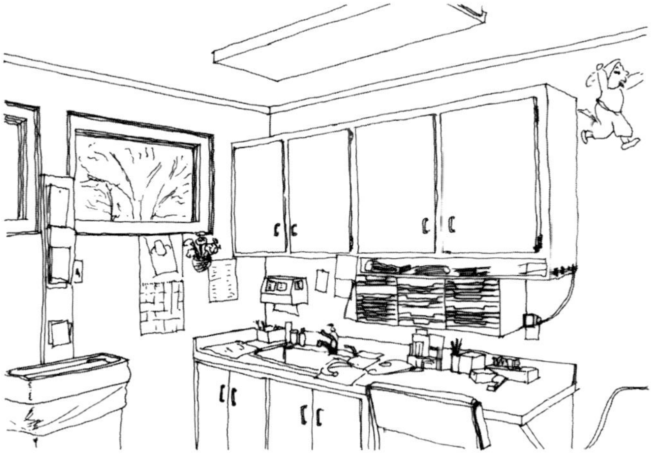

Fig. 1.6

staff had become fatalistic, with little control to influence one's physical work environment. In fact, in 1991 while visiting a clinic during the first stage of this work, a registered nurse burst into tears when asked to assess the physical state of her clinic. For the typical health unit, the playing field had become extremely uneven, with facility disparities perpetuated from the earliest facilities set up in orphaned quarters in parish courthouse basements in the 1920s (Appendix A).[23]

For the average patient, the situation may have been bad from the start, but the patients also persevered along with the staff, appreciative of the care received and the fact that it was provided at little or no charge. They frequently had no other care option. Complain they did, however, on crowded clinic days, for there was typically nowhere for them or their children to sit amid a chaotic, unsupervised waiting room containing as many as fifty infants and children. Witness the chaotic 1959 scene in the waiting room at the Madison Parish Health Unit in Tallulah (Fig. 1.9). The seats were so closely packed it would be difficult for anyone to walk between them. The children had to sit on their mothers' laps, sometimes for hours, on crowded clinic days because there was no subwaiting room to relieve the extreme overcrowding of the main waiting room. Among the most irritating persistent problems, besides sheer overcrowding, were a lack of air conditioning, making the building too hot in the summer, or, conversely, due to a malfunctioning wall or floor heater, too cold in the winter months.

Fig. 1.7

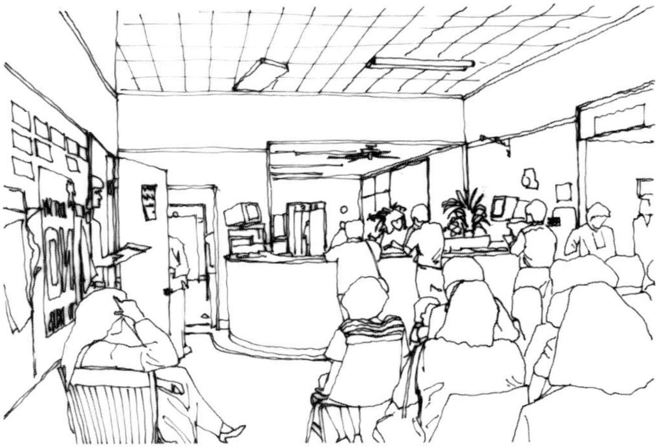

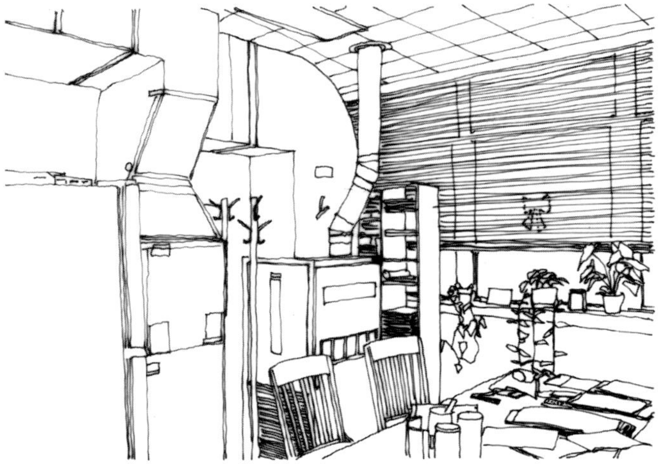

Fig. 1.8

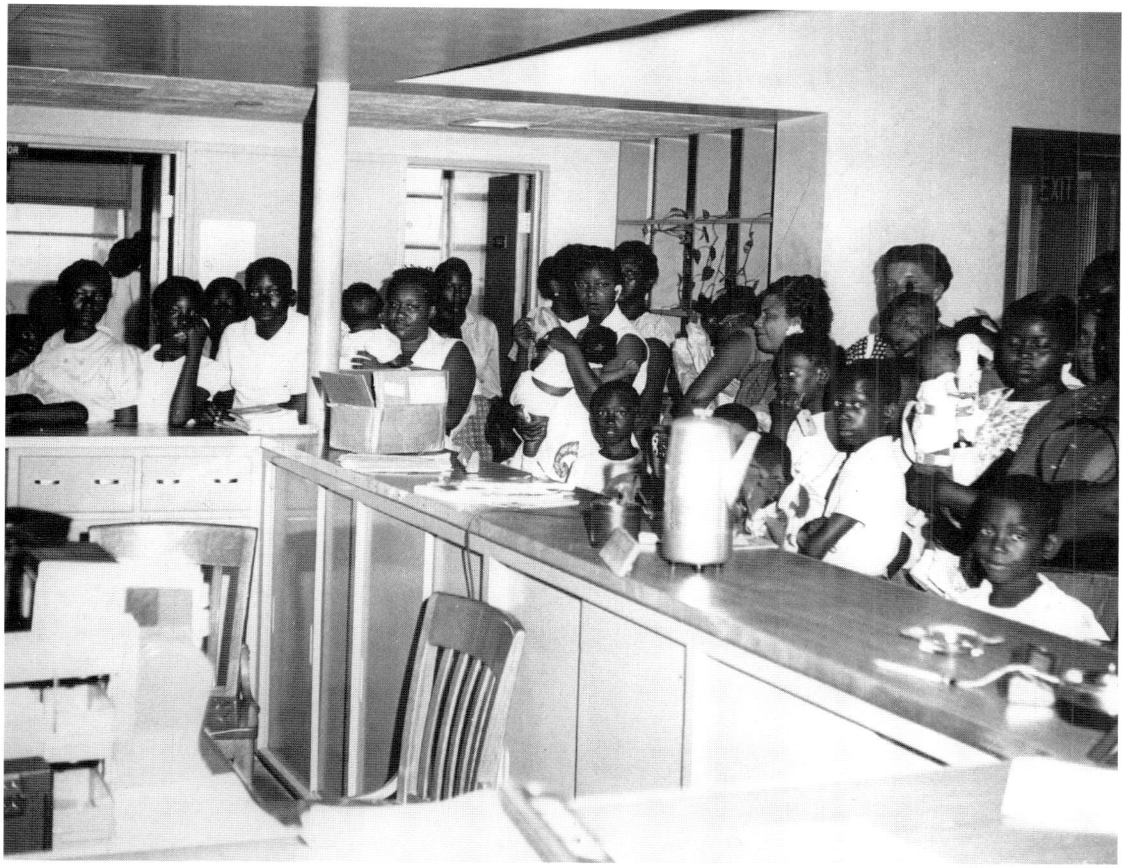

Fig. 1.9

Whenever a decision was reached by local elected officials to replace its antiquated Hill-Burton era parish health unit with a new one, the replacement facility often was exiled from Main Street to the edge of town in a "take it or leave it" scenario. In the case of Franklinton, Washington Parish, the health unit was relocated in the 1970s from a Hill-Burton International style facility in the center of town to a former bowling alley and bar. Some facilities, in other parishes, continued to operate in overcrowded former commercial storefronts on Main Street, such as in St. Joseph in Tensas Parish. Others were built on forlorn sites in desolate industrial manufacturing zones, as in the case of the Crowley facility in Acadia Parish (Fig. 1.10). And a few, remarkably, continued to operate in single family homes adapted in the 1950s or '60s into quasi-clinical facilities, such as in Farmerville, in the northern part of the state. The Tallulah health

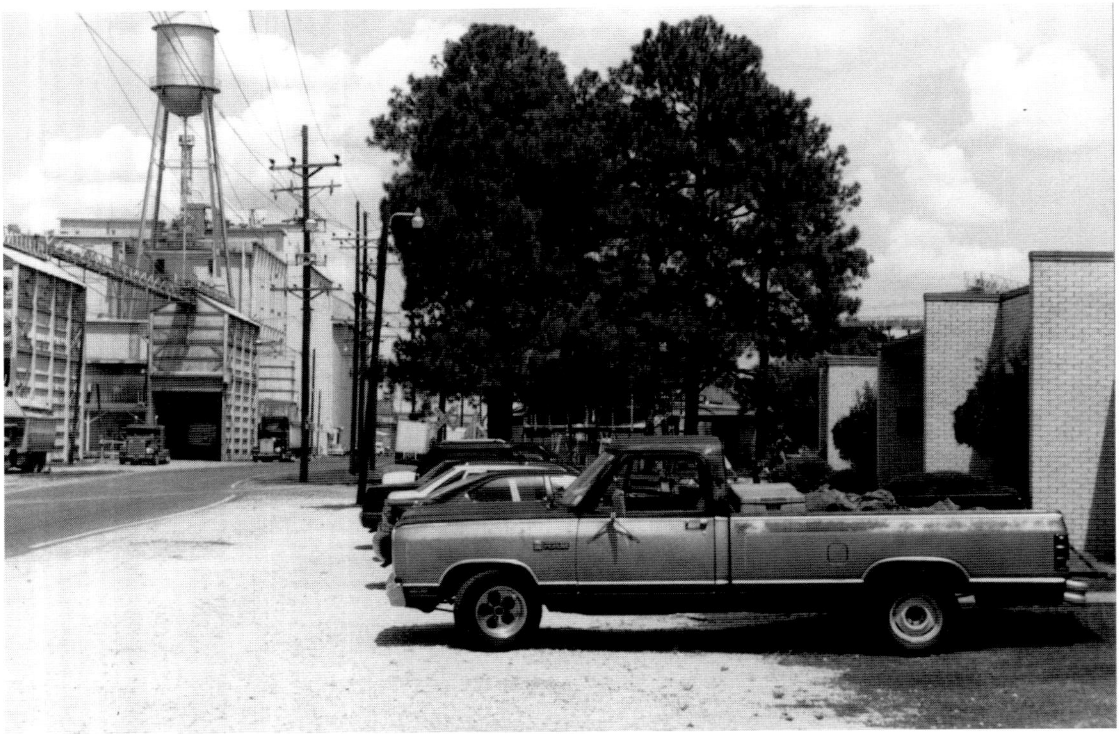

Fig. 1.10

unit's staff in Madison Parish coped at once with both the best and the worst of fates—it had been relocated to the town's stately, historic, yet poorly suited post office in the center of town. In the oldest, most obsolescent and overcrowded health units, a single room, such as an exam room, or a small kitchen for staff use, was used over the course of a day for four or more different purposes: as an exam room, then a staff meeting room, all the while in use as a supply storeroom, later in the day becoming a WIC classroom, followed by its use the next morning as the regional social worker's consultation room.

In the early 1990s, the Opelousas facility in St. Landry Parish was relocated for a year and a half to the showroom of a former new car dealership while its new clinic was being built nearby. From the street it was clear to motorists and passersby that only thin cloth curtains separated the drafty, makeshift "exam rooms," stuffed along one wall within a cavernous, drafty showroom. Suffice to say staff and patient confidentiality and privacy were nonexistent in such undignified conditions (Fig. 1.11 and Fig. 1.12). The situation at the St. Landry health unit was representative of the deplorable conditions existing throughout the system. And these conditions were exacerbated by a lack of adequate facility maintenance: when air conditioning systems or leaky roofs were repaired the work was often done in a makeshift, slipshod manner, and the problem soon reappeared (Fig. 1.13).

The Puzzle

In Louisiana, expect the unexpected in the everyday political landscape. Longtime residents understand this to be a fact of life. For generations, the reputations of various Louisiana politicians extended far beyond its borders. It can be difficult for non-Louisiana residents to comprehend this unique art form; in the 1990s alone, numerous scandals and bizarre stories were reported in the local, national, and international media.[24] Louisiana politics has a long and colorful history.[25] This legacy, combined with assertive individualism, geographic autonomy, and unusual local funding priorities, for decades functioned as an impediment to coordinated facility improvements. A state map with the parish boundary lines demarcated is analogous in this sense to an amalgamation of sixty-four distinct puzzle pieces. No two parishes, even adjoining parishes, behaved precisely the same when dealing with the same architectural, facility planning, or space management issue. In public and behind the scenes, debates on the merits of replacement versus renovation, for example, might create a political maelstrom, or, perhaps more appropriately put, place the health unit in the role of a punted pigskin in a hotly contested high school football game between two bitter rivals.[26]

The work began in 1990 with the commissioning of a five-part report. In Part I, OPH program staff completed a written survey. All 138 facilities in the care network were assessed with regard to the condition

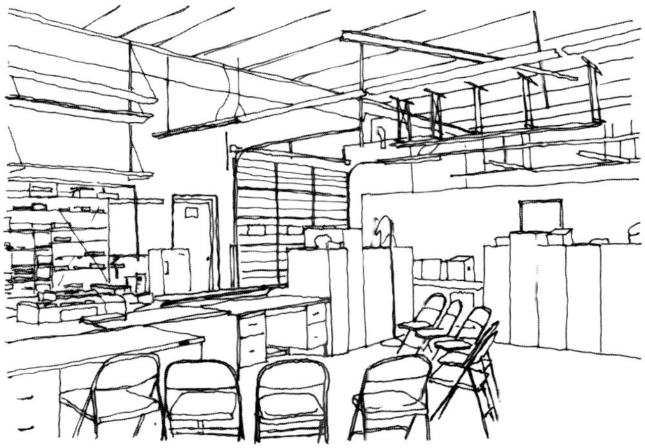

Fig. 1.11

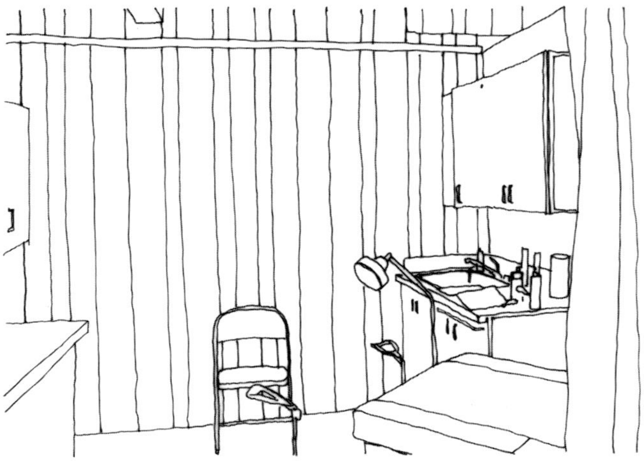

Fig. 1.12

and performance of each individual facility. Each was evaluated with regards to its aesthetic ambiance, internal patterns of occupant use, the record of maintenance and upkeep, the condition of its environmental control systems, its location within the community from the standpoint of access, and outward image. Survey respondents assessed the immediate site context, with questions addressing site security, parking, lighting, the surrounding neighborhood, and the availability of local public transportation (if any). An ad hoc architectural advisory committee of fourteen administrative staff was assembled at this time. This group provided critical input and guidance during the first year of the work and provided invaluable feedback on the compendium of 140 architectural and site-planning guidelines which were developed during the first year of the initiative (see Appendix C) amd which have since have been updated regularly.[27]

Part II reported the findings of twenty-five post-occupancy evaluations representing a cross section of the nine DHH-OPH administrative regions.[28] In Part III, the information obtained through the statewide facility survey, together with the post-occupancy evaluations, became the basis for the aforementioned compendium of planning and architectural design concepts. These concepts were developed for implementation by architects, and for use as a vehicle to elicit end user/occupant participation in all subsequent capital improvement projects (see Appendix C).[29] In Part IV, the results from Phases I-III were applied to demonstrate their amenity in the design of a speculative prototype facility for Slidell, in St. Tammany Parish. In Part V, a multi-step protocol was developed for the implementation of this participatory planning and design protocol in the field. These became the core ingredients, or tools, of what would soon be referred to as the Strategic Facility Improvement Initiative, or SFI.[30]

This protocol is rooted in organizational theory and social theory over the past forty years. Two fields—facilities management and environmental psychology—evolved from these debates. The former can be traced to the belief that the physical environment of work (extended to embrace the healthplace) via its impact in the healthcare workplace plays a significant role in the evolution of an organization. The work of Franklin Becker, among others, was rooted in the social science tradition and assumed the physical environment played a crucial role in human work processes. This concern for the "user" was not motivated solely by humanist concerns for the well being of people, but by a belief in the economic benefits of a better working environment.[31] Becker's position extended a humanist tradition in organizational theory that can be traced back to nineteenth-century industrialists such as Owen, Salt and Cadbury, who built utopian communities for their workers.[32] The growth of environmental psychology (often referred to as environment-behavior studies) in the 1970s carried these theories forward on a broader front in an attempt to introduce the behavioral sciences to the design professions.[33]

This humanist/behavioralist tradition represents but one strand of positivist, empirically-based organizational management theories.[34] Physical conditions, unless they are very good or very bad, are usually taken for granted. This anti-setting bias in organizational theory continues today in the mainstream literature. It is seen in the work of leading researchers as the relationship between the working environment and organizational creativity, although their definitions of the working "environment" do not include the physical environment, which is inexplicably considered a neutral factor.[35] This bias remains a serious limitation of the field of facility management. The field has been pushed hard to justify itself in terms of outsourcing and cost-driven measures (i.e. globalization and consolidation).[36] Its earlier focus on "user needs" and the benefits of a better person-environment "fit" that linked facilities manage-

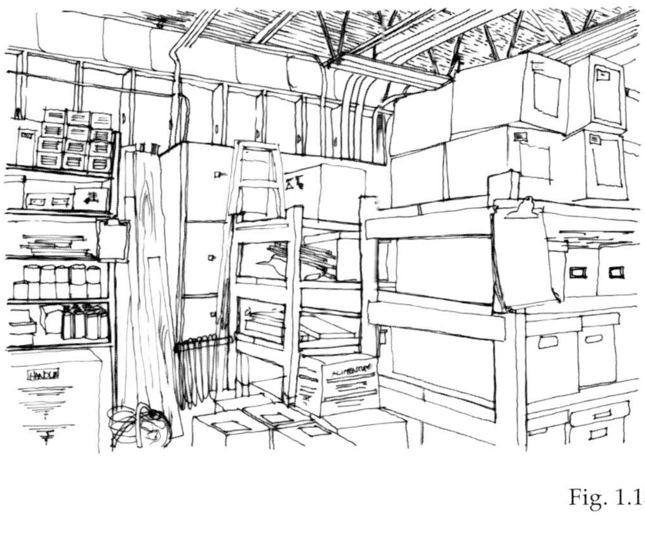

Fig. 1.13

ment via productivity to strategic facility planning became obscured, unfortunately, in favor of space (versus place) defined solely as a commodity to be bought or sold.[37] This preoccupation effectively cut out any serious concern for the role of place-making. A dispassionate view of placemaking therefore dominates the field's discourse. However, virtually all the mechanisms that govern societies center on placemaking.

Architectural humanists have recognized this insofar as buildings must not be viewed as simply props, containers or as inanimate backdrops for human habitation. Spatial syntax itself is a language onto itself.[38] Prior to being inhabited a structure is imbued with meanings reflective of its origins. Far from being passive and inanimate, space is an integral part of a dynamic social intercourse where the very configuration of space is meaningful in and of itself.[39] Architects who advocate this position come from a tradition that can be traced to the dialectical approach of Hegel and Marx. The occupation of space gives direct expression to social, economic, and political processes to deny or control its quantity and distribution. In this way, workspace/healthspace is no different from any other commodity that is expropriated. Most communities contain places of great significance, often associated with ritual.[40] In Western philosophy, the mechanisms that lead to the emplacement of some groups and the displacement of others is fundamental to striation in all societies. In the cultural landscape, place underscores the view that social change cannot happen without spatial change.[41] Traditional approaches to facility management have therefore been objective, top-down, rationalist, conservative, and rigidly functional. These same tendencies, if not carefully weighed, will also plague EBR&D if not fully taken into consideration at this time. This is discussed at some length in Chapter Six. By contrast, humanist approaches strive to express broad concern for the occupants of the workplace/healthplace. [42]

This latter view is more individualistic, subjective, and advocacy-based. It accepts the fact that a given situation will suit different people and organizations differently. This approach to attaining a balance between top-down versus bottom-up decision-making, design, evaluation, and space management is fluid and malleable.[43] Traditional rationalist and behavioral/humanist paradigms are therefore more or less diametrically opposed, as the effects of alienation, social disengagement, powerlessness, and exclusion persist as principal themes in how space, place, and human well being intersect in the architectural environment.[44] With this said, the central theme of this book is the dynamic tension between the rights of the individual citizen to freedom and self-determination, and, on the other end of the spectrum, the tendency of large healthcare bureaucracies to impose authoritative control over its constituencies.

A Rolling Stone Gathers No Moss

Consultant reports commissioned by government agencies, as is well known, frequently end up gathering dust. Once the client accepts a report and it is made public, the authors typically move on without looking back. Unfortunately this only serves to perpetuate the status quo. To counter this, four stakeholder constituencies to the success of the SFI were identified at the outset: locally elected officials, architects, engineers, and builders, health policy administrators and direct service providers, and patients/patients'-rights advocates. [45] In 1991, the five-volume report was accepted for implementation. The evidence-based design recommendations, the core of the SFI toolkit, have been implemented in forty-five projects. This is discussed at greater length in Chapter Five. New construction, renovations, and projects in planning at the

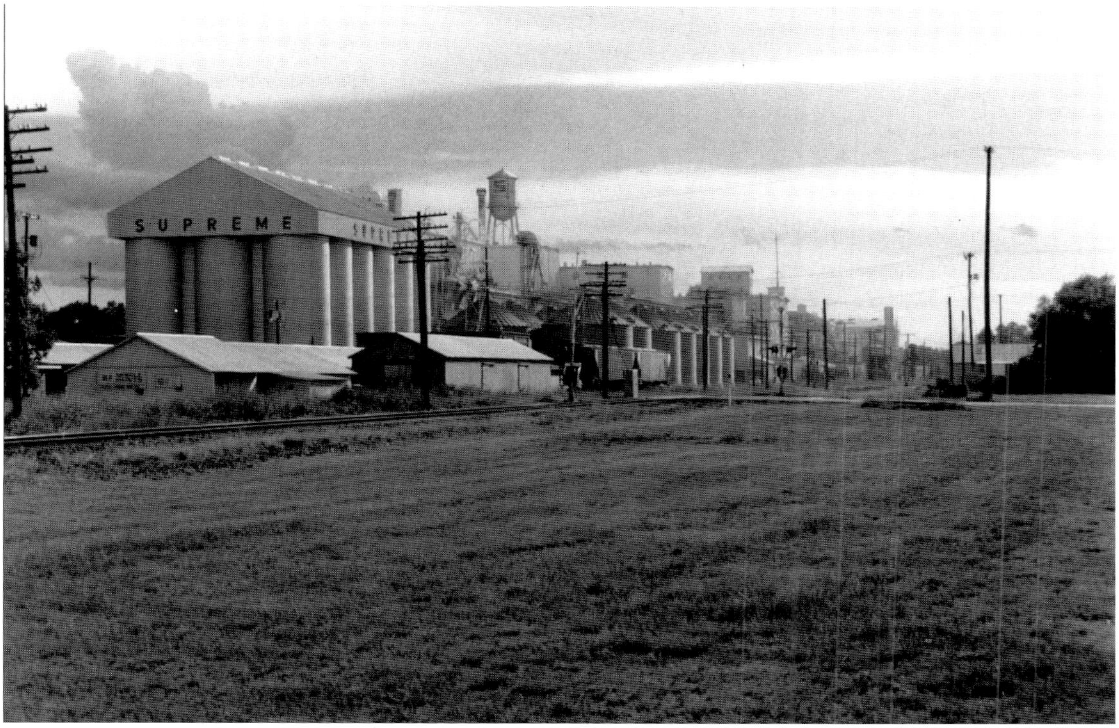

Fig. 1.14

end of 2004 exceeded $62.5 million. These spanned from the renovation of a waiting-intake area in a rural clinic to a $19.2 million replacement laboratory on an urban site. It is an understatement that bureaucracies, health related and otherwise, in the public governmental sector tend to move cautiously. Many years may pass before elected officials vote to build a new facility. In one case it took eight years to purchase a site.[46] The evidence-based design team criss-crossed an everyday landscape that at first glance appeared deceptively ordinary but was found to be captivating, even poetic, upon closer scrutiny: a rice-processing plant in Crowley quietly dominates the town's skyline at sunset (Fig. 1.14).[47] With each new or renovated parish health unit another piece of the larger puzzle would fall into place.

Fifteen years and running, the SFI Initiative in Louisiana is one of the longest evidence-based research and design projects of its kind in architecture in the world. Louisiana was the first state in the United States to adopt an evidence-based facility improvement strategy for its public healthcare network. The SFI attempts to bridge the often-disconnected realms of art and science, and to balance the organization's dictates with architectural humanism and functionality. There is a place in architecture for the fusing of aesthetic concerns, environmentalism, tectonics, and design therapeutics. Beyond this, this protocol and the central thesis it expresses has helped to sustain and further the aims of public health policy.[48] Verification—the translation of research into architecture and assessment of its performance—is not a dismissible extravagance.[49]

Chapter 2

The Setting

With Congress' passage of the federal Hill-Burton Hospital Construction Act of 1946 and subsequent amendments to this legislation, federal funds began to flow through the U.S. Public Health Service into Louisiana for the construction of dozens of outpatient community healthcare clinics. This massive federal public works program, in its early years, provided funding for the lion's share of construction on a matching federal-state grant basis.[1] Eventually, Hill-Burton dissipated, having become a classic, scandal-ridden example of pork-barrel politics, as the communities with the best-connected politicians received the vast majority of funds. In Louisiana alone, by 1959 approximately $4.2 million was spent on the building program for new community health units, with approximately half of this amount furnished by Hill-Burton.[2] Gleaming new minimalist International style clinics replaced obsolete dysfunctional buildings, with some second-generation clinics replacing programs that had been housed in the parish courthouse basements since the late 1920s. In cities and rural communities alike, gleaming new clinics were built. The 1950s generation of Hill-Burton clinics would soon themselves fall victim to poor maintenance by their owners (parish governments), overcrowding due to population increases, the expansion of public health services, and obsolescence resulting from new standards of diagnosis and treatment.

The typical Hill-Burton clinic was a one-level generic shoebox with a flat roof, and 1,500 to 2,000 square feet in size. Beige or orange brick was the norm, often with horizontal ribbon windows with sills high above the floor, presumably as a means to provide privacy to the occupants and to block views from the adjacent parking areas, such as at the former health unit sites in Slidell (Fig. 2.1) and Bossier City (Fig. 2.2). Opening day at a new facility was an important civic event. In 1958, the groundbreaking of Madison Parish's Hill-Burton clinic was featured in the town newspaper (Fig. 2.3). The site was prominent in the community, next door to the parish public library (Fig. 2.4). The large urban facilities in this era were 5,000 square feet or more. Some urban facilities were built two levels in height. As the range of programs and local population grew, so did parking needs at the local parish health unit. The best International

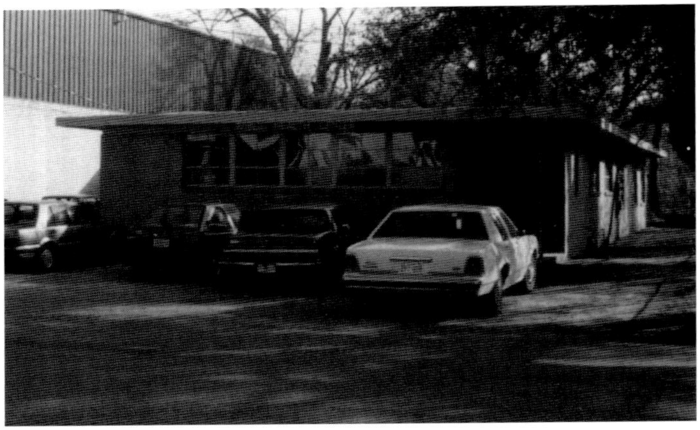

Fig. 2.1

style examples in Louisiana, such as the Hill-Burton clinics built in Abbeville (Vermilion Parish) Morgan City (St. Mary Parish), Homer (Claiborne Parish), Metairie (Jefferson Parish—see Chapter 5), Slidell (St. Tammany Parish), Oak Grove (West Carroll Parish), Springhill (Webster Parish), and Opelousas (St. Landry Parish), are worthy of designation as national historic landmarks. It remains worthwhile to preserve and adapt these second-generation buildings to new uses. In nearly every case the Hill-Burton clinic was built in a prominent location at or close to the center of town. The new clinic, which stood as a symbol of civic progress, was often across the street or behind the parish courthouse. A small staff of three to five persons cared for the residents of the parish, as shown in a photograph from 1940 taken in front of the courthouse in DeRidder, Beauregard Parish (Fig. 2.5). The core staff in the rural parishes consisted of one nurse, one sanitarian, and one clerk. An examination room at the health unit in DeRidder is shown in the accompanying photo, dating from 1940 (Fig. 2.6).

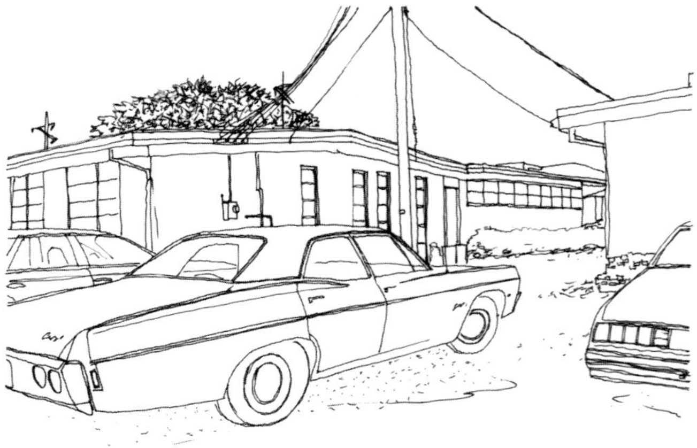

Fig. 2.2

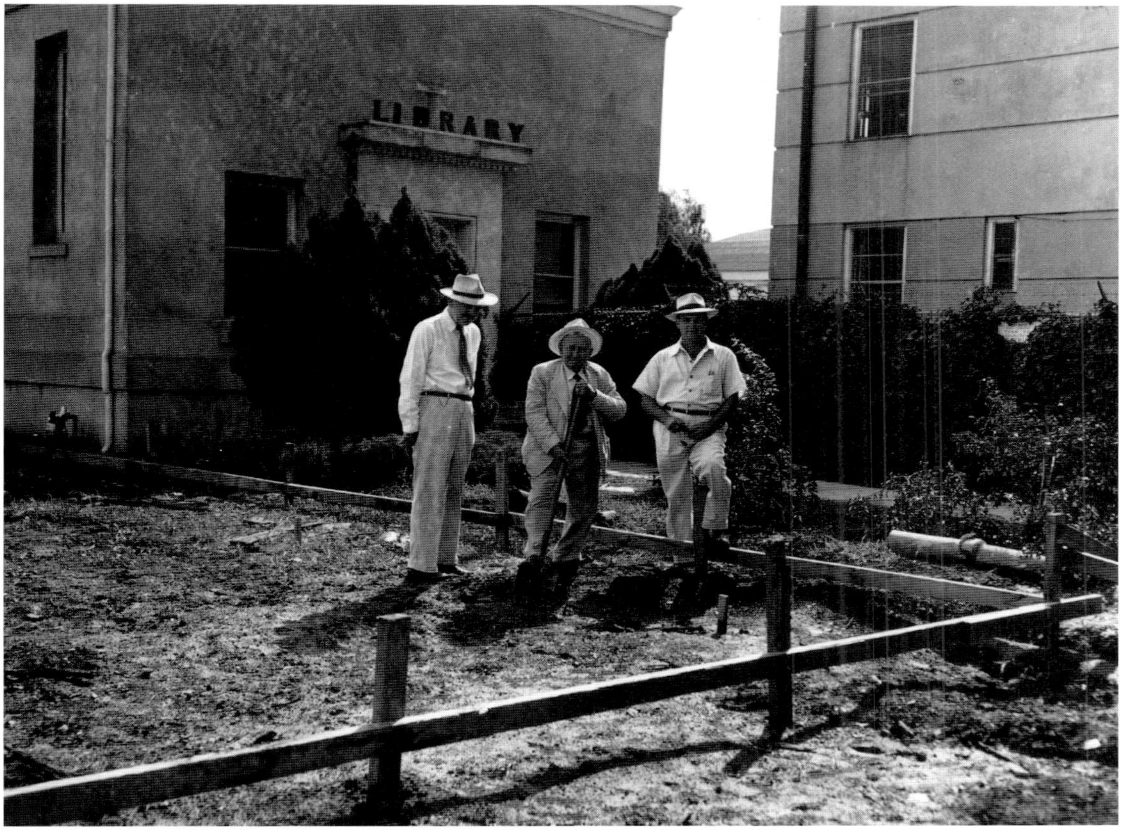

Fig. 2.3

Precursors to the Modernist Outpatient Health Clinic

The outpatient in Louisiana and elsewhere was traditionally held in lower esteem than the inpatient receiving care in a hospital. The history of the architecture of hospitals is filled with examples of compassionately conceived structures, which, in time, would disintegrate into uncaring, utterly dispassionate, hellish places. The portrayal of the hospital in art provides insight on compassion and its antithesis, as depicted in this scene from the Hotel Dieu, Paris, in 1482, from *Livre de la vie active,* by Jean Henry. In this painting, the administrative staff is perhaps identifying the least sick patients, to be expelled that night as outcast patients (Fig. 2.7). The hospitalized inpatient was held in

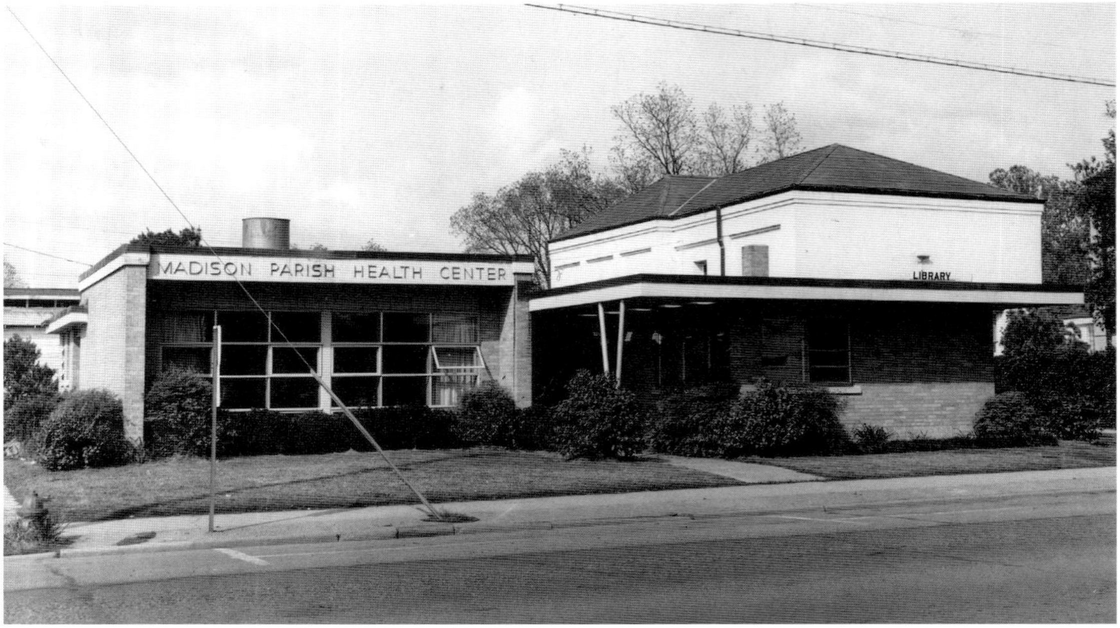

Fig. 2.4

higher regard, for the sicker the inpatient the more valuable he or she was to the caregiver, as a prospect for salvation in the afterlife, whereas the out-patient would be left to roam the streets (Fig. 2.8). The rise of the insane asylum in the eighteenth century, its eventual rejection on humanitarian grounds, and the current emphasis on outpatient care in mental health treatment, is a case in point. In discussing the nature of madness in Western societies, Michel Foucault, in his seminal 1965 book *Madness and Civilization*, discussed the power of passion and its causality in the everyday milieu:

> Before Descartes, and long after his influence as philosopher and physiologist had diminished, passion continued to be the meeting ground of body and soul; the point where the latter's activity makes contact with the former's passivity, each being a limit imposed upon the other and the locus of their communication . . . passion . . . disperses the spirits . . . that is, under the effect of passion and in the presence of its object, the spirits circulate, disperse, and concentrate according to a spatial design which licenses the trace of the object in the brain and its image in the soul, thus forming in the body a kind of geometric figure of passion . . . for when all the spirits are grouped around [it] . . . the mind can no longer ignore it.[3]

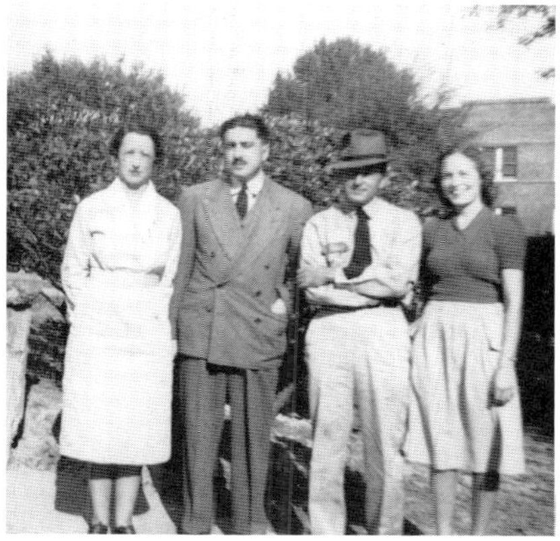

Fig. 2.5

The attainment of control over the less fortunate, aided and abetted by the all too willing support and at times even heroic guidance of a supposedly caring architect, represents a dark chapter in architectural history. At worst, blind arrogance characterized the conception and construction of buildings built for such "care." Around the world, glaring examples of this syndrome in the health milieu have been the vast institutional asylum complexes created for the warehousing of persons deemed socially misfit, deranged, or insane, or afflicted with a communicable disease. An individual faced the prospect of one of four scenarios. First, remaining healthy in the community, eventually dying of natural causes; second, falling ill and receiving treatment from family members at home with some slight probability of recovery; third, death caused by premature sickness and disease with the unfortunate soul never having set foot in a hospital; or, finally, death in a hospital, the result of a fatal condition and/or the unhealthful conditions within the hospital itself.

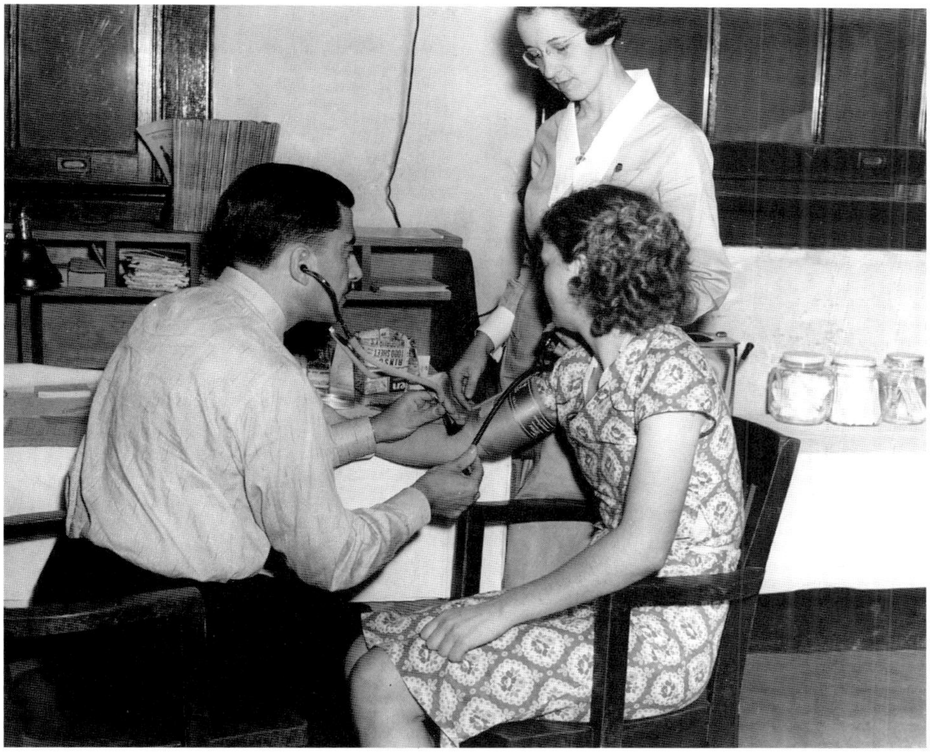

Fig. 2.6

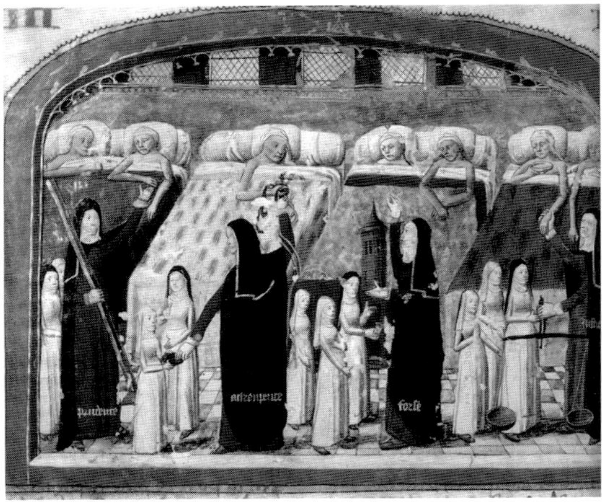

Fig. 2.7

From the standpoint of the outpatient, the hospital is perhaps the most complex and contradictory of all building types in history in terms of dispassion.[4] Psychiatric hospitals have long been conceived and built with the most compassionate of intentions at the outset, yet often resulting in edifices entirely contradictory in their scale, appearance, and inhumanity. Thomas Story Kirkbride's approach to the treatment of inpatient mental illness was considered in the mid-nineteenth century as progressive and compassionate.[5] Florence Nightingale, depicted here in the makeshift hospital at Scutari, Turkey, during the Crimean War in 1856, would transform the practice of nursing, as some inpatients were able, later, to be treated by her nursing staff on an outpatient basis (Fig. 2.9).

In times of war, armies are forced to improvise their accommodation of the sick and wounded, as depicted in this South African hospital ward during the Boer War (Fig. 2.10). The wounded often were, even in winter, deposited in open-air barns when hospitals became overcrowded. The hospital patients would die while the outpatients housed in barns and cold drafty tents often recovered, despite inadequate care. Soon, inpatients were carried outdoors every day as standard protocol.[6] This was also a policy in the tuberculosis sanitariums of the 1930s and 40s in America. By the early 1980s, hospitals were forced by revised third-party reimbursement legislation to focus far more on the quality of their outpatient services.[7] This would symbolize a paradigmatic shift in societal attitudes toward the

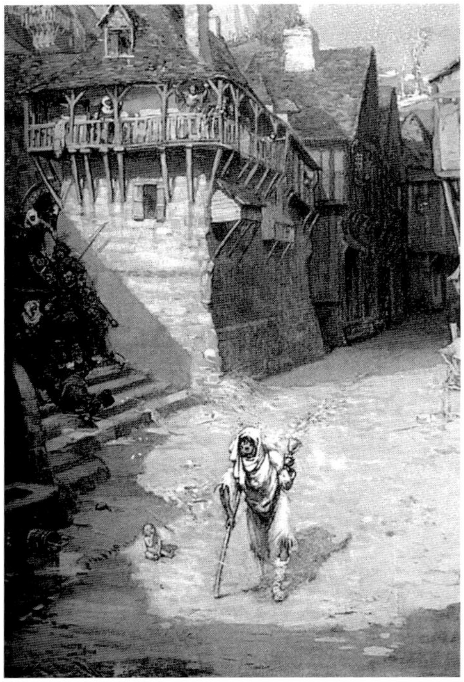

Fig. 2.8

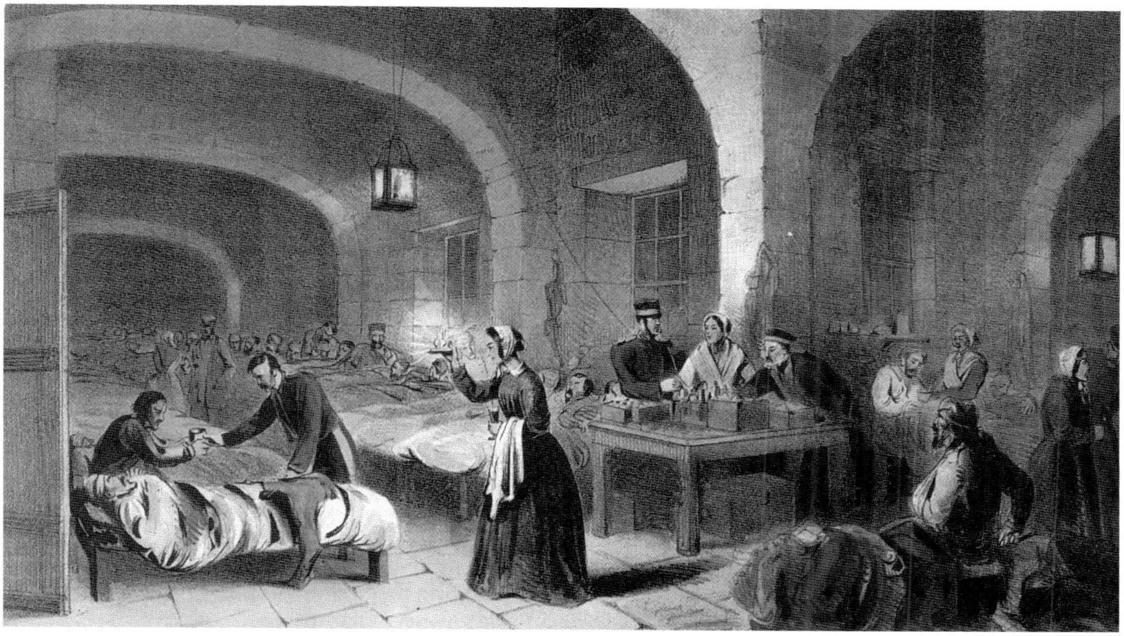

Fig. 2.9

outpatient (from second-class status to highly-desirable status), an emphasis on new diagnostic and treatment practices for the outpatient, such as laser surgery, and in architecture for outpatient healthcare, the appearance of new building types such as outpatient women's oncology centers.[8] In the medium of film, directors have depicted the experience of the hospitalized inpatient, in scenes of dispassionate, inhumane hospital settings spanning the spectrum of history. From the medium's inception, hospitals have been depicted as places to avoid at all cost, with the patient wishing to leave as soon as possible. Only in the past decade has Hollywood addressed with genuine empathy the experience of the outpatient, such as films about cancer victims, *Dying Young* (1991), *One True Thing* (1998), and *Stepmom* (1999).[9]

Historically, the architectural precursor to the Hill-Burton clinics in Louisiana can be traced to early-twentieth-century developments in public health and hygiene in Great Britain. There, the public health clinic had been invented in the then-fledgling International style. The Ministry of Health set up a council on medical and allied services with Lord Dawson of Penn as its chairman in 1920. In the Dawson Report, the outpatient community public health center concept is first mentioned as a discrete building type. When the committee produced its findings they were far in advance of their time. In effect, they advocated a merger of various medical services, preventative and curative, which were on the whole in a very rudimentary stage of development. At the time very little coordination and goodwill existed between the different branches of medicine and health care in the United Kingdom. Local authorities in the United Kingdom emerged with the best strategy in that they set up infant welfare, maternity and school health clinics free to the public, although this was not well received by local general physician-practitioners, who feared competition. As a consequence, little was done to implement the Dawson Report although the 1930s witnessed two notable exceptions which stand among the finest modernist clinics ever built.[10]

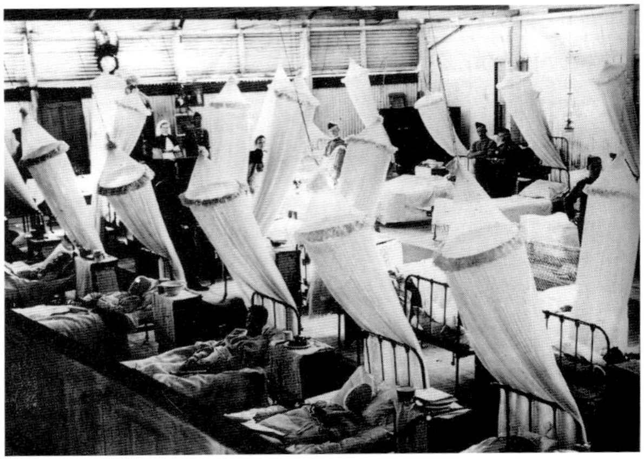

Fig. 2.10

These two landmark British clinics were the Peckham Health Centre (1935) and the Finsbury Health Centre (1938), both built in working class sections of London. Each targeted a geographically defined population and embodied a holistic progressive view of public healthcare, which included nutritional and social welfare assistance, psychological care, sanitary inspectors, immunizations, dentistry, midwife train-

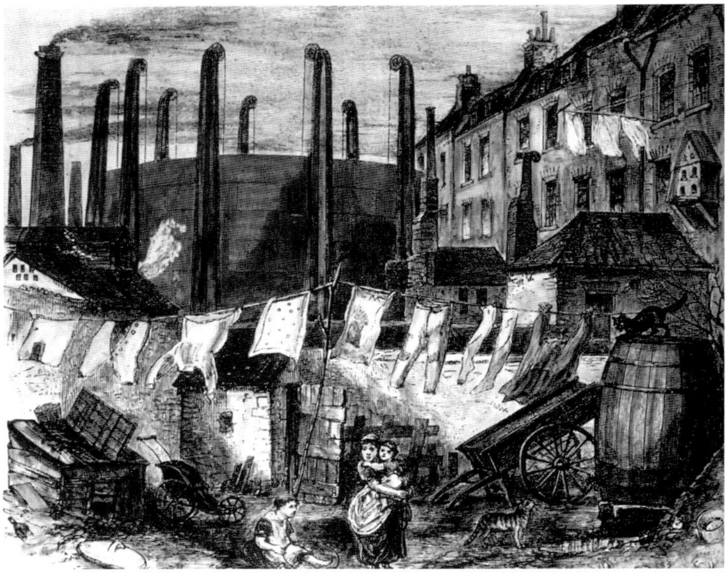

Fig. 2.11

ing, and treatment of conditions ranging from tuberculosis to sexually transmitted diseases. Also, large community rooms were provided to stage concerts, plays, and related cultural events.[11]

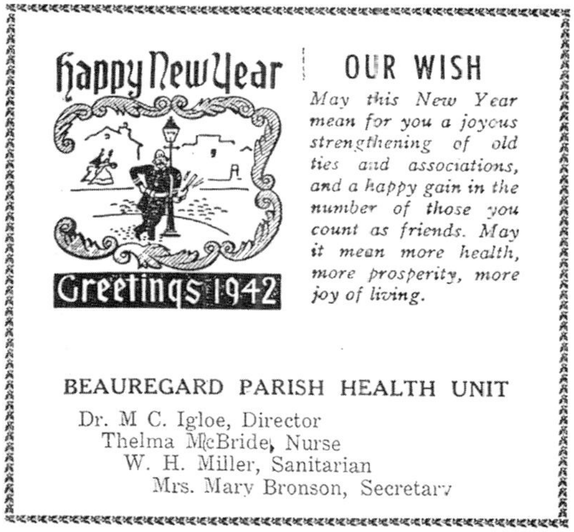
Happy New Year
Greetings 1942
OUR WISH
May this New Year mean for you a joyous strengthening of old ties and associations, and a happy gain in the number of those you count as friends. May it mean more health, more prosperity, more joy of living.
BEAUREGARD PARISH HEALTH UNIT
Dr. M C. Igloe, Director
Thelma McBride, Nurse
W. H. Miller, Sanitarian
Mrs. Mary Bronson, Secretary

Fig. 2.12

In England, young ambitious architects adopted public health as a proving ground for their modernist theories. And, at the same time, modern architecture provided a powerful implementation tool. To them, the medical and architectural professions could now work jointly to advance the cause of modern medicine and public health. These buildings no longer needed excessive ornamentation, deemed useless in the post-Victorian era. Nor were they to be places associated with the dreary miserable dullness of the bleak Industrial Age city, in its squalor and lack of sanitation (Fig. 2.11). Modernist clinics of the 1930s were simple and direct in appearance and layout. Public health itself, dating from horrific epidemics of the eighteenth and nineteenth centuries, now set the stage for the acceptance of this new mode of architectural intervention. Those who served were most appreciative of any gratitude on the part of the public, and this was no different in Louisiana, as the staff often reciprocated the appreciation of the community. In DeRidder, the staff extended this appreciation in their annual holiday message, this one from 1942 (Fig. 2.12).

Exiled From Main Street

In Louisiana, four phases occurred in the architectural history of the parish public health unit. The first coincided with their initial establishment, typically, in the basement of the parish courthouse, in residual spaces. Some of these spaces were formerly used as parish jails. A second phase, the Hill-Burton era, dating from roughly 1949 through 1965, coincided with the construction of more than forty new health units, nearly all designed in the International style. These clinics symbolized the emergence of the health unit as a bonafide civic institution, equivalent in civic stature to the local school, post office, parish library, and parish hospital. Having been designed in a progressive architectural style, they were also seen as progressive symbols of local government. Local civic leaders involved in their construction looked with pride at their health unit, and they immediatly placed a bronze plaque, prominently, at the main entry with the architects and virtually every local elected official's name on it. Not coincidentally, getting a Hill-Burton or Rockefeller Grant public health unit became a matter of keeping up with the Joneses. Competitive neighboring parishes watched closely who would build the next and nicest facility. This jealously, at its peak, was not unlike an intense high school football rivalry. Hill-Burton provided a construction boom statewide. The demise of Hill-Burton, in 1973, signaled a major shift in national health care policy. From 1965 on, with the enactment of Medicaid and Medicare, the emphasis shifted to new treatment programs, technology, and infrastructure, and away from brick and mortar capital investment.

A third phase occurred in the early 1980s, with the opening of a handful of health units built to replace the first wave of Hill-Burton facilities. This group included the health units in Marksville (Avoyelles Parish), Leesville (Vernon Parish) and Amite (Tangipahoa Parish). Each was planned and designed independently of the others, because, as discussed in the previous chapter, architectural "success" remained a virtual hit or miss proposition prior to the start of the evidence-based SFI initiative in 1990. A fourth wave of replacement facilities included, in addition to dozens of SFI-guided projects, the replacement of the four largest urban parish health units: Lafayette (2002), Monroe (2002), Alexandria (2003), and Lake Charles (2004).

Prior to 1983, the emphasis of the United States healthcare system was filling as many hospital inpatient beds as possible. During this period, hospitals had become ever-expanding monsters, with the largest labeled, by this author, as megahospitals. After 1983, however, with the advent of third-party cost-containment legislation such as the Tax Equality and Fiscal Responsibility Act (TEFRA), the unofficial emphasis shifted to keeping inpatients out of hospitals. Inpatient care itself was by then deemed too costly. Financial bottom lines for public and private healthcare providers had been redrawn away from inpatient care for all but the sickest. A corresponding radical shift towards diagnostic related groups (DRG) legislation took place, mandating new ambulatory and outpatient services, services increasingly provided at much less cost.

The parish health unit has remained relevant within this reinvented healthcare landscape. This is principally because public health has historically been positioned to provide wellness and sickness prevention services, i.e. immunizations, nutritional education, family planning programs, sanitation inspections, and the like. The subsequent movement of services away from highly centralized medical centers to community-based outpatient care centers has been referred to by this author as a process of "functional deconstruction."[12] By 1990, in Louisiana and elsewhere, the era of outpatient healthcare had hit its stride.

The Underserved Patient

In the waning years of the twentieth century the increasing cost of healthcare, coupled with the plight of the growing ranks of the homeless, the politically repressed, and the medically uninsured, had reached a critical point.[13] The scene of a makeshift shanty immediately across the street from Charity Hospital in New Orleans (Fig. 2.13) was repeated in cities across the United States. Unfortunately, the mainstream architectural profession, by and large, failed to rise to the challenge. The inherent elitism of architects' controversial proposals for the housing of the homeless only served to bring to light a glaring schism—between the bi-polarities of elitists and populist interpretations of the everyday built landscape. In one bizarre case, an upscale animal shelter for homeless animals in San Francisco opened to much fanfare and was touted in the popular press as an innovative intervention in the fight against animal cruelty.[14] Meanwhile, social, racial, and economic inequities in the United States persisted.[15] The Reagan Era fueled a culture of conspicuous consumption.[16] This continued

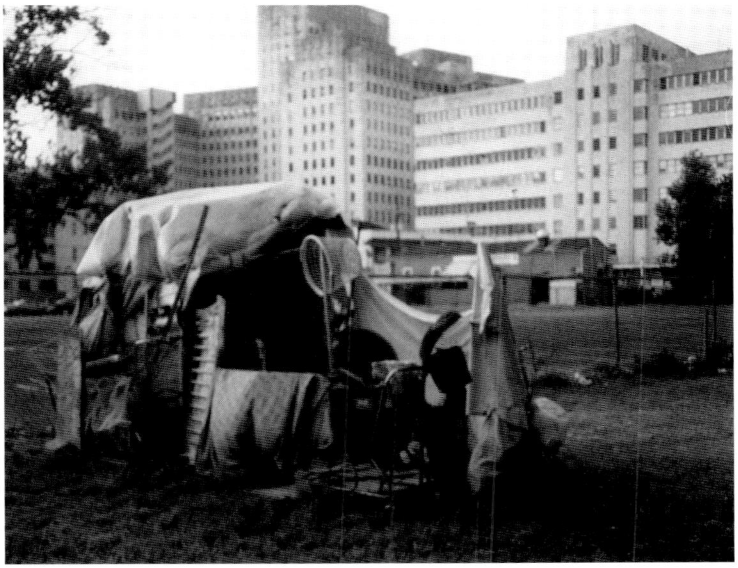

Fig. 2.13

until the bursting of the Dot Com Era economic bubble in 2000. Meanwhile, the ranks of the homeless and the working poor swelled and disillusionment among these underserved healthcare constituencies became widespread.[17] Compassion, in the eyes of a growing working underclass, had been reduced to little more than the insipid campaign promises of erstwhile politicians.

The plight of minority and medically underserved patients in Louisiana closely parallels that of a growing underclass as a whole in the United States. In 2005 it was estimated that as many as 47 million Americans lacked private health insurance. Budget cutbacks in government-operated health agencies resulted in reduced services, benefits, lack of access to care, inefficient or nonexistent public transportation, lack of knowledge of the options available, and learned helplessness among patients and would-be patients.[18] In the words of one young mother, D.H., in Luling, twenty miles from New Orleans:

> I been comin' here [to the parish health unit] for about a year. When I was pregnant I went to the one [the health unit] in Lafayette. Then I moved back here. I was goin' to school in Lafayette. If the health unit were shut down I'd have to pay for everything on my own. When I moved I called and they transferred my records here [to Luling]. I go to school in Thibodaux. I come in every three months. It is an important place worth keeping. It is as important as a school or a library, definitely, because if you don't have health [care] you won't be able to learn. You're putting kids at risk, otherwise. And schools won't let kids in without their health records.
>
> I think the waiting room is way too small. On most days there are not enough seats. And with all these kids it gets pretty intense sometimes. They have nothin' to do while they wait. Once, I missed an appointment and I had to pay about $120.00 to pay for milk formula. I get 31 cans of formula and cereal. Whatever you get, they put the check [voucher] through and just give it to you. All at once for the month. The nutritionist interviews me and gives out a pamphlet. Sometimes I'm alone and sometimes I'm with other people [in the interview room]. They have us watch a video. I watched a video and then they teach us how to mix the cereal and formula. The program is doin' fine for me.

Another patient, M.C., while having little success disciplining her rambunctious eighteen-month-old daughter, added:

I been comin' here for years. I came in four months after she was born. My husband comes in, too. This is the closest health unit to my house. I went to the one [the health unit] in Metairie since I was little for everything. My Momma took my sisters and me. I hope they never it shut down because these people don't have their own insurance, and that would be too tough on a lot of people. The children need to be healthy before they can go to school. I know that milk is very expensive. A lot of things the WIC people give you are very expensive Right now, she's [her daughter] is getting eggs, cheese, and cereal. They give you a recipe to show you how to do it. Sometimes if you don't have a job it gets real expensive. Especially when they're newborn. It takes 'bout fifteen minutes, unless we're watching films or whatever. When we're in there, there ain't nothin' for the kids to do but run around. Just like they are now. They need to put some color in and something up on the walls. That's one thing: maybe if they had a little play center. She [her daughter] doesn't have to come to every appointment. Only when they make me bring her in. When I'm just comin' in for another voucher or whatever she don't need to be here.

My house is right by the grain elevator. It [the health unit] could be a lot bigger, maybe. This room [is] way too small. We need a playroom for our kids. Some toys, books, next to here [the waiting room]. When you first come they call you 'round and you do your paperwork. You see that little thing [hole] in the window? I don't like that speaker 'cause I don't like to bend down to talk and I know they're not hearing me on the other side and I have to yell in front of everyone. But this is a pretty good staff. That's why I come back here. I'm 34 weeks pregnant now. A lot of people come for WIC and a lot of people come here for shots. Lots of my friends come here. One of my friends lost her insurance. Six or seven months ago.

On the absence of transportation to and from the clinic:

Well, see, my car is broken. And it's in the shop, and if my appointment is for 8:30 [AM] I don't have any way to get over here across that [Mississippi River] bridge. It's hard for me 'cause they done closed the health unit on the other side [of the river] some years ago. And my son is now seven years old. I been comin' here for seven years. I came to take my pap smears eight years ago. But I have to have my Medicaid card before they will see me here. I couldn't do it any other way. Cause it's only $5.00 dollars for me now. My ride today is waitin' for me outside. I can't get the transportation van now because I can't get certified. You have to apply. They said they sent the application to me. And I said 'I never got it.' So went to the doctor on the other side of the river and he said 'Your Medicaid's been cut off.' So I went back over here. We need two places [clinics] in this parish, one on each side [of the river]. A lot of people, you see, can't come in cause they can't make their appointment 'cause they don't have no ride or no car. My car's broken.

I even hitchhike to this clinic. My neighbor's husband has a truck, but if his truck is broken it's hard for her to get here too. A lot of people can't get here. That's all it is. Well, that girl's here with me now. It's hard for her and this is supposed to be the richest parish [in the state] and we don't have squat. If you call they say, you gotta come in that day. When you are able to go in the [Medicaid] van they come 'round to pick you [us] all up in the morning and we all gotta wait here 'til the last person is done, 'bout 1:00, 2:00 o' clock. I've been here waiting from 9:00 'til 2:00 o' clock. And everybody just sits around. They only got one van. When I come late and your appointment is cancelled, they say, 'Well, that's your fault.' If you can't get here you can't get your shots and then you can't get your kid's medical card for school. But who wants to bring you back and forth all the time? That's gas money and everything.

Why is this place so small and so hard to get to? Why is it this way?

If I miss an appointment [WIC appointment] it may be a month or two months 'fore I can get back in. Like me, I missed my October appointment and I'm just now getting' back in [December]. They say you have to bring your child in. I missed an appointment [WIC] for her last year and they rescheduled it and I had to buy milk for a month and a half, $115.00 dollars a month. You gotta buy juice, you gotta buy cereal, and you gotta buy milk. Whether or not you got your WIC voucher. When the days when everybody comes in here for their shots, you gotta see it. It is so noisy. On the days when its hot, cold, muggy. Everybody is standing outside in the rain, in the cold, in the heat. You gotta see it. I been standin' outside and don't get out [to return home] until 1:00, 2:00 o'clock. And when somebody leaves I run in to get their seat or else I be left out. And it's packed. And nobody [on the staff] wants to run outside, you know, to keep runnin' outside to come get 'ya. And you gotta bring 'em all in [your children] for their shots, and you 'gotta bring 'em in and sit 'em all down on that table and keep 'em from runnin' all 'round the offices.

We get to leave after they see us. We have to go see the health lady about the food and then they print the voucher right there. We need to put all the kids in one room, 'though we can't hear what they're sayin' when we're in there. Sometimes they [clinicians] need to see both the mother and the child. Other

> times, if you have a baby sitter that's fine, but if you don't, what do you do with your child?

She continues:

> For WIC sometimes we come in three at a time. She [the nutritionist] comes in and shows you how to set up and cook the food [in the WIC kitchen at the former site in Luling—Fig. 2.14]. She cooks whatever you get on your WIC [voucher]. Sometimes we see videos. It helps a lot, you know. Well not all the time. Yeah, I see videos, 'specially when I come in with a child. You only see one at a time, like when you come in for birth control, you know, stuff like that. Or on how to feed 'em. But other than that, you need those shots, you know 'cause otherwise it's $25.00 or $35.00 [per immunization]. If you [the child] gets a shot on Monday, and your child comes down sick on Wednesday, you 'gotta come pay for that [second] shot, too. Here, I can come in anytime I need to.
>
> It's hard on the kids, it gets aggrevatin' for 'em too. More than it needs to be. 'Specially for the babies whose tryin' to sleep. Because usually you got to hold 'em for a long while. Yeah. They want to run around and play 'cause they're kids. Sometimes the air gets real bad inside too with no open windows. I remember one day in the summer it got too hot and someone [a mother] with her kids [accompanying her] passed out. It's 'specially bad when you come in and the babies are all in their carriers cryin' on the floor and there's no place to walk.[19]

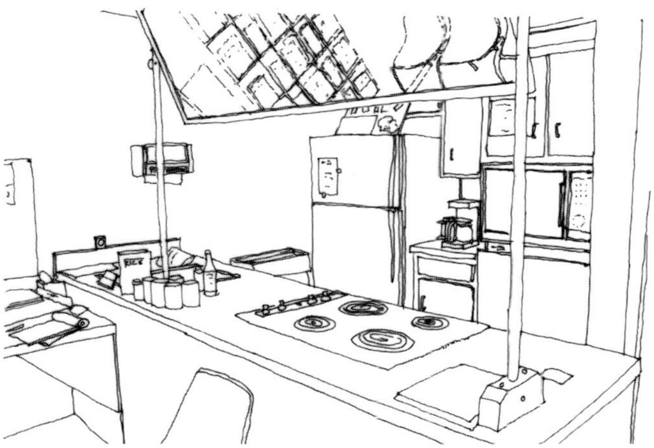

Fig. 2.14

An additional barrier would emerge, resulting in the further disempowerment of the uninsured and underserved patient in the everyday cultural landscape: the lack of access to online, virtual healthcare, a dilemma widely referred to in the popular media as the digital divide. The poor were now subjected to this new mode of marginalization compared to wealthier individuals on the basis of whether or not one had access to the Internet. Patient-rights' advocates are now calling for greater access to personal healthcare services for all in an era of virtual medicine.[20] Online sources of health information such as Web-MD, Medem, and other organizations have transformed the dissemination of healthcare information.[21] Besides the ramifications of the digital divide, social and racial disparities in the healthcare landscape are now receiving attention from critics of the U.S. healthcare system:

> Traditionally [researchers] have focused on health differences between rich and poor, or black and white people—unaware, in many cases, that race was serving as a proxy for socioeconomic status, since black people are overrepresented in lower income brackets. But the notion that a mid-level executive with a three bedroom, split-level home in Scarsdale might somehow be more vulnerable to illness than his boss in the five bedroom colonial a few blocks away seems to have finally captured scientists' attention. In the past five years, 193 papers addressing aspects of socioeconomic status and health have appeared in scientific journals, twice the number in the previous five-year period. The National Institutes of Health last year declared research on disparities in health related to social class or minority status [as] one of its highest priorities.[22]

This dilemma is compounded by the inability of many former so-called welfare moms, now statistically reclassified as the working poor, to obtain health insurance from their new employers. For the working poor, finding a job is no guarantee of obtaining health insurance.[23] As this occurs, inner-city storefront health clinics open and close at an alarming rate.[24] And even the construction industry has had a role in inhibiting equanimity in the built environment.[25] Four interwoven constructs are presented below to help summarize (and rectify) this situation. Each construct constitutes a transactional dimension of compassion (and its antithesis) as it relates to the built environment:

> 1. *The Empowered/Disempowered Patient*: This centers on the status and aspirations of the individual, seen from the viewpoint of the patient. The patient's well being, goals, and priorities are at one end of a continuum, whereas the well being, goals, and priorities of the healthcare system—the provider organization—represent the opposing endpoint. Comparisons and contrasts between these constituencies can be very illuminating for the architect. This is due to the simple fact that the care received (or denied), and one's perception of that care (or non-care) is typically the direct result of the funding priorities and policies of the provider organization.

2. *Perceptions of Provider Compassion/Dispassion*: This centers on the extent to which compassion on the part of the provider organization is experienced by the individual patient (low=discompassion; high=compassion). For example, an HIV / AIDS patient receiving care on a weekly basis in an outpatient clinic will naturally be interested in how other similar patients are faring in other similar care settings. The providers' degree of compassion is correlated with the quality of the physical care setting, although this is no different from what has been the norm for hundreds of years.

3. *High/Low Health Status*: This centers on health outcomes and the overall healthfulness of the individual patient (again, ranging from low to high). Low health status denotes a condition of discompassion directed toward the patient, as directly manifest in the architectural environment. Conversely, high denotes a significant degree of compassion as conveyed by the care setting provided by the provider organization. For example, a new clinic will symbolize a renewed commitment to offer a higher level of care. This has a ripple effect on the productivity of clinic staff, i.e. a well designed, spacious exam room allows the nurse to keep needed supplies on hand at all times, and he or she can therefore attend to a patient's needs uninterrupted. Outcome, presumably, in this context is measurable by assessing the patient's health outcome.

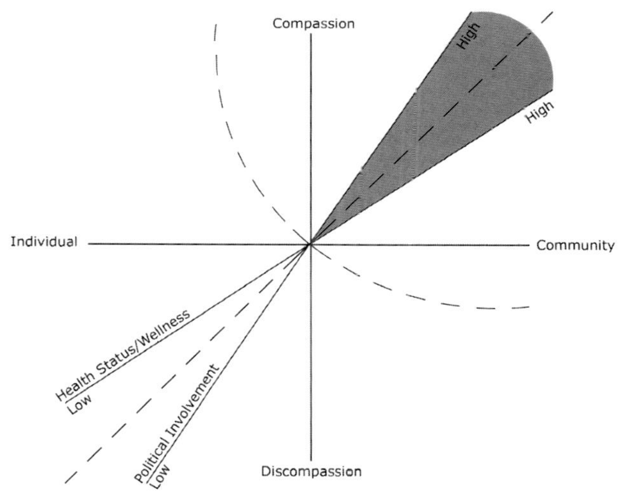

Fig. 2.15

4. *Patient Involvement/Apathy in Healthcare Policy Making*: This construct centers on the function of the individual patient in shaping the policies of the provider organization. This involvement can range from attending meetings to learn about and comment on proposed changes in federal Medicare reimbursement rates in the coming fiscal year, to overt advocacy as a representative of one's peer group (from a low to high degree of politi-

cal involvement) in the decision making process. Low involvement, in this scenario, is often attributable to learned helplessness, frequently a telltale symptom of dispassion on the part of the provider organization.

In an attempt to interpret this model in visual terms, and to convey the operative relationship between these four constructs, a diagram is presented (Fig. 2.15). The patient must strive to reach a point where she/he is involved in her/his care and treatment decisions, ensuring he will receive compassionate care in a compassionate care setting (shaded area of Fig. 2.15). Of course, seldom do we function solely as individuals, nor purely as members of a distinct social peer group. In reality, success in everyday life requires an ability to make sacrifices in order to satisfy our goals and aspirations and remain healthy in equilibrium with the environment. We endeavor to make sense of the places where we live out our lives in order to avoid negative situations we might find ourselves in. This amounts to a search for control over the course of events, and physical settings, and their consequences in our lives. The opposite condition, uncertainty, or the lack of control, is characterized by unpredictability in one's life and in the physical settings we occupy, and architectural settings have been shown to have a counter-therapeutic effect on well-being.[26] M.C. Escher's "Relativity" (1953) aptly conveys the stressful, dislocative effect of architecturally induced ambiguity and unpredictability in everyday life (Fig. 2.16).

The longer one is exposed to counter-therapeutic architecture, administrated by a dispassionate care provider organization, the more negative one's response to it will likely become. An architecture and urban environment centered on an "ethics of caring" is, by definition, one that is fully supportive of the patient who experiences health disparities.[27]

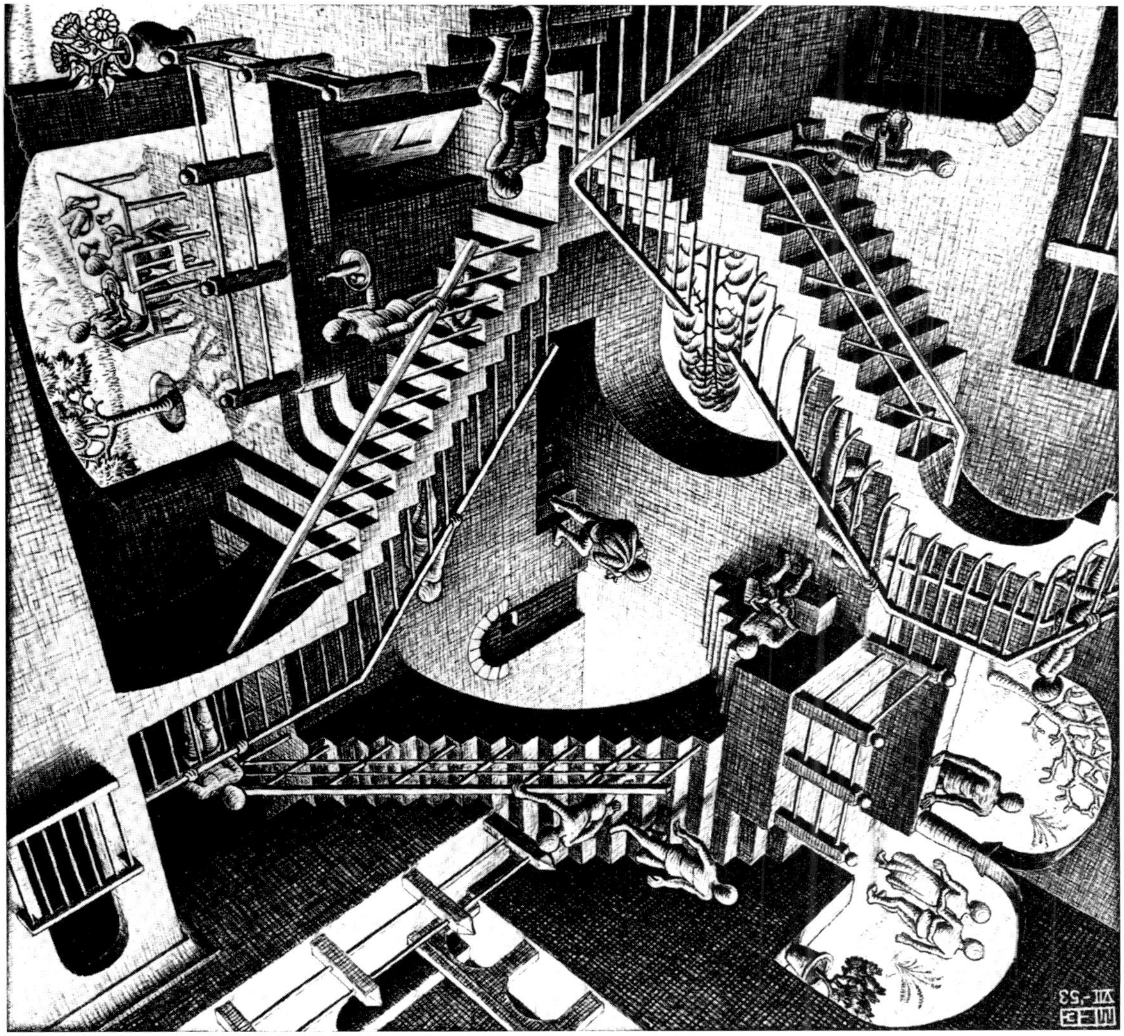

Fig. 2.16

CHAPTER 3

THE CAREGIVERS

The stories of three healthcare professionals are told in this chapter. First is that of the clerical administrative clerk. These persons are responsible for the day-to-day scheduling of clinic activities, work with patients to create and update their medical case history, and oversee the materials management aspect of the clinic's operations. This consists of ordering supplies and managing the limited physical space within the clinic to ensure that proper safety and security measures are maintained. This is followed by the story of the nurse, the professional responsible for the direct delivery of care, consisting of immunizations, examinations, check-ups, health education seminars and workshops, sometimes even home visits, and general consultation by phone, and related non-hospital types of care. For cases of broken bones, high-grade fever, severe cases of bronchitis, and the like, the patient is referred to either the local primary care clinic, if one exists nearby, or to the nearest community hospital. Nonetheless, many a patient has received this type of care in a parish health unit an on ad hoc basis over the last eight decades. The nurse coordinates and administers the following services: child and maternal health clinics, family planning clinics, communicable disease clinics, and children's health clinics.

The third narrative is that of the environmental health specialist, known as the parish sanitarian. Each parish is required by state regulatory standards to house at least one sanitarian specialist within its geographic boundary. This individual is also housed at the health unit. The sanitarian, of whom a growing number are women, are responsible for ensuring that all sanitation and environmental quality monitoring activities are carried out pursuant to all local, state, and federal regulatory statutes. The environmental health staff is the most autonomous in terms of physical spaces they occupy within a parish health unit. The only rooms they share with the nursing and clerical staff, in most cases, are the staff break room, parking lot, restrooms, waiting room, and conference room.

Usually, visitors to the health unit seeking approval of blueprints for a sewerage permit or a kitchen layout for a new restaurant will be instructed

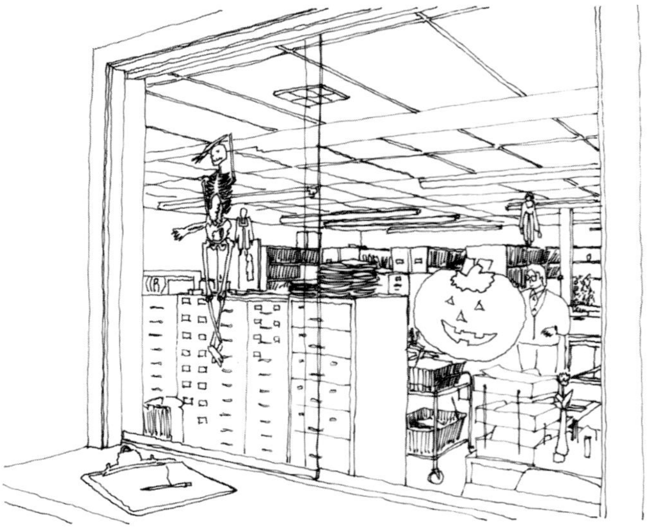

Fig. 3.1

to enter a side door, away from the clamor of the crowded clinic waiting room. Gender undoubtedly plays a role in the power structure within a parish health unit. Nearly all the nurses statewide are female, as is also the case with the clerical staff. And as mentioned, except in some situations the opposite is the case for the parish sanitarian. When it comes to interaction with parish police jurors on matters relating to the facility it is often the parish sanitarian, together with the facility manager, who function as spokespersons. This, however, can be a source of some friction between the nursing supervisor, clerical supervisor, parish sanitarian, and facility manager. It seems that no two locales are alike with respect to this decision-making hierarchy or the degree of influence exerted by any one of these individuals.

The Clerk

The clerk is usually the staff person with whom the patient first comes in contact. The clerk answers the phone, fields queries, provides referrals to appropriate staff locally or within the region, and provides information to the public. For the patient, the work of the clerk facilitates access to the state's community health care system. This process is called "intake." First, the patient signs in at a window or counter

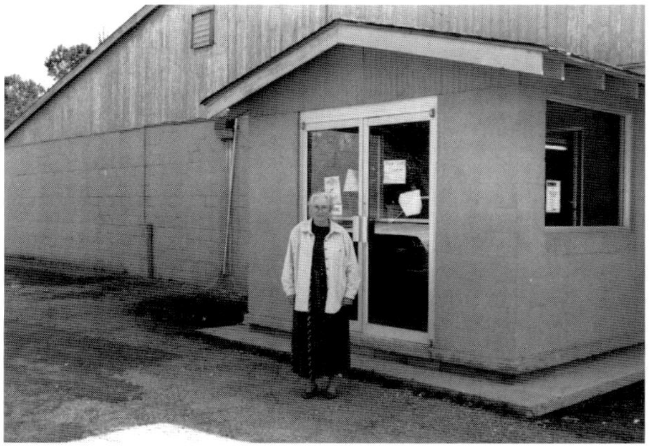

Fig. 3.2

(Fig. 3.1). Most rural health units have three or four clerks, working under the direction of a clerical supervisor. A large urban health unit might have as many as fifteen clerical personnel, as well as a coordinator and assistant coordinator. At the health unit in Franklinton, there are five clerks, including the clerical supervisor. Audrey Thomas is the clerical supervisor at the Washington Parish Health Unit, in Franklinton (Fig. 3.2):[1]

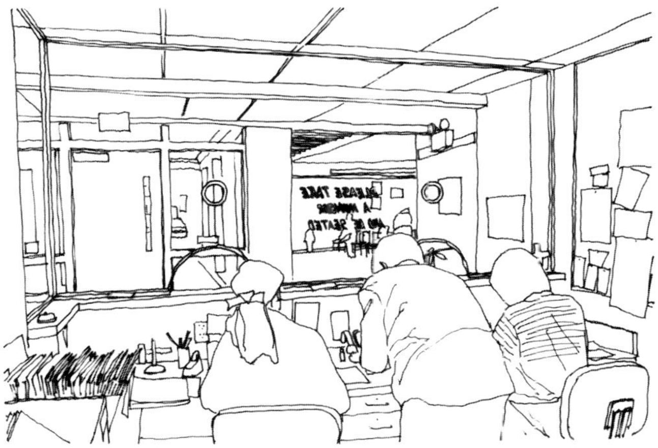

Fig. 3.3

I started in 1968 in the family planning program, with Dr. Beasley. But at that time it wasn't with the Office of Public Health. It [family planning] was a federal program. I think it must've come in 1967. The state had to pick it up when it fell into receivership. It went bankrupt. Something happened with the federal funds. The state picked us up in 1974. It [the clinic] was located down on the Main Street. We moved up here and they renovated it. I started workin' officially for OPH in 1974 cause that's when WIC started. We moved up here before the WIC program started. I was a Clerk 3 in family planning, you know, and after we got physically merged together I was a secretary for a while.

The main focus has always been on our clinics, on keepin' [patients] covered. Our charts are worked up and ready for the day's clinic and we set all clinic appointments, except on some "fast lane" days when we don't take appointments. When they just need shots or blood pressure [assessment], then they don't have to sit out and wait, you see. That has changed a lot, too, because the programs have changed. We're now doin' a lot more [screening] than we used to. We have a big clinic here on Tuesdays. We work together with the staff from Bogalusa [a sister health unit twenty-two miles to the east across the parish] as a team. Before, it was kinda like a rivalry, you know. So this has helped a lot because we all now feel like we're one. On Thursdays we have our big clinic over in Bogalusa. And we have the fast lane clinic here on Wednesdays so they can just come in and pick up their vouchers. A voucher is a WIC draft, you know. The patient comes into the program for three months and then she gets recertified for three more months.

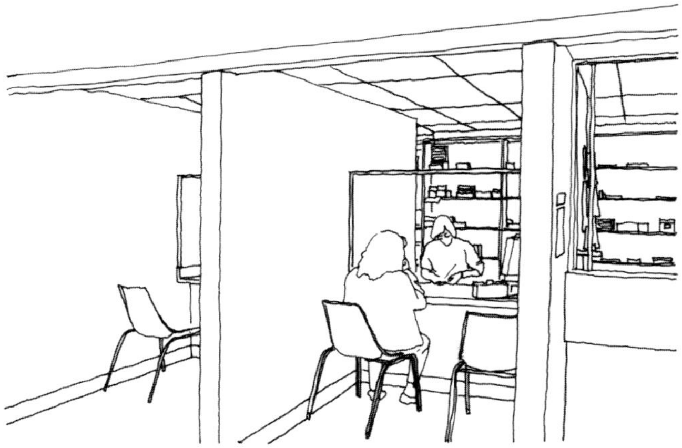

Fig. 3.4

When they call on the phone for an appointment, we then search to see if they've ever been here before. If they have, we have a record. Our numbering system goes back to '74. We have certain forms for STD [sexually transmitted diseases], and for every program, different paperwork. Oh my gosh. I don't know, but I believe there are more than 16 different forms. Sometimes all we give 'em is WIC. We have the form which records all the immunizations given. If they don't bring theirs [medical history form] we pull [out] ours [Fig. 3.3].

If they are certified under WIC, or child health, we set up a different set of appointments on different clinic days. And we have a special day for the family planning clinic. Usually we have to see our STD [patients] most anytime they call. And we have to see our TB [patients] anytime, too. When they come in we already got their chart pulled because our priority is to get the patient in so he or she can get cared for. When they are first interviewed they bring in their income information, and if they don't already have their Medicaid card we have to get 'em their card [Fig. 3.4]. When we get 'em in we send 'em to the lab and then to the nurse. And we give out to Medicaid patients a WIC-17 form—then they can kinda bypass the lab. We have different days for screening patients. Those days, it's usually from head to toe, so they're usually here for a long time. We have a couple of screenin' days per month. Most of the time, what's easy on the clerks is hard on the nurses, and what's easy on the nurse is hard on the clerk. On the screenin' days we don't appoint that many because of the time it takes, but on record days we do but then we have to print more vouchers and fill out more forms. We do all the personnel forms, keep up with purchasing paperwork, and fill out orders for supplies [Fig. 3.5]. With the budget freeze, we're always runnin' out, and having to borrow. Sometimes we bring in our own supplies. We wanted some blood pressure cups, and we had a time getting' 'em. Most of our patients come from the West Side of the

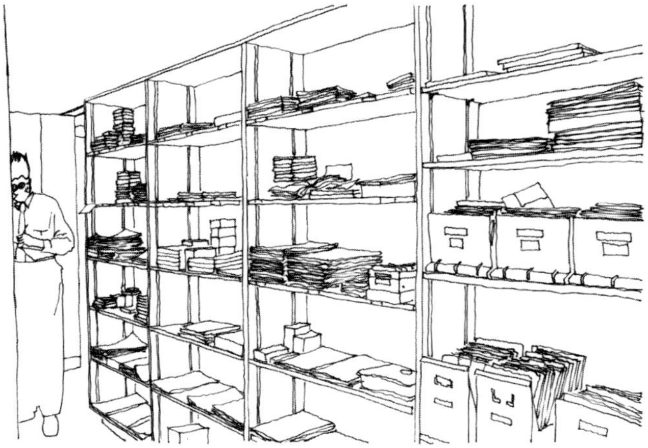

Fig. 3.5

parish. Our patients wouldn't have an option if there weren't this health unit. Even my children come in. Because you know even these birth control pills have gone sky high [in cost]. And they don't have to pay so dearly because of the sliding scale. You usually take their word, but with WIC we had to have 'em bring in papers to prove their income. In WIC you either qualify or you don't. For immunizations, you might have to pay $5.00 per visit. But not very many pay. The federal government pays for these kids' vaccinations. Ninety-five percent get free care. Most everyone. All the people who get Medicaid, we bill them down in New Orleans. The people who vote for our millage tax, we should just give it to 'em free. We need to help 'em [patients] get their Medicaid cards because we were told that we're [Louisiana] running neck and neck with third world countries in terms of infant mortality. We certify, start the files, and keep up with the appointments. We need to get them into prenatal care as soon as we can. With the card they can get care. It's good until they [the mothers] are six months post partum. WIC comes after the family planning program. WIC ends [for the mother] when the mother is six months postpartum, and when the baby is five years old. We [clerks] are the hub of the whole place.

As for patient privacy, in Bogalusa it's real good because of the [modular workstations and permanent intake] offices, but if we have somethin' such as a person with a communicable disease, then we have to find a room somewhere. And there might not be any open rooms. But the main thing is that we don't bring 'em in on clinic days because then they don't have to intermingle [with the children]. That would be unfair to everyone, and on the voucher pickup days patients don't have to bring in their children. If they bring their WIC-17 form with 'em then sometimes they don't even have to come in.

The police jury has been real helpful through the years. And now that we don't have to face fourteen of 'em it's been better [the present size is seven]. And Ron, here, our custodian, had to keep up both of 'em [the two health units in the parish] and it was too much for him. So we went to the police jury and we got 'em to pay for another helper and we got 'em to pay for it out of our millage. They [the police jurors] put you through it and I think that maybe the first time I did it [asked the police jury for a favor] I did it the wrong way. That's the reason they put me through so much grief, because I just hit 'em cold with it. And so the next time I went in I got all my ducks in a row. I went into the backroom with some of 'em and told 'em what I wanted, and that way it worked out real well. I didn't even have to attend the meetin' that night. So I think I learned the hard way. Sometimes, I have to write a proposal up [for assistance].

This facility was formerly a bowling alley and bar. The health unit has been housed there since 1974. On the process of getting a new facility built to replace their health unit, and the role of local politicians:

> Well, it's taken a long time. First, you have to get 'em to put it [a millage proposal] on the ballot [in order] to put it to bein' voted on. I went there and I spelled out what I wanted and said I want y'all to vote for it. But when I went to vote I could barely find it [on the ballot]. It lost. I went back and said we wanted something real simple and plain. But they told us that we had a good bit of money and we could do somethin' with it anyway [without a vote for a millage tax assessment]. You know, they've had all these elections [recently] because they'd decided to redistrict everything and change the form of parish government from a police jury to a parish council.
>
> I have a good rapport with them [jurors] because they know I've always been honest with 'em. I've never asked for anything I didn't need. I always asked only if I needed it and with my sales pitch already worked up. Nothing happens overnight. Nothing is problem free.
>
> And let me tell you somethin' about Sixty Rayburn [longtime, well known, irascible state senator from nearby Bogalusa, in the same parish]. We [the parish] would have been left out [of the state political landscape] without him. I went to a little community meetin' the other week, and it was all about a series of forums. They had a whole series of topics, and I signed up for the one on retirement communities. More and more people are beginnin' to move up here [from the New Orleans metro area seventy-five miles to the south].
>
> But Sixty, he meant everythin' to us. He was a real good person for the parish because he cared about poor people. He helped these [local] boys get good state jobs. He helped people. He never got above people's heads. They could call him up anytime. Two and three generations of the families knew him. You knew you could go to him and he'd talk to you. He was in office for nearly forty years. When this gamblin' thing [a scandal with Rayburn at the center of the controversy] came up [in Baton Rouge] he was voted out. I had a good relationship with his daughter. What I think did him in was all these young people who didn't know him. Us old people knew him. We knew he carried the purse [as head of the powerful state legislative finance committee] for years. But I guess he got tarnished with that gamblin' thing. So then Bill Sharp soon resigned [Rayburn's successor]. And a relative of mine is now the state senator [Jerry Thomas]. So that's good for the parish. His mother and my husband are first cousins. He became a doctor, and he first ran for coroner, and then as a representative for several years. Now Sixty, when he was the state senator and

we was buildin' the health unit over in Bogalusa [early 1990s], he got us about $60,000 in capital outlay money to buy furniture and all.

On information technology and its impact:

The parish government submitted a form as a [capital outlay] funding request. It is a proposal as to how it [the health unit] can be used by all the community. So now people can come in from outside for teleconferences, because we are gettin' into a big high tech world. I give 'em [parish officials] a list and, honey, if it [the requested item] won't last twenty years, it can't be on that list. The state legislator and senator get together, and there's a lot of visionary programs now goin' on, and there's federal monies for that. What we need is transportation, and if we can get those retirement people up here, and they bring their money, then we can get improvements up here. We used to have a bus back and forth from Southeastern [Southeastern Louisiana University in Hammond, forty miles southwest]. They took the [college] kids back and forth five days a week. But they took that away. They used to have a federal program for transportation to and from the health unit. If the people were on Medicaid, they could be picked up at home. But they don't have that anymore either. Nurses will, you know, go pick up patients in the rain if there's an urgent need, you know, to give a shot to a very sick infant. They'll go out. Sometimes we even treat prisoners at the health unit. When they come here an armed guard is with 'em. They'll all come in the front door but they're taken into a back room right away.

On loyalty and dedication:

We don't have a lot of [staff] turnover, you know, because we don't have no place to go to, compared to if we were over in Baton Rouge. Or Livingston, or some of the larger places, because they [staff] there just use it [experience acquired] as a training ground. I feel sorry for those supervisors. Staff take their experience away [when they leave] but here we get to keep our clerks a good while. At one time we had thirteen clerks. That was a time. Back then everything was a paper world. But with everything being computerized now, I still tell 'em that a clerk's work is never done, just like 'a woman's work is never done.' We always handle paper charts. All the time, every day. I don't know how many in a day but our charts, all 20,000, are housed here. We now [in 1999] have eight clerks, with one out now, Penny, the Assistant Office Manager. She's been here now almost twenty years. Penny's out now with her back, and, uh, with a paid medical leave she will eventually roll over into a family medical leave. Her doctor sees somethin' on her tailbone, and she may need surgery. We had a girl [clerk] here that, uh, died, but she was an Old Faithful, she never missed work, but she got to feelin' so bad. She had come down with liver cancer.

She died. And then that same year, we had about five people who retired, and two more died, and they were only about 52, 53 years old. We had a rash of deaths. That was, probably, four years ago. We used to not have that hard of a time replacing 'em.

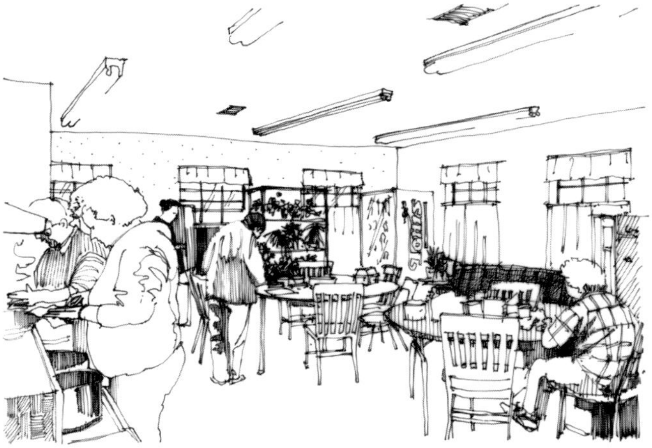

Fig. 3.6

You know, public health is somethin' you just love. You may wonder why I say that because we're often dealing with a lot of screamin' kids and irate people and all that. You don't want 'em [new clerical staff] to first come in on a hectic day [during training]. But I tell everybody I hire its somethin' that you just get in your blood. Is it maybe because of the sense of satisfaction that maybe you helped somebody that day? And I guess you'd have to. I've never had to fire anybody. Most either retire or die. They don't switch [jobs] much because once they've got the state job they really think they've got it made. I see 'em [patients] as infants and we follow 'em all the way through. Those girls [the nursing staff] that work with 'em know way more than I do about 'em [the patients]. They go way back, too. You know, we had a very sick baby here recently and we had to handle her [case] different. The mother has cancer, and, you know, she and the baby needed special treatment. 'Course we can't ever do *enough*, but when she came in we sat her and the baby in a private exam room right away. We do whatever is needed.

During times of hurricanes the health unit becomes really important. When the hurricanes come up through the Gulf [of Mexico] up through Mississippi we always get some of it. When [Hurricane] Camille [1969], came up one Labor Day I remember I heard that every tree in Bogalusa was down. And all the nurses came in and the sanitarians were real busy delivering food, especially milk, to all the stranded people. We were open. When we have [staff] parties, I like to do a lot of the cookin', but we all pitch in. We're like a good family here [Fig. 3.6]. And I hope this [the health unit] never gets torn down, because we

> used to have crawfish boils in the spring, and we used to have a lot of things [social events]. We used to pay for all that ourselves. Take birthday parties, for instance. Somethin' like that would happen during the day and it would pick us all up. We still have a big Thanksgiving and Christmas party.

The parish's only health unit for many years was in Bogalusa, twenty-five miles away. That health unit first opened on a full-time basis on November 1, 1921, and was one of the first six in the state. On growing up in the rural South:

> When I was a girl there was only school nurses. There was no health unit. The parish health unit first opened in the basement of the parish prison downtown [in Franklinton] in the early 1940s. I'm 69, so I go back a long ways. When the polio and TB vaccines came out they were given in the health unit, that's when all these vaccines were first given out. They used to do skin tests on everybody. Polio, flu, measles, TB, and everything. The sanitarians have put up with us, I think, as a marriage of convenience from the beginning. They didn't have milk [quality control] inspectors back then, before World War II. In ten years, '45 to '55, everything changed. See, I remember us not havin' electricity 'cause I lived out in the rural area. We had kerosene lamps and a well with a hand pump. We had a big cement culvert and the cows would just come over and drink until they would just about pop on a hot day. But that hand pump was a tough job all right. I think about my momma so much. We didn't have any money because we just about raised everythin' we lived on. And she did not have a lazy bone in her. She always had somethin' on the stove for us.
>
> We would come into Franklinton for food, and to Warnerton to the little general store north of here. But there was really nothin' there. Just a railroad track [station]. We lived about a mile from there. We came in to do our trading, you see we didn't purchase back then. When we came in for our eggs, we would ride the school bus in, 'cause we didn't have a car. We would have enough money left over to go to the show, to see maybe Will Rogers. I was maybe 13 or 14. I was a big girl pumping water when we got electricity. We used firewood for our heat. We walked to a small country church. Oh God, has this parish changed. But you know, I wouldn't change anything for being born and reared in the area that I was, and, of course, y'all don't know anything about what I'm sayin' but it's real to me. I try to tell my kids but they don't pay any attention.
>
> My dad worked real hard. They had three girls and I was the middle girl. I guess I was the black sheep, the baby for twelve years. My oldest sister, I guess,

she had it hardest, workin' out in the fields. One day we went to the health unit and Dr. Hollis passed us and said 'boy, them girls must've really been dropping some sodium because their backs are so bent outta shape.' Nitrate soda, you put around the corn, for acres and acres, by hand. We probably farmed about eighty acres. There were no fences, and the cows would always come up to our lot. The roads were horrible. That was the worst thing. Old gravel and dirt roads. Every Saturday we came into town. But when I was a little girl we went into town to that little grocery store that had everythin.'

That's another thing. See, these peddlers would come around. The peddlers would come by and they would stay at the house. And the next day they would open their suitcase and show us all these pretty materials, fabrics, washin' products, health tonics, and Momma would buy some and he would give us a gift for lettin' him stay overnight. They came along in cars. All year round, I guess. [They even sold] burial policies. They would then come by and collect the fees every so often. Mine was 15 cents a month back then. Just the other day I was thinkin' 'bout my policy and I called about it, and the fee for the next year [2000] is $1.65. Before there was a health unit here, the mommas did all the doctoring.' If I had a broken arm it might've just had to heal on its own. I remember old Dr. Hollis, because there weren't many. There were usually these old midwives. Aunt Collie was one. Everyone was born at home back then. When we had pneumonia they would wrap us all up in these 'stinky bags.' They would towel us up and cover us with all kinds of ointment for I don't know how long. We slept in them bags. We were kept in them. I remember my sister had tonsillitis real bad. I remember the midwife told her to fry some eggs and put them in a cloth poultice. She tied it around my sister's neck and she then slept in it. The next day when she took it off, those eggs were *green*. And she then threw 'em out into the yard and the dog ate 'em, and he died. But she [my sister] got well. The nearest hospital [fifty miles away] was in Tylertown, Mississippi.

Reflections on racial segregation in the South, the health unit, and its future:

Everybody comes here now. Before integration [1964] the patients at the health unit were mostly white. And, uh, blacks would be allowed to come here only for maternity clinics. I don't know if there was much prenatal care for 'em. There were separate restrooms and waiting rooms [for blacks] in health units, including here, when it was in the jail basement. I never will forget when they [blacks] started comin' to the clinics in larger numbers. One white woman said one day, 'Look at that colored woman, why is she in here?' The doctor said, 'this [place] is for everybody!'

I think the health unit has a good future in this town. It will come to a point when more and more people will depend on it. For a while we were worried [in the 1990s] that they [private providers] were goin' to take away our jobs. But the federal government audits all these private programs real carefully, and I don't think these people [private providers] want to deal with all that [bureaucracy].

On the perception of the health unit within the local community:

> Before all this other private [primary] care came in [in the 1990s], this was the only place available. And as for all the people who went to these private providers, they're now comin' back to us. When we built that new health unit in Bogalusa, they said 'we're gettin' a new health unit.' They're proud of it, and they think of it the same way as a new parish library or school building. They take pride in this health unit. Now they'll say, once in a while, that they would like the place [facility] here [in Franklinton] to be better. But they know they can call on us for practically anything. If they want a number for a related social or health service they can just call the health unit. Even on things unrelated to health. We like to call it the *help unit*.

The Nurse

Cynthia Sloan is the nursing coordinator at the Tensas Parish Health Unit in St. Joseph. St. Joseph, a once-prosperous parish seat, was the economic and cultural hub for the surrounding cotton industry and associated processing plants. The parish has been losing population steadily in recent years, from a peak of over 20,000 in the late 1950s to a current low of only 6,000. Cynthia and one other full-time registered nurse staff the clinic in St. Joseph (Fig. 3.7). In addition to the nurses, there are two full-time clerks and one parish sanitarian.[2] The parish provides custodial and rudimentary building maintenance services. Cynthia begins:

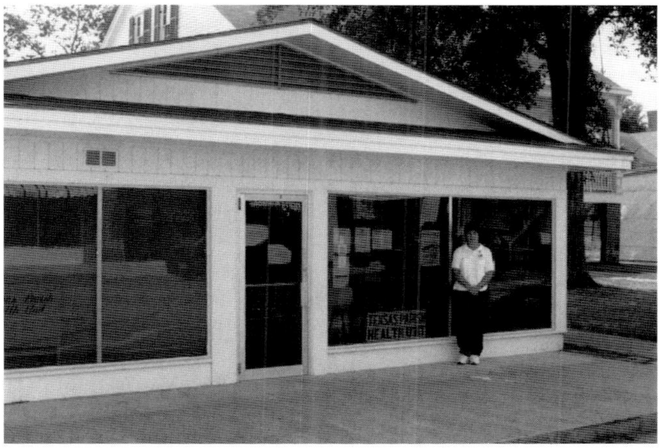

Fig. 3.7

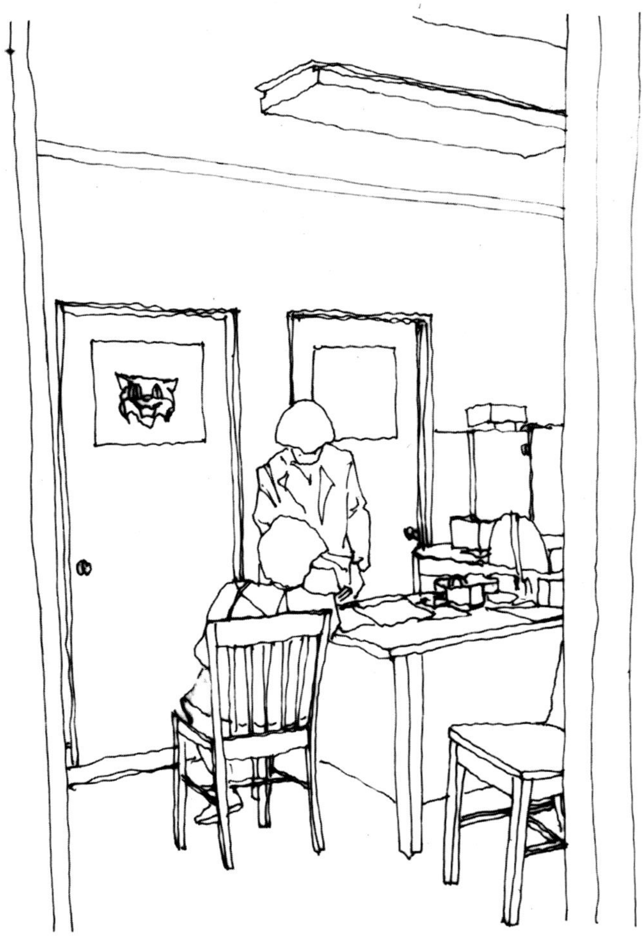

Fig. 3.8

Our parish doesn't have a hospital. Well, we have a doctor in town, but if somebody doesn't have a medical [Medicaid] card they know they can just come in here and get our opinion and ask questions like 'Do you think this is somethin' I can just take care of on my own at home?' Or 'What should I treat it with?' We guide them to the right place. Sometimes, though, it gets kind of scary because I might be out of my realm. But I then just refer them to the local doctor if I'm not sure. Like, on Friday afternoon, a lady came in here with a swollen throat and I told her 'Just go get some Benadryl and if you have any trouble go to the doctor.' In fact I was tryin' to get her to take a shot.

I've been here for nineteen years [as of 1999] as a public health nurse. We have as many as three [nurses] here at one time. But one is part-time three days per week. Well, you just get to know 'em [patients]. The nurse I replaced had been here for twenty-five years, and the other nurse replaced one who had been here for twenty-nine. This goes back to the 1930s. You start out and you just get to know 'em and you know when their kids have kids, and you [eventually] know 'em all. And that's what's great. And through nineteen years I've seen the kids grow up, through age five with WIC, and then when they come back in as teenagers to either get their shots, if it's the guys, or the girls, when they come in for their family planning. I say 'I haven't seen you in so long.' And they say to their Momma, 'How does she know me? She's actin' like she knows me.' And I go '*cause I do know you*. I used to take care of you when you were a baby!

I can keep up with 'em though family planning, or if I'm readin' the paper and I see that's so and so playin' basketball or something. I watch 'em, you

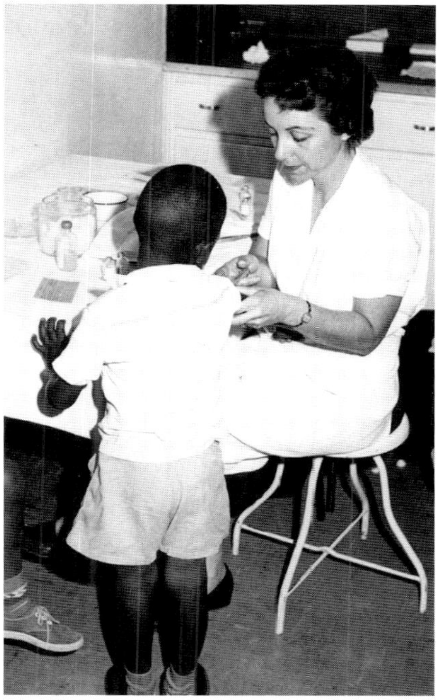

Fig. 3.9

know, if they're goin' to college or whatever. I know the kids, the parents and when *they* become parents or even grandparents. We know the families that care of their children and the families that don't take care of their children. And that's an advantage to us in a small town, with a small health unit. We'll call and ask 'Did you get that baby to the doctor?' I pretty much keep a mental list of all that but I also have a referral list I check up on. But mostly mental. I say if they can't get me at least get to somebody.

Everybody knows what we do. I give a lot of flu shots [Fig. 3.8]. A lot of people come in here to get their blood pressure monitored. Everybody knows everybody in this parish. We know people that in a bigger parish we wouldn't know, out and about, like at the grocery store, and we can 'cuss 'em out to see that they get proper follow-up care. We see about 300 patients per month. We do not make 'em have a medical [Medicaid] card to let them get their shots here for free or for five dollars, versus $350-400 dollars. We see a lot of WIC patients here. When a mom comes in with their baby for shots, I'll say 'Have you heard about our WIC program?'

We have a hard time having 'em keep their appointments because of the lack of transportation. I only have the Council on Aging, and the St. Joe's neighborhood center. I think they're federally funded and they provided transportation. And then they cut out the Medicaid funded transportation 'cause it was bein' abused [statewide]. The biggest problem is the lack of [public] transportation in the parish. Often, you may have somebody walk in and say 'I didn't have any way here yesterday.' They really don't. And even if they come in on their day, they might miss their appointment for that day.

The Office of Public Health has for generations provided immunizations for young children, as illustrated in this 1963 photo from Tallulah, Madison Parish (Fig. 3.9). In the 1950s and early '60s a mobile chest X-ray unit made the rounds in the state's northernmost rural parishes, and its itinerary included scheduled screening for tuberculosis on scheduled clinic days in St. Joseph and in the neighboring parishes (Fig. 3.10). Regarding nurses' dedication, in emergencies Cynthia has frequently ventured during clinic hours and on evenings

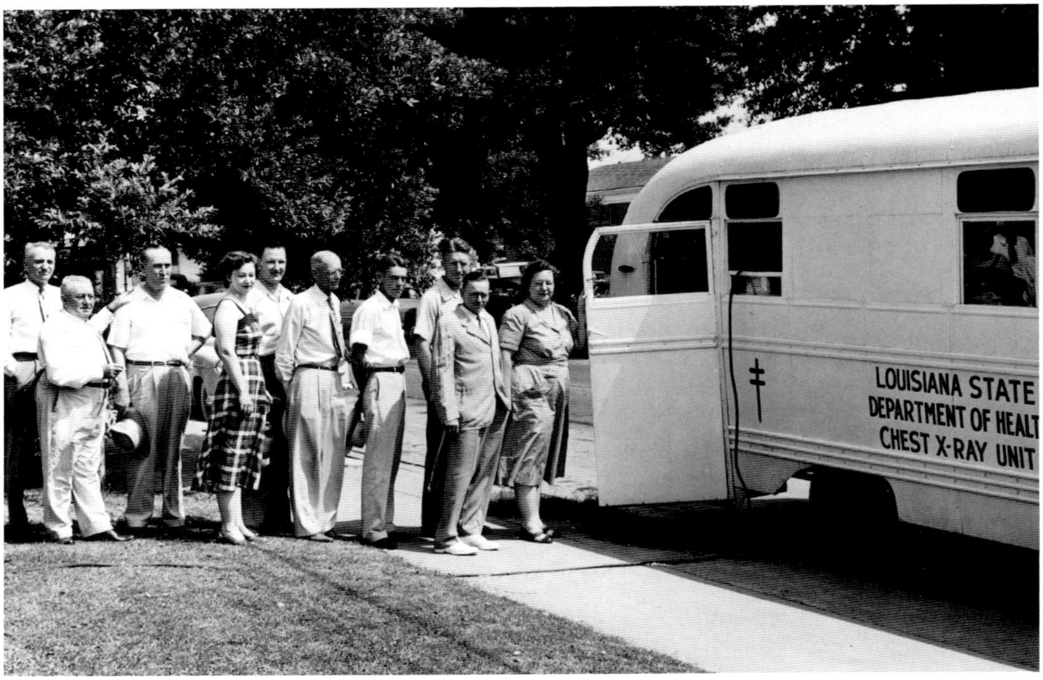

Fig. 3.10

and weekends to the rural countryside to make house calls. One such case involved a small baby.

> Once, there was a case of a sick baby in Newellton. I had to go out and do some checkin' up. The little baby was here from Texas. They were visiting over the holidays. We had to get the names afterwards of all the relatives to see whom the baby had been in contact with. There were *lots* of relatives in that house over Christmastime. If there are accidents on the schoolyard, the school nurse calls me for a second opinion. The nearest hospital is forty-five miles away [in Ferriday] and an hour way [Vicksburg]. One place here in town does take x-rays. We have a nurse practitioner in one clinic, in Newellton, and she has a doctor come in from Winnsboro four hours a week. Then we have an old doctor, Dr. Whitaker, who comes in one day per week. And we have two family physicians that work clinic part time in town. They'll be between Ferriday, here, Newellton, and Vidalia.

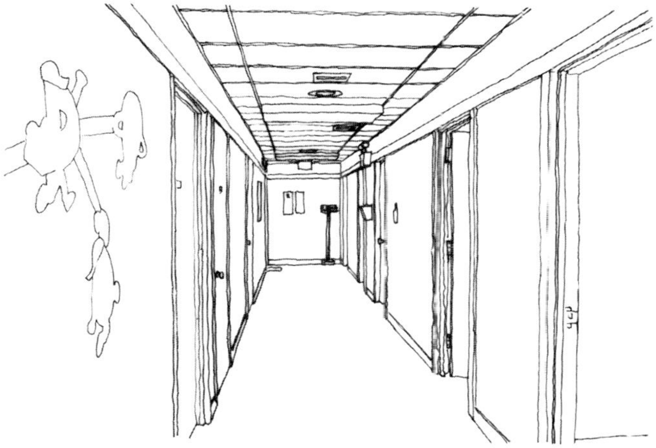

Fig. 3.11

Many new programs have been started over the twenty-one years Cynthia has worked at the health unit. One of these is called Healthy Communities:

> It [the program] is about collaborating with people in your town to help solve issues and work on projects to help your town. It doesn't have to *directly* relate to the heath of the community, just to the overall betterment of your community, whatever that takes. I set up the meetings. Most of the meetings are across the street at the restaurant at lunch-time. We've been havin' 'em once a month. We're workin' on the St. Jude rock-athon and sponsoring the St. Jude's coalition. The other project we have is for some type of beautification, because I know there used to be funds for some of that stuff. Workin' on old buildings, plantin' flowers, trees, whatever. I don't think they think it's too unusual for a nurse to do stuff like that. They accept me because they trust me and because I'm from here. I've been here the whole time. That's why they [community leaders] are workin' with me.

On the then-current location of the health unit on Main Street (a replacement facility designed by Waycaster Architects of Natchez, Mississippi, opened in 2002, one block away), and its civic importance in the cultural landscape:

> But even to those who don't use it [the health unit], I think they think it's a real good thing that it's here. It used to be down the street in an old building on the corner, an office building or somethin.' Where we are now was once a dress shop. I'm not sure how long it was a dress shop. The health unit has been in here about twenty-one years. This was, before that, a family planning clinic, before public health merged with 'em. This was considered a big step up then. They had done some renovations for us [Fig. 3.11]. They had put in a WIC kitchen, some sinks in the exam rooms, and they purchased new file shelves. It is important that we're in the center of the parish, next door to the library and near [one block] the parish courthouse.

On the current physical condition of the health unit and the political pressure to remain in the old location:

> We [are] not all on top of each other but storage-wise we are, and the clerks are [very crowded] up front. But at least we do have *a little* bit of space to move around. We need to purge our record files. Emily's nephew owns the health unit building because it was his daddy's. He rented it out to a dress shop for years. When I most recently talked with the police jury about the tobacco monies, I was asked 'if y'all had given any consideration to just renovatin' the building you're in?' I've been asked if that would be a possibility for us. I then asked [them] 'Have you been asked that by the owner?' And he said 'I can't divulge that.' Well, he's [the owner] a bigwig in New Orleans. The owner would never spend a penny of his money on this building. So I'd like to take those cabinets and anything else out of the kitchen because they're *ours*. We paid for 'em. The rent is about $600 per month. We just renewed the lease 'cause we don't think this [new facility] is gonna be done anytime soon.
>
> We were lookin' at that house down the street [three] years ago. It still hasn't sold. We looked at the social services [building] site, the residential house, the vacant lots in the neighborhood back in there behind us, and the residential house that abutted right up behind the town attorney's house. He really wanted me to look at that. Some of these sites I knew weren't worth pursuing. Land sellers sometimes come out of the woodwork. I even ran an ad in the newspaper '*Looking for a health unit site, at least an acre, within city limits, please call.*' Why? Because I thought it was never gonna happen. It's been just awful. And I was gettin' desperate. You can't just find any land without a buildin' on it. Unless it was somewhere out in the middle of a field. And we're lucky that the police jury can tear that mess down [existing dilapidated structures on the site finally purchased] without chargin' us for it. The attorney general's office told us that you could not offer more than the appraised value for a property unless somebody approves it. Well. I think they're goin' ahead with it anyway.

On the era when Main Street separated the white and African American sides of town:

> During the fifties it was booming, but I don't ever remember it booming. On Saturday nights, according to the old nurses aide who used to work here.

> She told me that on Saturday nights you wouldn't believe how many people were out on that street. Well, the movies, the bars, the vacant corner right here—that was a bar. Downtown was all white during those years, though there was a white bar down across there [in the colored section], now called the 'Walking Pig.' Blacks couldn't go to the movie theater, and there wasn't much else for 'em. The theater closed down right after integration.
>
> I don't know if they [the blacks] just chose not to, or couldn't [come in the front door], but blacks just came in the back door of the saloon. There were just two rooms. The night I went in there, heck, half of the people I knew were on the other side and they were callin' me by name 'cause they knew me. I mean, everybody in town knows everybody. I wanted to go see. So, my daddy said 'I'll take you to see.' It had swingin' doors, and mounts in there. See, at the end of the street [at the levee], when you made the loop, see, if anybody was goin' there the doors, you know, would swing open and you could see what was on the walls. And there were mounts of deer, buffalo and all these different animal mounts, bobcats and everythin.' They [the field workers] came in through the back door where, he [the landowner] already had it all set up to where they were taken care of—drinks, whatever, on the other side of that wall.

Each fall the Louisiana Sportsman Festival takes place on the vacant lot across the street from the former saloon. Earlier, it was called the Turkey Festival. Up and down the street the vendors flank both sides. Vendors come in from many states: Texas, Arkansas, Mississippi, Alabama, other parts of Louisiana, and other parts of the United States. From noon on the day before the festival the health unit does not schedule appointments. Instead, the nurses offer free screenings for blood pressure, counseling on flu shots, and general sickness prevention advice, just as though it were a health fair. Local residents call Cynthia before the local pharmacist: "Adam has a bad fever, tell me what I need to do."

The staff waited years for a new facility, and it finally became a reality through the receipt of "capital outlay funds" from Baton Rouge. These funds, from the state's general appropriations bill, were dedicated for construction of a replacement health unit facility and represented a small fraction—$550,000—of the State's settlement of its $300 million lawsuit against the tobacco manufacturers. The total budget for the new health unit would be $800,000:

Senator Jones obtained the money to build a new health unit building a year ago last July. The money was to be spent to choose and appraise the site we were considering for the new building. We wanted a big site and the one we first wanted down at the corner [four doors down from the existing facility, on the site of an old gas station and furniture store, which had burned down in 1990] had old oil tanks under it. The owner did not want to take 'em up himself. It would have been at our expense. But we had to legally bid on it as well as the one [finally chosen] across the street even though we had no intention of gettin' it. We had to attend a number of meetings to get them [the police jury] to vote for the one we wanted. The first appraiser, his piece of property was appraised higher than the other properties around it, and then they had to hire a second appraiser. He used the same exact land measurements as the first appraiser, and he came in with the same figures. Then they hired an architect from the outside [from nearby Natchez, Mississippi] to help because one juror said 'this is not our area of expertise.' So they hired him and he said the property measurements and the plot size don't match.

He [the architect] had built the new bank here, so they knew him. He thinks [the site chosen] is great. When the bids came in, Ronnie had put a clause in that it would be binding only on the architect's approval. Some of the surrounding owners were thinkin' 'Well, I can get more money for my property with a higher land appraisal.' And 'why is he gettin' more for his land than I am for mine?' That's when things got hot. The first appraiser, from out of town [Columbia] was the mayor's friend. He appraised the mayor's land higher than anybody else's. And the mayor, conveniently, wasn't there, but he was gettin' fried right there. And on the larger site [of the two finalist parcels] there was a lady who wanted her big white house moved someplace else. Well, I sat at that meetin' on needles and pins because my husband is a contractor, you know, and he said once a bid is accepted [it] is legally binding. And the attorney said to Ronnie, 'I'll get you all these titles and good bids if you don't shop 'outta town for an attorney.' So then, when they decide that they wanted it, the president went around to all the surrounding owners to see if they would sell. All will sell except for one. Turns out there is a lien on the title. Turns out the parish president has been paying the taxes on it so the property could be kept in the family. See the family couldn't afford to keep it up anymore on their own. The parish attorney, who has to get all the titles together, said there would be a problem gettin' a clear title.

So after they get the bids, the attorney [hired from the public health funds allocated from the state] goes 'Cynthia, do you realize there's another piece of town of St. Joseph land in it? I say, 'No, I didn't know it.' So he talks with the mayor, and he [the mayor] says 'That's OK, we'll let that go for the same price.' See, legally, the parish had to bid on the two properties we were lookin' at. Even through the one we're gettin' is smaller than the one on the [gas station] corner, they agreed to buy it at the same price [as they would have paid for the larger parcel]. Can you believe they done that? That should have been the town's priority to say, 'Why should we pay the same for that little piece [the smaller parcel which was eventually purchased]?'

The police jury was split on whether to hire an architect. They decided they needed a professional. They just needed some help. There are seven on the police jury. And the mayor and the president are really behind this. Of course, both own pieces of land involved. There was one [juror] who was always causing problems. He questions just about everything. He says 'All the state agencies have to be next door to each other.' That's the first thing we had to hear. He wanted us out on the edge of town next door to the social services unit. He wanted us down there by them. We said 'Please don't stick us down a side road. You know, where no one can even see us 'cause we might have to share driveways and all that. Well, at least we haven't had to hear any of that for a while.

Well, I think, when the building starts to go up, woe be us. He will stay on us. A lot of times it is due to bad blood, things I don't know anything about. I just feel I'll have all kinds of trouble from him once the building starts to go up. It won't be the right color. It won't be the right size. The point is that he's got another agenda, because he wanted a committee for the health unit's construction, and they didn't do it.

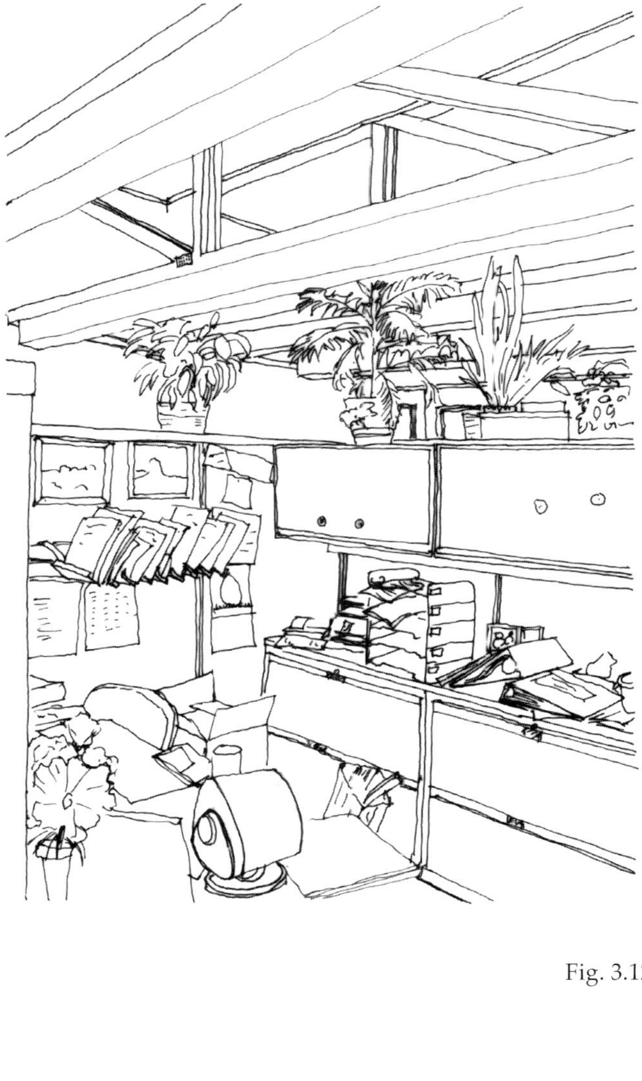

Fig. 3.12

The Parish Sanitarian

The term protector, versus caregiver, is perhaps more accurate in describing the work of a parish sanitarian. The sanitarian provides a wide spectrum of services to the community quite apart, at least on the surface, from those of the clerical and clinical staff. The origins of sanitarian services date from the 1890s in Louisiana. The sanitation specialist had become a key staff member by the late 1920s and remains integral to this day (Fig. 3.12). Ricky Mahaffey is the regional sanitarian in Region V. He administers all the environmental health programs in the region monitored by the Office of Public Health[3] and he coordinates a staff of eleven inspectors.

> There are some newer programs that have been instituted such the lead programs and other monitoring [programs] that have come about. The older programs are basically in three categories; these are in general sanitation, retail food, and laboratory. Those programs have been greatly expanded upon in many areas. In other words, what we used to do ten years ago might seem superficial compared to the way we do it now and [everything is] much more detailed now, with all the [new] regs [regulations]. Much more detailed, much more involved. The federal regs have gotten much bigger and it's all filtered down, especially in general sanitation and in general food. General sanitation encompasses your general sewage program. In other words, many years ago people used to just come in and fill out a permit and put in a sewer system before you [they] did anything. Now, with the ordinances we have in place, no matter what you do you have to come in and get it checked out by us, whether it's to build a new house, trailer, a motor home, whatever. Used to be you just told us what was out there. Now, we've got to send an agent out to the site before we can ever issue anything. We have to check out the discharge points. So when we see a person come in to fill out that permit we have to see what we have in place. So if there's not there when we go out there they have to come back. We might see them three, four times before we can issue anything. Used to be we used to see 'em once in the office and once in the field.
>
> Now, with the *stress* that they've put on environmental factors, and stuff, with the population growth you've got more emissions from individual sewer systems. So therefore, we've got to worry about those emissions being of an approved standard. We've also have now a greater populace utilizing more and more retail food service outlets, and this can cause a great deal of damage

to a lot of people. Also, since 1988, we've implemented fee programs, where all these establishments now must have a permit. Fifteen years ago there was a lot of establishments operatin' by means of a permit that each individual parish gave out, and if you didn't have time to fool with retail food, you know, there was some of those places that may never have gotten looked at for two or three years, or business places. This is a statewide program. Now, because of the fee process and with the feeding [WIC] programs and all that kinda stuff we've to get those programs on our fee rolls. Those businesses are tied to our WIC programs [and] to our alcohol and beverage control programs. In other words, those agencies won't be allow 'em to accept WIC [vouchers] unless they have a permit from the health department. They won't allow 'em to sell alcoholic beverages unless they have a permit from the health department. So, we're tied in to a lot of other state agencies, on businesses. And every year we get more and more businesses because business follows the growth of the population. One fee increase was considered recently but it wasn't passed by the legislature.

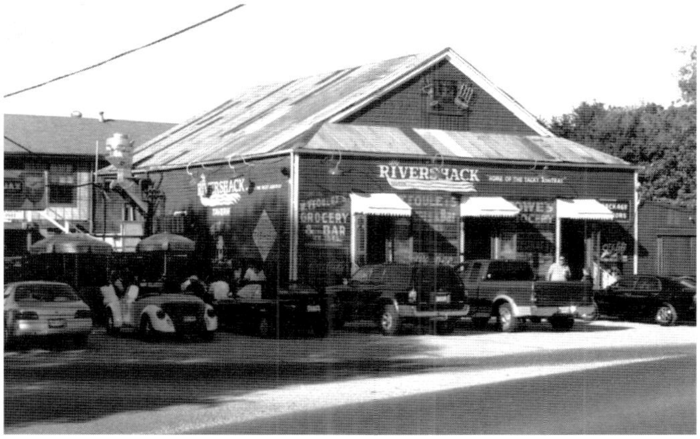

Fig. 3.13

The role of the sanitarian in the event of a local environmental health emergency:

Well, in most cases anything that happens locally falls under the environmental health and nursing programs [at the health unit]. And of course we'll rely on assistance from the local region office and the central office. But it depends on the type of emergency. They may not be able to assist us in anything other than general information. I mean, as far as the actual collection of data, and the home site investigations and stuff, that would be handled by us, and of course it would be handled in accord with protocol handed down from the central office. But the manpower itself most often comes from here. And that's gonna involve anything from—we went through an ice storm here a couple years ago [1997] where it was probably anything as bad or worse as any hurricane that could've hit because we lost power throughout this whole parish [Calcasieu]. When those lines started breakin' from that ice it virtually leveled all the major power lines in this area. So, for a day we were virtually shut down, ineffective, for a day because the red light were out, the phones wouldn't work and we couldn't travel. Course, once the red lights came back on, and we could get around to see what happened, and the phones came back on, we were surveying establishments to see how the long they had been without power. We went out to see what kind of damages we had to food products, [and we were] giving 'em [businesses, schools, etc.] information about food damage for certain products and information bout how long you [they] could keep it [the food]. You know, if it had to be destroyed.

We lost power to water supplies and so they were in need of monitoring. We lost power to the sewerage system so the sewerage was not bein' fully treated. All we could do was stay abreast with those people and tell 'em, 'Hey, look, you know, this is what you need to do to keep these things goin' and take these precautions.' And of course, on the major water supplies and major sewerage systems you [we] were getting information provided from the regional and central office level. But all the local retail food stores and eating and drinkin' establishments, we were takin' care of those and keeping information on all that [Fig. 3.13].

Also, anytime you have a food borne outbreak, in other words, you may have a school population that is infected by salmonella, segalia, or staffocaccus [*sic*] or whatever it is, whatever microbe might be the causative agent, then we get involved with food sampling and interviews which also involves the laboratory. There's a lot of times when we do interviewing, and the nursing corps is with us. You know, it depends on if we can isolate the organism. Once these people go to the hospital or whatever they [hospital biotechnicians] will help us isolate the organism. The hospital will call us and tell us what they suspect is the causative agent and then what has been cultured as the causative agent. That gives us a little more information, a little better idea if it's strictly food borne due to a food handler, if it's a disease where we have to call the nurses in, or a carrier type individual. A lot of times they'll do the interviews of the food handlers or whatever while we're takin' the food samples. They're [nursing staff] also interviewing the people who are ill. The rural parishes all have a rabies control program where you have an instance of actual contact between a wild animal or an unvaccinated domestic animal [and a person] and you have a bite or a scratch occur or a skin break. The rural parishes will end up havin' to submit the animal heads to the [region] laboratory. Fortunately, in this parish [Calcasieu] because of the size of it and everythin' there's no way this office could even make a dent in tryin' to do that because you've got to respond immediately. So, here, there is an animal control program that is operated by the parish, but, operated under the Calcasieu Parish Health Unit direction and [its] budgetary [control]. Because of the metropolitan [nature] of this parish, you've got a titnus control program—which is your rodents and rats—you've got a mosquito control program and you've got a rabies control program.

In a rural [health unit] the parish sanitarian has also has to respond to all those things. In the cases of rodent control, and mosquito control, there's hardly no positive effect at all because if you can't spray, [and] don't have the sprayers, or can't spray, [you] can't do anything other than contact the local police jury 'bout it. You have to say "Hey, look, you know we need somethin' for the drainage out here and can you help us out on it?' Or, 'If you don't mind can you look into puttin' in a mosquito control [program]?' Of course, the rural parishes don't have the money to do that. The rodent control program is almost nonexistent except for the issue of roadsides, and hopefully then you can get some volunteers to disseminate 'em [traps] once a year or somethin' like that. But it's difficult.

On the monitoring of water quality, Mahaffey continues:

Fortunately, in this parish all the water supplies are groundwater supplies, and not surface water supplies, [however] all the surface water is monitored in the parishes all along the Mississippi River over there [the eastern side of the state] but over here its groundwater. We have to monitor—we pull the actual samples on these water supplies except for the city of Lake Charles—they do they're own monitoring 'cause we don't have the manpower. They send us a report, but for the rest of the parish we sample the water districts based on only a certain number of samples per population which will range from one sample on the smallest systems to very many. In [the town of] Sulfur, we've got to pool twenty samples every month—that's every month. So we probably sample at least 100-150 water samples every month through the lab next door. When the population grows the number of samples naturally increases.

From time to time, the parish sanitarian becomes embroiled in disputes and lawsuits with developers, business establishments, and private individuals:

Well, I'm in one [lawsuit] right now. I can't really go into any great detail on this. There's a case where there's a dispute between our agency on the handling of an individual sewer program. Due to some competitive forces out there with the mechanical plants, and so on and so forth, there's some concern over whether everybody's bein' treated fairly with regards to their units and the components that are supposed to be going on. The one I'm in right now [lawsuit] is the biggest one ever. This one is for a lot of money. I definitely do get caught right in the middle. There are always disputes with homeowners and landowners in non- compliance with the requirements. And of course you know when you're dealin' with business clientele. Their bottom line is money. Sometimes they didn't do things because they didn't know, and I can buy that, and sometimes they do things just to be saving the bottom line. And, you know, we run into those issues with developers, who want to take subdivisions and develop 'em with house lots—to utilize individual sewerage in this parish—because the ordinance states you can go down to a lot as small as 80 x 200. You've got to have 80 feet of road front and 16,000 square feet of area. Now, [for] an individual who has a large tract of land our code says that after 124 units you have to have to go to community sewerage. So, we get into those disputes a lot because those people want to develop 200-300 acres of land with 300-400 lots all using individual sewers. Because if they use an individual sewer and he sells the homeowner a lot, the homeowner builds a house and puts his own individual sewer system [then] the developer's out of the picture. But, if he [the developer] has to put in a community sewer, somebody has to be responsible to the [community] system not only from the time of implementation, but *forever*.

It [regulation and monitoring] all falls onto us. As far the initial recommendations and so forth, now the final continuous operation of a community discharge system is all caught up with DEQ [State Department of Environmental Quality] discharge permits. But those developers don't want to go through community sewerage. It probably cost 'em a half million dollars for the system, and another million to put in the collection lines and everything else and they have to pass that cost on to the purchaser of the lot. This would make the value of the lot go extremely high, so they'd rather try to do it with individual sewers and what you'd end up with would be 400-500 individual homes on an individual sewer each producing around 400 gallons per day of water per resident. Now calculate that out. You've got 400-500 emitters with 400 gallons a day of water. Rather than *one* central community sewer collection system which would be maintained by a maintenance provider. And having to follow strict DEQ discharge permits, which would be, environmentally, much more sound, but, economically, extremely expensive. Well, to get around it they try a lot of ways—by sending subdivisions through in phases. They would send in a phase of lots, say, 60 or 70 lots. And you approve a phase for individual sewer development. Then, later on you get another phase and it's 60 or 70 lots and you're lookin' at it—it's all fewer than 124—but when you total 'em all out they have gone *over*. And, man, when you try to stop that, you know, you run into a lot of . . . flak . . . you don't want.

But the developers, they don't want to understand it because it costs 'em money. See, as long as they have 124 [unit lots] they're on the same playin' field as everybody else. But when they go over that and they have to go to the community sewer they'll say, 'Well here's a developer over here that's got only 60 lots. He's gonna sell his 60 way faster than I am because he doesn't have to.' And they just don't want it. They don't want the legal ramifications and responsibility of having to continually maintain that system.

On flood control, drainage problems, and rapid population growth:

Each parish planning a development operating through the FEMA [Federal Emergency Management Agency] program has to file the flood elevation [data]. The only thing we have to worry 'bout is that with the use of mechanical systems and with the use of compressors. They have to be located above the flood plane. Because if it floods, it's a legal question and you've gotta' remember, your rural areas are developing much faster than the municipal areas because most of 'em are already developed. So, they're sort of stymied with [rural] annexation, because every time they annex they annex rural property [and] this increases their expenses with community sewerage and community water. This often means that not only is there more expense in providing those services to allow the extra flow goin' in but also they have to upgrade their entire system. And they depend on grants and so on and so forth, and that takes years. So, as our local population grows it grows out into the country, it grows into the rural areas that need individual water wells or individual sewer systems. Well, these people are migrating from the city to the country. They don't know. They gettin' used to flushing their toilet and turnin' on their water faucet. And, you know, the waste is treated—they never see it—they don't know or really care how. They don't know if that plant's working or not. They're able to get the electricity off of it, and you know, and the breaker's liable to throw and they'll never know if the compressor's not runnin' or [its] burned out. They don't know. They'll go on vacation, turn it off, and it's not gonna work, so . . . if we didn't have all this *growth* we wouldn't have all these problems. We're 175,000 and still growin.'

On the issuance of construction permits for the renovation of existing properties:

> In the older neighborhoods most big parishes have construction ordinances requiring permits before they can do anything. That means we can go back in and do somethin' about making 'em upgrade those old sewage systems. We still got many, many places on what we call 'postage stamp lots,' meaning 50' x 100.' In the city that's not a problem but in the country it is [a problem] 'cause those lots were created prior to 1967, when there were no true mechanisms to force people to connect to larger sewer systems and we're taking 'bout lots of situations like that. And even as they come through [the permitting process] we try to catch 'em. In those situations it works because they're trying to do somethin' with that property. The money's there. But on each side of 'em there might be ten non-compliant sewer systems. So the only other way you can do it is through attrition. When they're developing or when a house burns down in a neighborhood, we require the upgrade. They usually have some sort of loan or federal grant so we can capitalize on that. Otherwise, if we just go out there and try to make 'em do it we would flood the court system with impoverished people claiming they have no money [to upgrade]. You're lookin' at $1,600-1,700 per lot it it's a mechanical system with gravity flow and if you add a sump pump it's at least another $300.00 dollars.
>
> They have to come here first. If they [the public utility] turn off the electricity for 90 days, or it's a rent house or your own house, you've got to go through us and we'll go back out and inspect your existing system to see if it's compliant. So, we may review some systems many times. And others we may never see in a lifetime. Some of those rental properties—we got some files two inches thick. You know, the worst problems are those outside the municipal limits.
>
> We are in a big bind right now 'cause I'm down to a staff of five. We can't run around too much because time is such a factor. See, what we've got to do is just delay their services. I just can't send one guy to Fenton and then send him to Thompson because he'd travel 200-250 miles just inside the Parish. Well, each person here has a geographical area he covers. When I came here I developed areas for each one [of the staff] and, you see, one only goes to 'Area 7' so it would be cost-efficient. Also, we devised it such that we developed a balance of a certain number of food establishments. Each supervisor has subordinates under him. Each person serves roughly 20,000-22,000 persons in their area. But each [area] contains from 140 to 190 food services permits, requiring that many inspections within each three-month period. Those people do anywhere from 40 to 60 food service inspections in a month's time. And with all the sewer in-

spections and applications, each [sanitarian] has approximately 8-10 of these per week. Then, we have to do plant inspections at least once a year, in conjunction with the state Fire Marshall. And we have to do the incarceration facilities twice each year. These are 100 to 200 bed facilities.

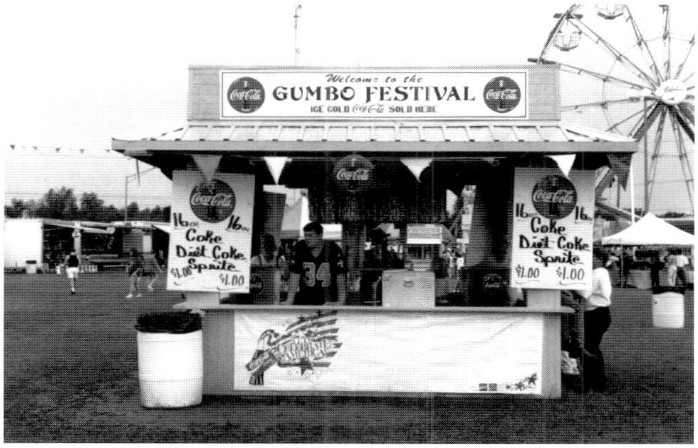

Fig. 3.14

On having served as a sanitarian in a rural parish:

I was the parish sanitarian for fourteen and a half years in Allen Parish [a neighboring parish]. I came here in February of '96. When I was in Allen that prison [Allen State Correctional Facility] kept over 1,400 inmates. That was a three-day job, with at least three days office follow-up work the next week. You have to go in and ask the inmate to turn on all those faucets in all those cells and check everything, even the ventilation and all that. You sleep well those nights. There's over a mile of catwalks up and down. You check the kitchens, bakeries, all that. You try to do it once in the hot weather, and once in the cold weather, per year. And when I made suggestions, I had no problem [with compliance] because some years ago a federal judge [Polozola] laid down a consent order on reasonable living conditions—that they had to meet certain standards. Then they came up with new standards. Now the state leases the buildings to a private concern and the State is out of actually running the facility. And without ACA [American Correctional Association] accreditation, they lose their lease. They've got some stringent standards and in fact they say that in an incarceration facility there is no reason why something shouldn't be clean, fixed, and workin.' All those inmates [1,440] are sentenced to hard labor, so they [the administration] has all the help they need to get anything done. You walk through there with maybe a couple of correctional officers and a safety manager, and you see something that needs repair, sometimes by the time you make the walk back [to your on-site office] it's done. If they need a part, in most cases they can get it right from their warehouse. And big parish hospitals, nursing homes, they're most all like that. As I said, the most difficult thing is to deal with individuals, their money, and mom and pop operations.

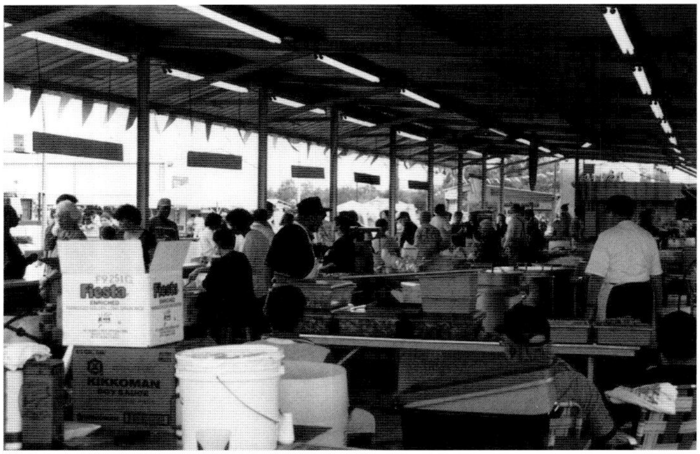

Fig. 3.15

Many parishes hold annual food festivals. Most are held in the fall or spring and take place in the parish seat. Examples include the Bridge City Gumbo Festival (Fig. 3.14 and Fig. 3.15) the Louisiana Rice Festival in Crowley, the Ponchatoula Strawberry Festival, and perhaps the most well known, the annual New Orleans Jazz and Heritage Festival in New Orleans. The festivities revolve mostly around a particular local food legacy—crawfish, shrimp, rice, and tomato, to name but a few delicacies. These culinary traditions are typically celebrated in consort with a local community's indigenous music. The parish sanitarian tends to adopt a unique, and, some would say, unorthodox, stance with respect to these popular events:

> Fairs and festivals in the state of Louisiana are exempt from [DHH] Health Department jurisdiction, unless they apply to us at least thirty days in advance for us to monitor 'em. The way I understand [how] this all happened was that one or two of 'em went back to the legislature, and, well, I was on a board, and I didn't have to participate 'cause I was in a one-man parish. The World's Fair in New Orleans [1984] was how all this happened. We were told that we would all be put on two-week shifts to help out. We were all put on alert. They were goin' to put us up in dormitories or whatever. And when it came down to it I didn't have to go 'cause I was in a one-man parish and if I'd left we'd have nobody there. So, a lot of the sanitarians started servin' over there [New Orleans]. I think that when the fair started strugglin' financially, and they had a lot of those little food booths, that was when the problems really started. Those people were paying their fair share for their operation while they weren't exactly meetin' our criteria. So they were gettin' shut down. They were goin' broke. So it got to a point that the Legislature convened and passed a resolution to exempt the World's Fair. That was soon challenged in court by the others [some other fairs and festivals statewide] and so they had to exempt *all* fairs and festivals thereafter.

> But the Jazz Fest [New Orleans] right away went back and said 'Hey, we want to be in [health] departmental jurisdiction. We don't want to be exempt.' So they said 'OK, now we've got a request that this particular entity wants inspections.' So they said, 'fine.' So when some of the others heard that they said 'Well, we'd like that too.' Some of 'em were worried about the liability. Some other parishes, cause they had had so many applicants, were lookin' for reasons to exempt [deny] 'em. Using the health department is therefore a good way to restrict the number of parties who want to participate. They then passed that thirty-day resolution, saying they [applicants] had to submit their site plans, sewage plans, water plans to go along with the application. Some times, some years they'll do that [apply], some years they won't. But out-of-state traveling carnivals or circuses—they're not exempt. We inspect 'em. They have to be declared an official event, by the mayor or the Department of Tourism. For instance, we have a Red, White and Blue Festival day in July. The mayor declares it a festival and it sneaks in without any regulations. But if a bunch of people just want to get together and say they want to hold a Red, White and Blue Day picnic or get-together, then that doesn't exempt 'em. Every parish has a parish fair. Beauregard, Jeff Davis, Allen—every one of 'em has a parish fair. And they're all exempt, by law: The Rabbit Festival, in Iowa, the Rice Festival in Crowley, all kinds of events statewide. In Cameron Parish there's the Fur Festival, where they skin muskrats, and alligator skinnin,' with contests for the fastest skinner. And they cook up all that stuff in gumbos and all that. They're all exempt. Nobody's gotten sick out here during my tenure. No. I think God takes care of those people. You know, you're drinkin' and havin' a good time and not eatin.' And the few people who do eat are probably the healthiest 'cause they don't drink [laughter]. You take a guy who's drinkin,' he's worried 'bout poppin' the next top or shootin' the next shot.

On taking the word of the food preparers that their products are safe and properly prepared at the myriad festivals and fairs that take place annually across Louisiana:

> But with those big vats of gumbo, you've got to get 'em real hot to boil 'em so to maintain proper temperature you'd have to have big heat source. But most festivals take place in mild or hot weather, so you don't have a real rapid loss of heat like you would in cold weather. So when you're cookin' stuff like gumbo that's a big plus. Crawfish, things like that. Well, again, boilin' usually takes care of most of your biological microbes. Now, some chemicals, no one has a way to check if someone's putting something in at night. With alcohol,

> no one knows the difference when they're drunk. Now even with that old Jax beer, that was the worst tastin' stuff you could ever want, but even after a few of those . . . [laughter].

The roadside bars which dot the countryside, many of which have a gumbo or crawfish boil one night of the week, pose a potentially serious public health threat:

> Well, there is a lot of concern about that. When you have a drinkin' establishment, that's a violation because that's not technically a food establishment. If you want to look that the other side of the parish festival—that is an event that occurs once per year. But for the places that do it every Saturday night, now you're getting' into a different situation. You don't know where the product came from, you don't know how it was handled before it got there. In bars and stuff, you never know who you are encountering. Some people might have TB or a lot of other things. But if you have that kind of employee even if it [the problem] isn't food-borne, preparing these foods unprotected can be a real problem. But then I'll come along and I'll see 'em passin' round the spoon [tasting] and I'll say 'Hey, Joe, how you doing?' Now you go try and regulate that. That's a custom that's been goin' on in this state for over a hundred and fifty years. You're going to run into opposition. Politically it's going to be very difficult, you know? And I can understand the politician's standpoint, I mean, here's all there people [voters] out here havin' a good time. Now, you can say 'Look, it's OK out at Joe's duck lodge, but let's not do it at Joe's lounge.' But they don't see the difference.

Many rural eating and drinking establishments evolved over the years out of private residences, as places of informal gatherings. Perhaps someone's grandma had a great gumbo recipe. Social customs and profit making imperatives are first and foremost:

> Momma always said, 'Just taste this, what do you think?' A main reason is the culture, but another is business. I try to look at all the underlying reasons. The problem started when liquor was pitted against liquor. When the drinking age was raised to twenty-one, and when the additional taxes were passed on liquor for health care [federal and state alcohol and tobacco taxes] that put the bars at a serious disadvantage with the package liquor stores. The bars became legally liable if someone got drunk and in an accident. It was now cheaper

and safer to just buy it in the store and take it home to drink on somebody's front porch. So, the bar owner, in order to compensate for his losses, he had to do something than just sell liquor. He's now got to do more than just have a band and other enticements in order to get people in there: 'Let's have gumbo as a benefit for some poor guy who got hurt in a wreck. So and so got hurt so lets get together.' Or, 'Some poor guy got cancer so let's have a benefit' Well, he's doin' a benefit, all right, and it might benefit that person, but he's doin' the biggest benefit for himself. He's going to get all that extra business. So that has changed the philosophy of lounges and that has made it even harder to regulate 'em.

It becomes a political thing when you go and try to stop that stuff and he's got a license to operate from the Police Jury as the bar owner, and he's payin' all the state and local taxes. He's a businessman, a proprietor. He's providing tax revenue for your rural parish. In mean, he's already been squeezed from all other ends by the liquor taxes. The costs of liquor licenses are goin' up. For him to set up a kitchen like in a restaurant . . . you know . . . if he sets up the three compartment sinks, the proper sized cooking area and all that stuff he's now got a much bigger expense. And he'll say 'I'm not doin' this every night. I'm only doin' this on Friday and Saturday nights.' He now can't afford to pay the band anymore. He can't afford to buy all that stuff needed to stock the kitchen, and *then* he can't just *give* it away to sell a drink. He's gonna have to sell it [the food]. But again, these things happen after hours. So we don't know about a lot of the stuff that happens. And if you're a participant, watch out! Are you gonna drink and eat and then shut 'em down? [Laughter] But seriously, you usually don't know 'bout all the after hours stuff. But, you see, if they start advertising that stuff then I have to cite 'em. I say 'Well, I can't help you, man, if you want to do the food stuff.' When you get into those little rural parishes, and those roadside lounges, instead of being competitive with one another, they set it up so you can go to one on Tuesday night, one on Wednesday night, and a third on Thursday night. And Friday night you go to the one with the band. Friday nights and Saturday nights it doesn't matter that much because they don't *need* the clientele. The clientele are in there anyway. The problem is the weeknights. Now, as for the Parish Sanitarian, on weeknights he's hone with his wife and kids. But this is what goes on in most all the parishes.

And there are your church organizations. It's not just about bars. Their doin' the same thing except they're not servin' liquor. They've got food at the Bingo night. Football games. School events. We're trying to do the best we can. We're concerned first and foremost with the public's safety, over enforcement: 'If you want to do this, be careful, and take the necessary steps.' The biggest problems come up a lot of times when you have benefits—maybe Aunt Ruby needs an operation—and she's been an outstanding lady in the church, and they're goin' to give her a benefit. There may be 15-20 different people makin' dishes, comin' from 15-20 different homes. Now, out of that many, all it takes is one. But at this point we're getting away from the public [arena] and into the private [arena]. If you've got a hundred people and 25 of 'em end up in the hospital from food poisoning, that is an investigative event for us. We just try to do our best, you know? And when to try to regulate 'em who knows who you'll get a call from, it might be the Governor. I mean, it's a *serious* problem.

I'm not sure now, but for a long time the CDC [National Centers for Disease Control and Prevention] listed food poisoning as a reportable [public health] event. But most food poisoning events don't make it to us, because more than anything people are afraid of gettin' shut down, or, they may just try to call it a virus. In actuality, if they call me I really can't do anything for 'em unless they've been to the doctor and he's confirmed it.

On the difficulty in determining whether some events are "public health" in nature:

It can always ultimately be termed a public health event whether you regulate it as such or not. Common sense, and tremendous people skills, are essential. I know every code verbatim, but if you can't take a common sense approach—knowing, in other words, when you've got to step hard, when you've got to step light—you will have a hard time. Why? Because public health is something that has to be *sold* [to the public] rather than regulated or enforced. You've got to almost *sell it*. In fact, we had a medical director here, Dr. Connely, who said that preventive medicine was the hardest medicine to sell. And [sickness] prevention is the single issue that binds us all together in the health unit.

On differences between the rural sanitarian and the urban sanitarian:

Well, first of all, there's really two different types are plan reviews. There are those that are drawn by architects, and then there the ones by local folks. You've got to have a place where you can lay those plans out, in a conference room or someplace, and determine by code if all the plumbing fixtures, laboratories, sewage lines, grease traps, ventilation hoods, stainless steel fixtures, and so on are goin' to be compliant. Most of the time the ones drawn by architects are goin' to be pretty much on the money. We may have some comments such as the location of the handwashing sinks, the laboratories, to make 'em a little more convenient. Construction hasn't begun, so that's not a problem. Next, you make a site inspection once the facility is almost complete. Of course, you assume that everything is in there but they might have overlooked some important details [in construction].

Now the mom and pop operations are totally different because you're dealing with a sketch. You don't have any finish schedules. You don't have anything like that. All you've got is a floor plan with holes drawn for sinks—it's gonna be on a piece of typing paper, you know, hand drawn. Here's one for a duplex. All you can do is take that little scratch and hope that when they've roughed it in you can say 'Yeah, it looks like you're gonna have all the sinks you need, lavatories, restrooms and all that kind of stuff.' But you're gonna have to make periodic trips over the course of construction because you don't get a full set of drawings. So you're gonna have to go out and meet with people, and the owners, especially if you go back just when they need a permit [as a food service establishment] and they're ready to open. They want to get started makin' their money. Well, if you go back tagging a bunch of stuff to re-do, that's not gonna go over. You've got to remember that your dealings with this person are not just limited to the review of this plan and the issuance of a permit. You're gonna be inspecting this individual four to six times a year for as long as that person's in business, and as long as you're a Sanitarian. If you establish poor rapport your job is gonna be very, very difficult from that point on.

If you can't get off to a good start with that individual and I mean in a manner that shows you want to work with him without letting him get off on any regulations, or causing any great burdens, as time goes on and as times come along and things might deteriorate, you're goin' to have an easier time getting him to make needed corrections. You are serving the public's health more by not havin' to be confrontational. If he hates you, you can make him to something, maybe, if it boils down to it, in ten days: 'You are in violation of this and this. I'm comin' back in ten days and if you don't have it corrected I'm shutting you down.' Well, on the eleventh day he then goes back to just how he did it before. So, now, two and a half months later—for two and a half months—he's been doin' it the way he wants to do it. And when you go back unless you can prevail in what you told him not to do in the first place, he's gonna stay in business. My job is to have these people do what they're supposed to do *every day*, not just on the day I come in or on the day I write 'em up. But, if you don't comply I'll give you a notice. If you don't comply with that notice I'll call you in for a conference and try to work it out amicably. If you don't comply with that my next step is to call you in for an administrative hearing. Then I have no choice but to shut [you] down. The same happens with fee collection notices, which are sent once a year from Baton Rouge. If they don't send back their money then they get a second notice. Then they get on the delinquent list. And after a period of time they send me a letter to be delivered telling that person to report to an administrative hearing on a certain date. If nothing happens then the sheriff can padlock the doors [of the establishment in violation of state sanitary code statutes]. That's [the] enforcement [process].

In a rural parish, we have go out and pick up the drawings and other information 'cause we don't have time nor the staff to make appointments [at the parish health unit]. In a big parish with many agents people can just drop off the permit documents for review. For a rural regulatory agent it's not like a nurse setting up a patient's 10:30 appointment at the clinic. For us, that's hard. It's not like an office appointment. If you're fifteen minutes late that person's still [sitting] out there [in the clinic waiting room]. But [for us] when you make your field appointments you may get tied up longer—you may have to take a photograph, write up a notice of violations—so, by the time you get there this guy might have left, or he's fuming. So when we've got business people we make 'em the first appointments in the morning. After 9:30 they [parish sanitarians] are out in the field doing inspections.

On events which solidify the entire staff in a common purpose:

As I said before, [sickness] prevention is the common thread that binds us all together in the parish health unit. But the main difference is that we're [each parish sanitarian] a regulatory branch while they're [clerks and clinicians] a service branch. We're regulatory whereas they're not. Because somebody is coming in there in need of care: 'I need to get my child's shots for school.' The *nurse* is not forcing that mother to bring that child in for that immunization. By the same measure, if they [patients] want WIC [services] the public health nurse is not forcing 'em in [to the clinic]. Those people are coming there voluntarily, even if those patients have to wait for six hours. They might complain, but they can get up and walk out. Now there is one exception—communicable diseases. STD and TB carry regulatory authority, because the patient can be forced to come in for treatment and to take one's medicine [a program known as Directly Observed Therapy]. Or, they [the nurses] can have the patient confined to the [one's] house. Now [by comparison], *all* my stuff is regulatory. I don't deal with anything that isn't [regulatory]. Either you comply, or you *don't* comply.[4]

CHAPTER 4

THE POLITICAL LANDSCAPE

> A man with a watch knows what time it is, but a man with two watches is never sure.
>
> *-James Gleick*[1]

Distinguishing "fast cultures" from "slow cultures," Gleick, in his 1999 book *Faster*, delineated a scenario which certainty rings true with respect to the political landscape in Louisiana. It is a place where the past often holds the future hostage, unwilling to let go for fear of the unknown road ahead. Things can, and often do, move slowly. Although it can be said this is a characteristic of any political system, this modus operandi at times reaches new depths in Louisiana's sixty-four parishes. This attitude persists in the parishes, especially in the face of the Information Superhighway. By the late 1990s the rural populism and cultural autonomy of the parishes, a loose collection of identities nurtured since the 1920s, was undergoing change. As a result, and against stubborn resistance, the fiercely guarded home-rule independence of the parishes had begun to show signs of diminishing. Various scandals, the escalating cost of running a political campaign, increasing voter disenchantment with new taxes, and a negative perception of all politicians everywhere (greatly reinforced in the national mass media), was resulting in a higher rate of turnover among parish-wide elected officials. Moreover, the chronic fiscal constraints exerted on parish government, combined with the shifting budget priorities from one gubernatorial administration to the next, were omnipresent obstacles to contend with.

Louisiana's parishes, like counties in other parts of the United States, are political and geographical subdivisions of the state. They comprise a middle layer of government originally established to administer state policy and serve local needs. The parish remains, for the most part, a child of the state. This parent-child relationship is a meaningful analogy to describe the parishes as they evolved historically from state control to home rule.[2] Writing on the origin of Louisiana's parishes, June S. Rowell explains:

> Louisiana parishes, although middle levels of government, preceded the formation of state and municipal governments as we know them today. A form

> of civil rule in Louisiana can be traced to the Crozat charter given by the king of France in 1712. Local administration began to take form later in the 1700s when, after the [Louisiana] territory had passed into Spanish ownership, Alexander O'Reilly, captain general of the Spanish armies, reorganized the territory, dividing it into eleven rural districts and one somewhat urban district, Orleans. Twenty-one ecclesiastical parishes were also established although only nineteen were headed by a priest. In 1804 after the purchase of Louisiana by the United States, the territorial legislature again set up twelve counties, which were similar to those formed by the Spanish under O'Reilly. The counties, however, were found to be too large for proper administration, and the population was growing rapidly at this time. By 1806, for the purpose of civil administration, the state had been redivided into nineteen parishes. Because these districts resembled the nineteen Spanish ecclesiastical districts that had been headed by priests, the name *parish* was retained.
>
> Early local administration was very much a part of state government. The first territorial legislature in 1804 did, however, give inhabitants of the county of Opelousas the authority to maintain a road . . . [as] determined by the county judge, the justices of the peace, and a jury of twelve inhabitants. This jury was the predecessor of the current parish governing body known as the *police jury* [author's italics]. Although some autonomy existed in the management of local affairs, parish officials were appointed by the governor until 1811, when police jurors were first elected. . . . Thus, the parish was considered a quasi corporation [and] the institutions of parish government that had developed by the mid-1800s are generally those found in parish government today.[3]

A police jury may levy taxes in accord with state-level constitutional stipulations, call elections for the passage of local bond issues to raise revenue for specific purposes, such as the construction of a new health unit facility, appropriate its funds for general purposes, and incur indebtedness. In addition, regulatory powers include establishment and enforcement of parish zoning ordinances and health ordinances, police, the licensing businesses and amusements, emergency preparedness management in the event of hurricanes or other natural or human-made disasters such as, in the aftermath of 9/11, acts of terrorism, and oversight for the general well being of the residents of the parish.

The legislature, together with the parish police juries, holds control over the entire system of parish health units. Pursuant to Section 8 of the 1973 state constitution, Louisiana "shall establish a system of economic and social welfare, unemployment compensation, and public health."[4] This wording closely follows that of the populism espoused by Huey P. Long in the 1920s. The parishes, on the other hand, act as the implementers. They hold power in terms of the facilities. It is their prerogative, as empowered by the 1973 Louisiana state constitution, to maintain or not maintain, to build or not build a replacement facility. A parish or municipality, as stated in Section 27, Article VI, is empowered to levy two types of millage taxes: dedicated and undedicated. Dedicated taxes are collected annually for a specific purpose, such as roads, the parish health unit, schools, fire protection, the parish prison, or parish SPCA program, to name but a few specific benefactors. Undedicated taxes, by contrast, may be applied to any facet of parish government as determined by the parish police jury or parish council (many parishes have adopted a council form of government in recent years, and others have reduced the number of members on their local police jury).[5]

The police jury is a parish's legal governing body. Authority is divided among the elected police jurors and several other elected parish officials, including the sheriff, assessor, clerk of court, school board members, and the coroner. Governing authority also extends to the parish district attorney and to those district judges whose jurisdictions lie within the boundaries of a single parish. As mentioned, the police juries were first empowered in 1807 to meet at least once each year to take up matters regarding local roads and levees. By 2000, all parish police juries met at least once per month. In addition, subcommittees may meet more frequently, sometimes as often as once per week when urgent decisions must be reached. The position of fiscal director, or administrative manager, is a full-time position, with this person answering directly to the police jury. The parish courthouse remains the legislative and symbolic center of local government, such as in Lake Charles (Fig. 4.1).

The maintenance of parish roads remains perhaps the most politically charged campaign issue in most, if not all, parishes. The subject of roads can be a very emotional political issue, along with the parish prison, the overcrowded courthouse, the parish library, schools, and other parish institutions, with the parish health unit significantly further down the list of political priorities, in many cases. But it is this tradition of building roads and their maintenance, dating from the earliest police juries and the dirt roads of rural communities,

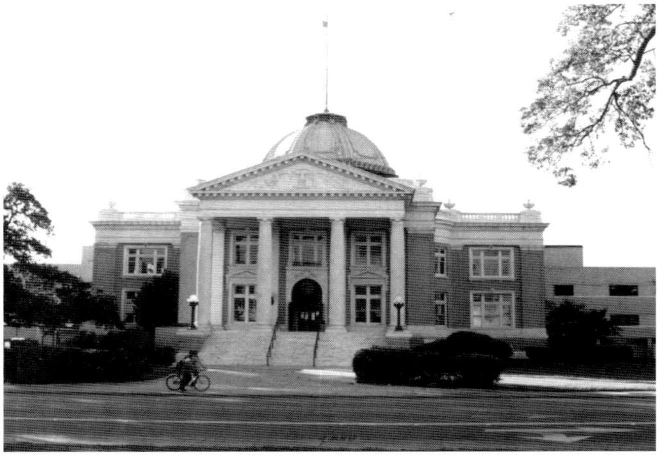

Fig. 4.1

which remains a top priority to this day. And, historically, jurors have promoted their reelection campaigns by focusing on roads. Recent federal and state legislation has added additional layers of legislative and oversight requirements. Wetland loss protection and the need for wetland and coastal erosion restoration projects emerged as a significant public issue in the 1990s. Also, during this period, various charges of environmental racism by environmental advocacy groups were leveled against police juries in parishes where the petrochemical industry sought to expand its presence. This has been a particularly resonant issue, and one, which has drawn considerable national media attention in the *New York Times* as well as in poor communities, nationwide, inhabited by large percentages of African American residents.[6]

Police jurors are elected to a four-year term in the state's general election. Many parishes now have term-limit statutes allowing no more than two or three consecutive terms in office. Some parishes show little change in jury membership from one election to another, while others may experience extensive turnover. Of the 663 jurors who took office for the 1976-1980 term, 261, or 41 percent, were new; in one parish all members were newly elected. On several of these juries, black and female members took seats for the first time. In 1976 there were fourteen women, seventy-two blacks and seven Republicans, all of whom can be considered minorities on the predominantly white male juries of Louisiana.[7]

This pattern has continued in parish-level elections across the state, with an increase in the representation of women and African Americans.[8] Most police jurors, traditionally, were drawn from the families of wealthy landowners, farmers, or successful local businessmen. Others were self-made entrepreneurs with little formal education beyond high school. An increasing number are licensed attorneys. And, as to be expected with this development, the level of formal education has increased. In the earliest days, the many possessed only a few years of formal education. Today, many jurors are university graduates and graduates of post-baccalaureate professional schools. By the end of the twentieth century the typical police juror was less likely to be a construction road crew foreman, contractor, or farmer by day. Their oversight authority, as mentioned above, includes their parish health unit, such as the Acadia Parish's facility in Crowley (Fig. 4.2). Citizens who live inside as well as outside city limits demand water systems, animal protection, sanitary code compliance, garbage disposal, police and fire protection, and a growing list of services. Since the 1960s, federal legislation has deeply involved juries in the local administration of federal programs, such as vocational work training and community block grant projects. The more active juries have also initiated social programs for juveniles, the elderly, and other special interest groups.[9]

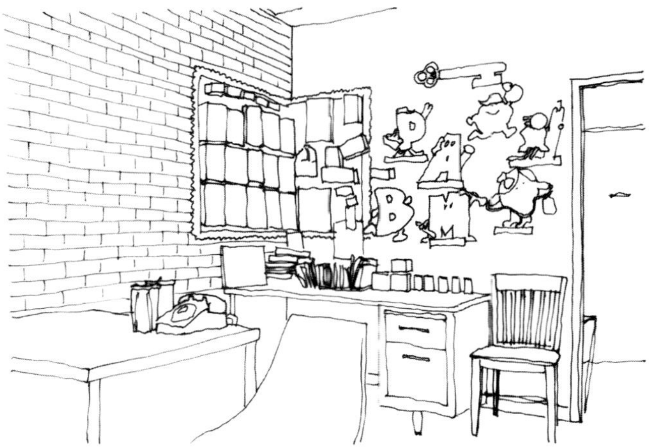

Fig. 4.2

Larry Richard served as the region administrator of the Office of Public Health Region IV through 2002.[10] His seven-parish region is centered around the city of Lafayette, in the south-central portion of the state. It is the cultural, socio-political, and economic epicenter of what is called Acadiana. For over 200 years this highly French-influenced region has been home to the Cajun people and a unique culture steeped in closely held traditions. Richard's considerable experience was indispensable to the agency over the years. He (as do the other eight region administrators) devoted significant time and energy to interactions with parish police juries on all matters concerning the operations of his region's nineteen health units.

On his years of experience with the agency:

> I have been with the Office of Public Health for twenty years, in the role of Region Administrator. Before that, I worked six-and-a-half years in the disease control program. I have always worked in this region from the start. I have

> oversight for the seven parishes [here]. About fifteen years ago the people in [OPH] Central Office [New Orleans at the time, it has since been redesignated as Baton Rouge], including the director and various administrators and the budget director, would come out once each year to meet with local staff. They worked with us on the preparation of the next year's budget. Police jurors were invited [as well]. We were at the St. Landry Parish Health Unit one day, and the director [the assistant secretary of the agency] made a comment about how the disgusting physical condition of the health unit. It was an old building. And he was correct. He said 'We should try to do something with our local juries to get new facilities or at least renovate some of them.' Based on that one comment I said to myself, my goal in the next fifteen years would be to try to get every police jury in Region IV to construct a new health unit facility. So, that day prompted me to get the juries to make a concerted effort. The first one was in Opelousas. First of all, I don't live or vote there. I don't care if it's completely new, or an addition; the people who have the most influence are the elected officials and our staff personnel in that community. They live there, vote there, and pay their taxes [there]. Basically, what I did was persuade the staff and our clients to become advocates to persuade local officials.

On elected officials' unawareness of the dilapidated condition of their health unit:

> In some places they were counseling patients in a janitor's closet. Sometimes the staff [at the health unit] literally begged us to do something to try to help. In other cases it came out of a meeting I had initiated with a staff where I would ask if anyone would refuse to help if we made a request [to the police jury]. I remember in Jeanerette they had a hot water boiler room with some very old rusted pipes. It was just a matter of time when it would have blown up in the faces of the patients and their children who were receiving care in that room. The buildings were terrible. That one was an old converted building on Main Street. When the police jurors were politicking they came in and the staff took them around and showed them the terrible conditions—no privacy, no curtains, no space for anyone—eventually enough people said 'We really *need* to do something.' It often takes four or five years just to sit down and start talking.
>
> When a police jury is getting ready to spend a million, or even a half million, those things aren't decided overnight. Unfortunately, it takes a long time to persuade the key individuals. And even when they have the funds, a lot of times they don't rank a new health unit as a priority. Let me give you an exam-

> ple. A certain parish decided that they needed to divert dedicated funds from the health unit to other more important issues. And we'd gone on the public record to disagree with them. It's particularly a problem because the voters voted the taxes [for the new health unit] and that's what they said they wanted them spent on. Back in the '80s one of the parishes had 1.5 million dollars in escrow in funds dedicated strictly for public health. They were donating to the Office of Public Health $27,000 a month to help out with daily operations. Basically, they wanted to stop taxing their constituents so they rolled the health unit millage to zero. They continued to give their $27,000. They eventually depleted their reserve, and when they did, they rolled their millage forward and started taxing the people again. If they wouldn't have done that and they had continued to earn interest on their savings, a brand new building would have been possible [years ago]. Today [2000], that same parish is having to *borrow* 3.5 million to build that facility. At the time they were more interested in saving some of their [wealthier] constituents $50.00 in tax dollars per year versus building something that *everyone* could use for perhaps thirty or forty years. That decision wasn't wise, but it's history now.

Over the years, many parishes developed special financial arrangements with the Office of Public Health. Some parishes have been allowed to withhold their monthly payment to the state on the condition that those funds would be reinvested directly in a replacement facility. Others have been rather generous in providing parish salaried staff in return:

> Another parish right now has approximately one million in escrow for a new health unit. They recently discontinued making their monthly contribution to our agency, a total of $218,000 a year. Their plan is to continue to save their dedicated funds for public health until they have enough saved to construct a new facility. That's the official position. Now, the truth of the matter is that a disgruntled retired employee, someone unhappy at the local level, and who disagreed with many policies of the Office of Public Health related to its environmental programs, has a strong relationship with many on the parish council. Over time I think he's persuaded them to not build a [new] health unit facility, and he's even made comments to the current staff to the effect that even though he is retired he is going to control how the health unit millage funds are spent. Now that's what *he's* saying, but I think there is some truth to it.
>
> The key in overcoming this wall is for *them* to develop a relationship directly with the elected officials. The facts must be stressed, including the fact that this is not for the employees, but for the entire population. For me that is

just about the only way for things to happen. Being candid is essential in telling them that the voters need and deserve a new facility in the long run.

When one person speaks for the entire staff as a unified entity, that's good. If the point person, no matter who it is, goes of on his or her own agenda and disregards the total needs of the health unit, that's bad. But sometimes that is human nature. Some just don't want to be team players. Sometimes it's a power or control thing. Then it takes more work on the part of the others to convince them [parish officials] of the need [for capital improvements].

On group dynamics and the unpredictability of local elected officials:

Here's an example I heard of only moments ago: earlier in the day [that same day] I met with members of the health unit staff and with a newly elected police juror. I just heard that there's another jury member, one who has been on the jury for years, who advised the new member *not* to vote to construct a new health unit. And I don't know why. But what I like is that the newly elected juror came to the meeting. He told me himself 'I'm just here to learn and educate myself.' I think he was telling me that he was willing to hear both sides. He was listening to us and he asked pretty good questions. Then he'll make his decision. That police jury needs to establish a building committee. The committee cannot vote to construct a new health unit; they only make a recommendation. The parish president selects the members of all the committees. It can be stacked one way or the other. The best strategy of our staff is to meet with the members of that committee individually before their meeting to vote. Why? Because if I were sitting on that committee, I would like to know as much as possible *before* the official meeting. Only the full jury has the authority to vote to build. And yes, most of the time they do follow the committee's recommendation. I can't recall in Region IV a committee making a recommendation to build that was not approved by the full police jury. But it has happened in other regions.

Usually, when everyone has done their homework, there's very little discussion in the full meeting.

It's wrong to hit people cold in a public meeting and then force them to make a decision on the spot. The worst thing that can happen is that if all the pertinent information isn't available or if there are still unanswered questions then the issue might be tabled for two or three months, perhaps longer. That's why full disclosure is essential prior to the public meeting of the full police jury. A few months ago we invited all twelve of the jurors to the health unit for an open house for them just to see what we do. Only two showed up. Some

> have absolutely no interest [in us], some have some interest, and a few are strong supporters.

The socio-economic and racial background of the elected official has an impact:

> I think the awareness levels of police jurors and their educational levels vary. It helps if one of them is a next-door neighbor or a fishing buddy. The president of the police jury in one of the parishes in this region, which recently built a new health unit, had grown up with the parish sanitarian. They went to school together. They built on a relationship that had existed for years and years. One of their employees' mothers, whose son was now the chief engineer of the parish, had worked as a nurse at the health unit for years. There were some strong ties. This goes back twenty, thirty years. There was only one juror who was against building that new facility. But in my experience, through attending the meetings over time, I noticed that he voted against the majority at all times. He just wanted to be different, and sometimes you just run into such individuals.
>
> In Ville Platte, once they had voted to build, they specifically stated they did not want three individuals representing the health unit. They did not want the confusion of a nurse, a clerk, and a sanitarian all with equal say. They wanted only one person designated to communicate with at all times. This was because during the prior period when they asked a question they would get two or three different answers. Sometimes, I don't have to designate a contact person because someone says 'When the call comes, I'll take the question and we'll all sit around and talk it over. Usually, people work together to streamline communications between the jury and the staff. Sometimes this goes on for four or five years. I think that with a large [health unit] staff it is a lot more difficult than with a small staff. In Lafayette, the architect, or the parish government official always calls me with questions. Sometimes I might refer them to someone to call at the health unit if it is a highly detailed question.

A region administrator's job is filled with unpredictability. Some days require a crisis mode of management, with pressing personnel matters to address, issues of staff turnover and recruitment, coping with chronic hiring and expenditure freezes, maintaining the delivery of services, responding to lawsuits, and even private family matters related to OPH personnel in the various parishes. For example, late one summer evening in 1999, an estranged husband burst into the Alexandria home of his former wife and shot her to death. The murdered woman had been a long-employed clerk at the health unit in Rapides Parish. The region administrator dropped her scheduled duties for two days to grieve with the victim's family, and the staff. Who has the time to devote to facility matters?

Richard's response:

> First of all, is it part of my job? Yes, it is, even though it's not mentioned in the job description. If we—and this includes my entire staff in the region—can do whatever it takes to successfully administer the programs of the Office of Public Health in the field, than this is part of our work. Our work can include anything from disciplinary problems, working with architects, hiring people, firing people, to determining what services should actually be offered in the face of budget cutbacks—a multitude of issues are involved. So is this [architecture] part of my job? Sure. We can't operate without adequate facilities. Is it enjoyable? Yes. I would rank it in the top 5 percent of all the things I do in my job. It always brings out important issues and healthy discussions. Today [in an earlier meeting at the Acadia Parish courthouse] we were discussing the philosophy of public health. For instance, take yourself [author]; I don't think we would have ever met you, or anyone who would specialize in this area, on our own. Working with someone like you [author] has been a win, win situation for us. We were in dire need of someone to take a look at all the health unit facilities throughout the state. The person from OPH who asked you to step in did us all a service.
>
> Before 1990, it was a hit or miss situation. Before—and I'll just state my thoughts on this—we just sat around and tried to come up with our own floor plan, without any architect. We pretended to try to walk through a clinic from the viewpoint of patient and staff flow. To me, it was the most logical way to at least come up with the first idea of how it might work: Where do you sit? Where do you work? Here's the patient at this point in the visit. Let's try to follow that patient through the entire visit from beginning to end. And from there, most of the time, we put together a rough sketch. We could then sit down with an architect and have an intelligent discussion. It started out with common sense—putting a few lines down on a piece of paper. But there were a lot of things we never thought about and we made a lot of mistakes. My point is that bringing a professional [author] in from the *beginning* was the most appropriate way to do it. Take, for example, patient confidentiality. I specifically remem-

ber Jeanerette, and the walls between every exam room; you could hear every conversation. You had the waiting room right next to the exam rooms. It had been that way for twenty-five or thirty years. Patients had to yell their information through a small hole in the glass at the front counter. The addition of computers—the Passport [WIC] computers—had a major impact on that facility. When I started [with the agency] there wasn't a WIC program, and the facilities did not have WIC kitchens. The WIC services were often done in the staff lunch-break room [Fig. 4.3 and 4.4]. I was amazed whenever I found a facility that did not have hand-washing sinks in the exam rooms. Also, we had an x-ray machine in every parish health unit. Now we have the family planning program and we have discontinued the x-rays. Facility needs are always changing.

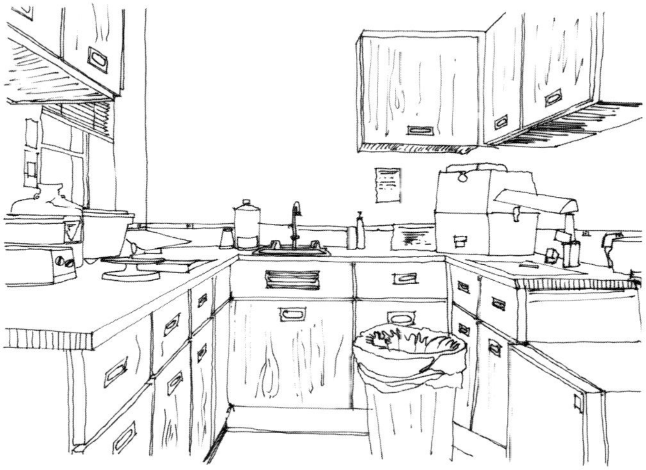

Fig. 4.3

On the importance of forging personal relationships with elected officials and community leaders:

I don't go to the police jury meetings in my own parish unless there's something of special interest to me. It's good to spend time with them [elected officials] if you can find the time for it, or if you're even invited. I shy away from that, and this is why and I've been asked on several occasions to go to their [someone's] hunting camp, or to a barbecue, and their intent was probably to get me to turn my head on a certain issue. One of them actually told me, months later, that they wanted me to talk to a certain sanitarian who was

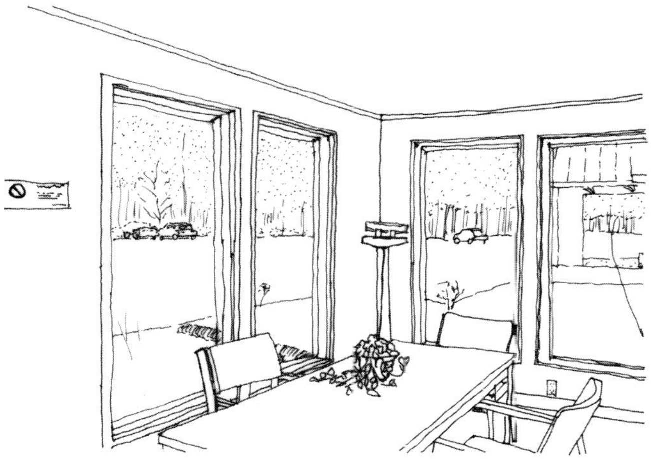

Fig. 4.4

trying to make them comply with certain regulations related to sewerage. And they didn't want to [comply]. So their approach to get me to tell my staff to look the other way was to wine and dine me. So you have to be careful. Now, I can attend every function and I can say no. But I chose not to go at all. It's just a matter of how one handles it. I went to a few in the beginning so I quickly learned what was going on, and they [the jurors in that parish] haven't invited me since.

Government in a sense is a business. I try to apply basic business management principles in my work. I'm not saying it's about profit or loss, but too often people just don't apply sound business principles. Some [region] administrators come from backgrounds in nursing, some from social work; one had worked as a parish sanitarian for years. The credit should go more to the local staff because they're the individuals who live here, vote here, and pay taxes here. They can attain much more success, and should rightfully receive the credit. They should be at the forefront, and I'll help them in dealing with the elected officials. But, if I'm an elected official I'll tend to listen more to the people who put me in office. I'm an outsider. It's a team effort.

A police juror's plate is very full, usually. You go there with the local staff and if the answer is yes, it's yes. But if you go and you sit and wait and nothing happens, then someone dropped the ball. They have other full time jobs and small staffs. Sometimes it seems like you've been waiting forever. But that is probably because they have so many other concerns. Then you have to light a fire under them to get things going once again. As a priority, they want to look good to their constituents. They want to make the most popular decisions to the largest number of people. Every jury has a different agenda. And there are competing agendas between the districts within a parish. They have to sort all that out first. You almost have to live there and get to know the people involved [the decision-makers]. Here's an example of one individual: on just about any issue that could ever come up at a meeting he educates himself and takes a stand—he represented the whole parish. But his eyes were on the parish presidency. Or, eventually on a state representative or senatorial seat. I could see why he was conducting himself in such a manner [and he is] now well on his way. And right next to him I could see someone who only cared about doing something positive for his little district. He had no larger ambitions for statewide office or anything. So it all goes back to what their goals are, if they want to use that as a stepping-stone to move on. It's a plus if the local state representative helps. This comes up sometimes when the facility is going to be moved [to a different part of the parish], or built in a different district.

The state constitution mandates the presence of a full service health unit in every parish, yet between 1992 and 2000 the agency decreased by nearly 1,000 full-time employees:

> I think you're going to see some health units specialize in some programs and other health units specialize in other programs within a region. Also, as we receive less and less state funding for our programs some parishes are going to find alternative providers within their community. For instance, we might no longer be involved with family planning. Our remaining staff may just provide immunizations, and communicable disease control, such as TB, HIV/AIDS, and STD. But what happens to the rural parishes where the health unit is the only provider, the only game in town? Those health units may continue to do a little bit of everything, but never meet the total needs of the parish. There are pressures to cut services back. We already in a few places contract with private providers to do WIC. But they want to get the biggest bang for their buck. It doesn't make sense for them to see only ten or fifteen patients a week. The endangered species programs over the next five to ten years might be the Medicaid program, and we may once again become the only game in town when the feds keep cutting the Medicaid reimbursement rates to the private providers. It depends on what part of the state we're talking about. It all depends on what's available in these different communities. And I don't ever see parishes cooperating across parish borders. These programs will continue but probably continue to be downsized. As for environmental health, government will continue to have a role in terms of inspections. That should always be part of the role of the state public health agency. It is not a service where you can go down the street and contract with a private service. This involves the public's food and water. We need to rank in priority all the things we do; if we're bare-boned we cannot do all that is required of us. This is about the public health of the *entire* population. We *have* to remain involved in disease control.

An emerging role for public health at the agency level in Louisiana is assisting communities prepare for, and respond to, natural disasters and acts of terrorism. The aftermath of a hurricane includes threats to the food and water supply, the spread of disease, and massive flooding. The agency's role is expanding in this area:

> The [emergency preparedness] effort in recent years in this part of the state has gone from zero to one hundred. Basically, in years past when shelters were

opened the staff were called and asked 'If you want to help out, this is where you should report.' It was strictly voluntary. We've changed from voluntary service to mandated service. If a shelter is opened for people with special needs they will not be placed in a local general shelter. These people need round the clock nursing, in a different location. If a nursing home is evacuated, some will be relocated to a local hospital. Others will be relocated to a special needs shelter. The nursing home may send some of their nursing staff there but the public health nurses will most likely coordinate the services provided. You might have four or five hundred special needs patients in a special need shelter. Our role is not to open it or to run it. Our role is to provide care. However, if there's an 18-wheeler that tips over on the interstate [I-10 or I-49], we will use the health unit as a staging area, or even shut the health unit down to send nurses out to the site or to the local hospitals. If the nurses have to come down from northern Louisiana to help out after a hurricane the health unit could house them. It would be good to have a generator and showers and some sleeping accommodations. Being able to keep the refrigerators going and the lights on is important. A given parish's refrigerators typically store between $75,000 and $85,000 in vaccines alone.

If we're going to start thinking about designing a health unit as a special needs shelter we're looking at $5 million instead of $1.5 million [see Chapter 5]. I think that the police jury will say that would be good to have, but how often will it be needed? If we have generators and other support needs during emergencies, who will train the staff? It's a lot of trouble to transport vaccines; this is what happened during Hurricane Andrew [in 1995]. A lot of health units lost their power then. This is worthwhile, but it may only cause more political headaches.

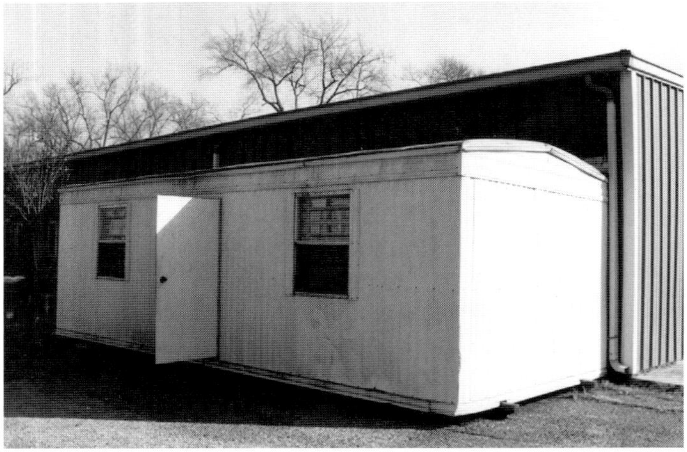

Fig. 4.5

Regarding the use of the parish-wide millage tax, a parish has the option to pursue funds for renovating an existing health unit or constructing a replacement. However, as recently as 2000 twenty-two parishes lacked any form of millage tax revenue dedicated for local health units. There, facilities existed in a "hand to mouth" manner. The windowless prefabricated metal building in Mansfield, DeSoto Parish, remains a prime example (Fig. 4.5). This had been a particular problem in the case of Catahoula Parish, formerly housed in an adapted schoolhouse (Fig. 4.6).

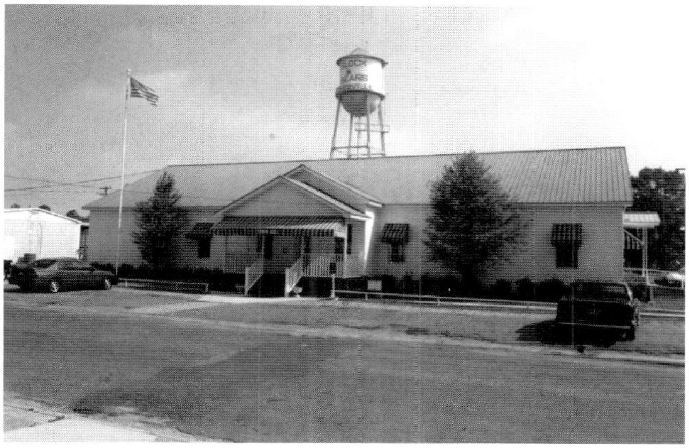

Fig. 4.6

One increasingly popular alternative source of funding exists. This is known as the capital outlay process.[11] It never hurts to have friends in high places. In Louisiana, as elsewhere, upper-level government officials have often had prior experience at the parish level of government.[12] In this respect a given parish may have a built-in lobbyist in the state legislature. These persons share common backgrounds with local police jurors and empathize with their local elected counterparts and voter constituencies back home. Between 1988 and 1998 a number of parishes had been successful in obtaining this type of funding. Success is predicated upon a mixture of one's gender, experience, and the ability to build broad-based coalitions at the local level among parish police jurors, state representatives, and state senators.[13]

In wealthy parishes, or those not genuinely committed, recalcitrance, or "foot-dragging," takes root. This manifests in an attitude, publicly at least, of indifference. Consider the case of a newspaper account of the situation in St. Charles Parish, which, until its replacement facility opened in 2003, operated one of the state's oldest, most obsolete clinics.[14] On the other hand, a parish may simply be insolvent, and the beautiful, historic courthouse itself may be obsolete and dilapidated, in need of renovation. Such is the case in DeSoto Parish (Fig. 4.7). Out-migration to urban areas also continues to have an adverse impact on all civic institutions in the rural parishes, including the demise of the 1930s motion picture palace in the town of Many (Fig. 4.8). For the politician, the disappearance of the health unit from the civic landscape would represent one less tax-supported institution to sustain, one less leaky roof, one less lawn to maintain. As Rowell states:

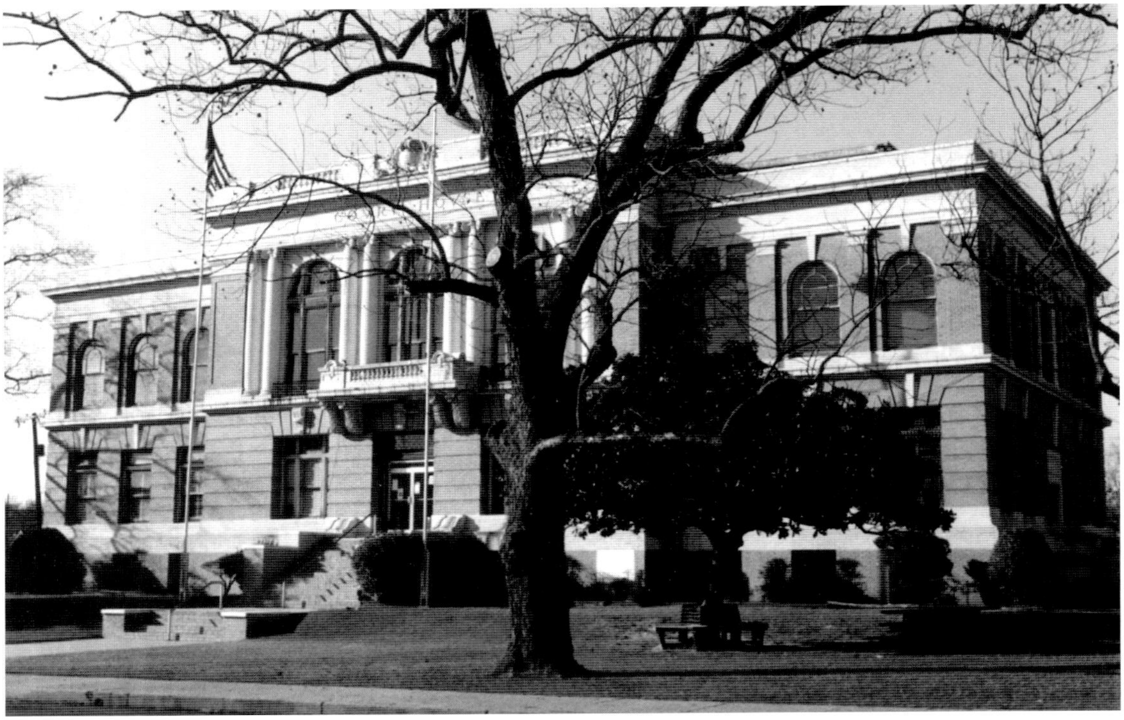

Fig. 4.7

> Parish government in Louisiana has not been known for policy innovation whether through imitation or otherwise. This is evident in its reluctance to take advantage of home rule, its lack of professionalism, and its lack of merit-system employment. Generally, it has been the municipality, rather than the parish, that has exhibited innovation . . . the possibility exists for the parish to emerge as the pivotal unit of intergovernmental cooperation linking local-municipal, state, and federal governments . . . modernized parish government could assume the role of prime surveyor of those public services that are best performed for areas larger than a municipality, including . . . public health.[15]

Fractionalization at the local government level is definitely not unique to Louisiana—it exists nationwide and as urbanization continues, city-parish consolidation may by default transform the face of local government. However, resistance to change remains strong. Rowell concludes:

> What then are the prospects for parish government in Louisiana? Probably more of the same structurally but with a tendency toward increased governmental activity and professionalism especially as the result of expanded federal-local relationships and the demands for services from culturally urban constituencies . . . (with) a move toward leadership in parish administration. This specifically involves the addition of executive officers to juries, a change that has been slowly occurring through charter provisions in home rule parishes and the appointment of professional or jury-member managers in several others . . . (in) a move away from parental confines and toward a position of near autonomy. . . . The progress that parishes make toward effective self-government now depends upon the desire of their citizens to see this accomplished.[16]

Historically, local, somewhat idiosyncratic, rural political traditions throughout Louisiana have been deeply rooted expressions of its cultural landscape—not at all different from the unique food, music, outsider art, architecture, and folklore to be found in these communities—and these traditions are unlikely to disappear anytime soon. Although parish government in the rural districts preceded centralized state government in Louisiana, the centrality of the parish government will continue, even in the face of coping with the complex, contradictory challenges of urbanization, suburban sprawl, and coastal erosion.

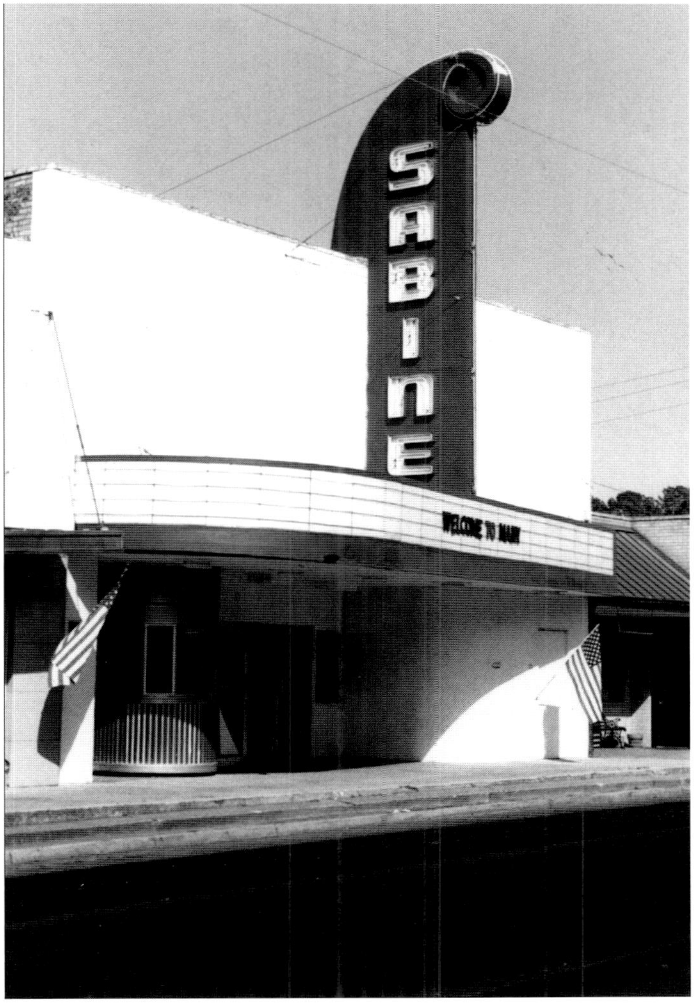

Fig. 4.8

Chapter 5

Case Studies

In this chapter, eight case studies are presented, spanning a period of thirteen years. They reflect a strategic mixture of renovation and replacement facility projects and represent a mix of rural, suburban, and urban contexts. This design work has been shaped by the evidence-based paradigm expressed in the SFI protocol. This perspective has informed, and has in turn been informed, by the compendium of 143 design guidelines developed, modified, and updated as the SFI initiative has evolved.[1] The guidelines evolved as new programs emerged and existing programs were restructured.[2] The research findings (see Appendix C) were applied to all eight case studies presented below and to all SFI projects completed to date. For these eight, not every guideline is called out for a given case study, although the entire compendium was influential in its development. The guidelines function as a datum line for architects and care providers—the case studies represent a blend of indigenous vernacular architecture with the "subculture" of a particular place, its staff, its composition, local patients, and the idiosyncrasies of the local political landscape.[3] Post-occupancy evaluations have been completed for all fifty-five completed SFI projects including the eight presented here. Following the case studies, a summary of the SFI initiative is presented.

The evidence-based research findings are summarized as eight provisos: (1) there is no single optimal, easily transferable floor plan or site plan configuration. Cross plans, box clinics, courtyard clinics, and multi-level clinics were studied, and no ideal footprint emerged although semi-enclosed courtyard configurations have been found to most clearly express the three programmatic domains; (2) It is preferred, from a staff and patient flow perspective, for these domains to be distinct and somewhat autonomous from one another; for example, waiting areas should be zoned to control patient flow to the clinic, control the random movements of children, and minimize noise; (3) Natural daylighting design strategies are preferred and considered by end users to afford therapeutic amenity, i.e. full height exterior windows and room-to-room windows along corridors afford openness and transparency, and views of nature are highly preferred; (4) Residentialist imagery is viewed as symbolizing an inviting patient-centered community care environment; (5) Flexible—or flexive—rooms designed to be easily converted into a second (or even third use) provide more amenity than uni-functional rooms, i.e. a play area/mother's breastfeeding alcove, waiting/health education areas, nutritional education (WIC) kitchen/seminar room, exam room/seminar room, and conference room/health education. Additional provisos include the finding that children, in some situations, benefit from having their own dedicated space, i.e. a playroom within or adjacent to the main waiting room, and an adjacent outdoor supervised play zone; (6) Innovative approaches are encouraged to maximize patient confidentiality within the total care environment in the digital age, i.e. a private intake space which doubles as the clerical office, opening into adjacent open plan workspace; (7) Provide clearly identifiable entrances and parking areas for staff and patients, i.e. environmental health program staff prefer a separate entrance distinct from the main entrance to the clinic realm. The eight case studies are presented below.

Ouachita Parish, West Monroe

This facility afforded the first opportunity to apply the SFI methodology from a project's inception. The evidence-based team conducted a feasibility analysis, site selection, programming, the budget analysis, and served in the role as lead designer.[4] From this point on (1992) every SFI initiative was benefiting from the compendium of site planning and architectural design guidelines. In this case, the evidence-based team worked in a joint venture of R-2ARCH with Hugh Parker Architects of Monroe, with the latter firm commissioned by the Ouachita Parish Police Jury who served as architect of record for this 12,500-square-foot replacement facility and provided day-to-day onsite supervision during construction. Total construction cost was $1.2 million. The clinic was housed since the early 1950s in an art deco building on Main Street in West Monroe. No renovations had been made in many years and the programs and staff had long ago outgrown the facility.

A 2.5-acre site was purchased, allowing for future expansion options. The site is adjacent to an east-west interstate (I-20) allowing for future expansion and a minimum of sixty-five parking spaces. The building's components were arranged as a series of parallel bandwidths, with adjoining functional spaces.

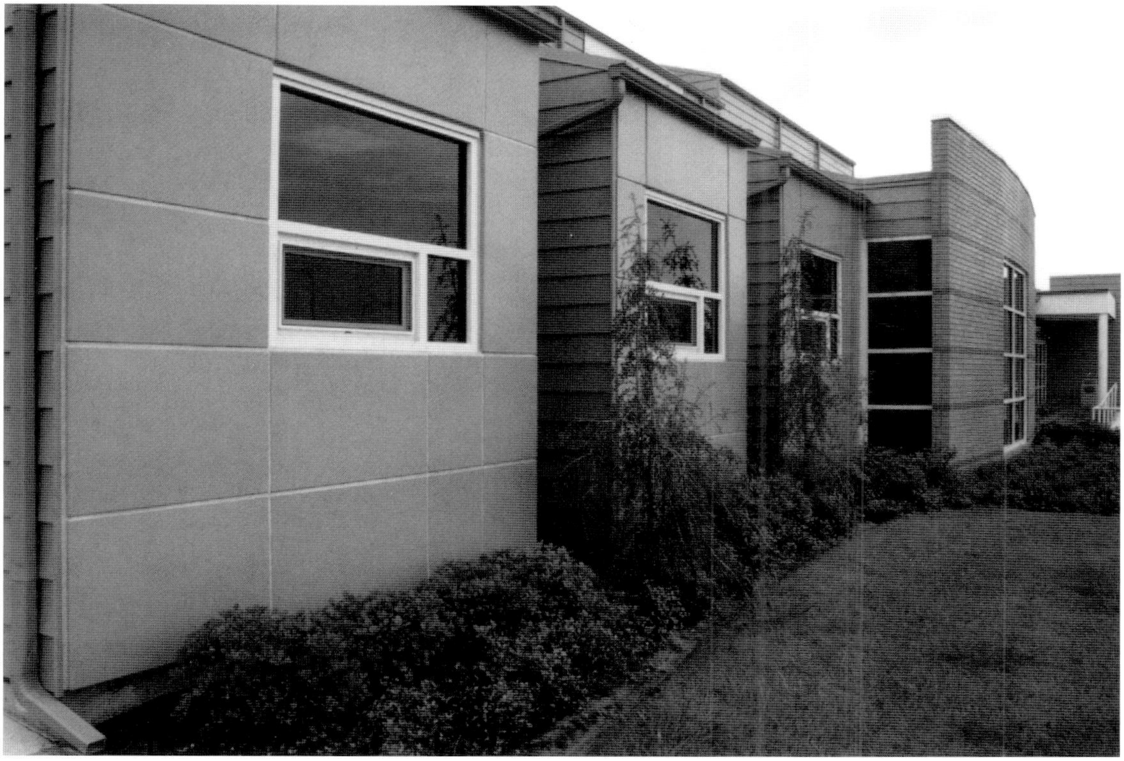

(Fig. 5.1) These bandwidths were variously shifted: left to right, the main waiting room and adjacent multipurpose room (this included an interior and adjacent outdoor play area for children); the main arrival/departure axis, running north-south throughout the entire length of the building, connecting a porte cochère at the front to the main parking era to the rear; the clinic administration housing the regional environmental health program in a second-level "loft;" the core bandwidth at the midsection housing medical records, nutritional education programs, and subwaiting; a clinic support space bandwidth; and a nursing administration and support bandwidth. (Fig. 5.2) Fig. 5.1

The program called for six exam rooms, a laboratory, subwaiting area, nutritional education kitchen, staff offices for nursing and clerical personnel, including five intake stations, environmental health offices and support spaces, social work office, and related clinical support spaces in support of communicable disease and family planning programs. (Figs. 5.3 and 5.4) The completed

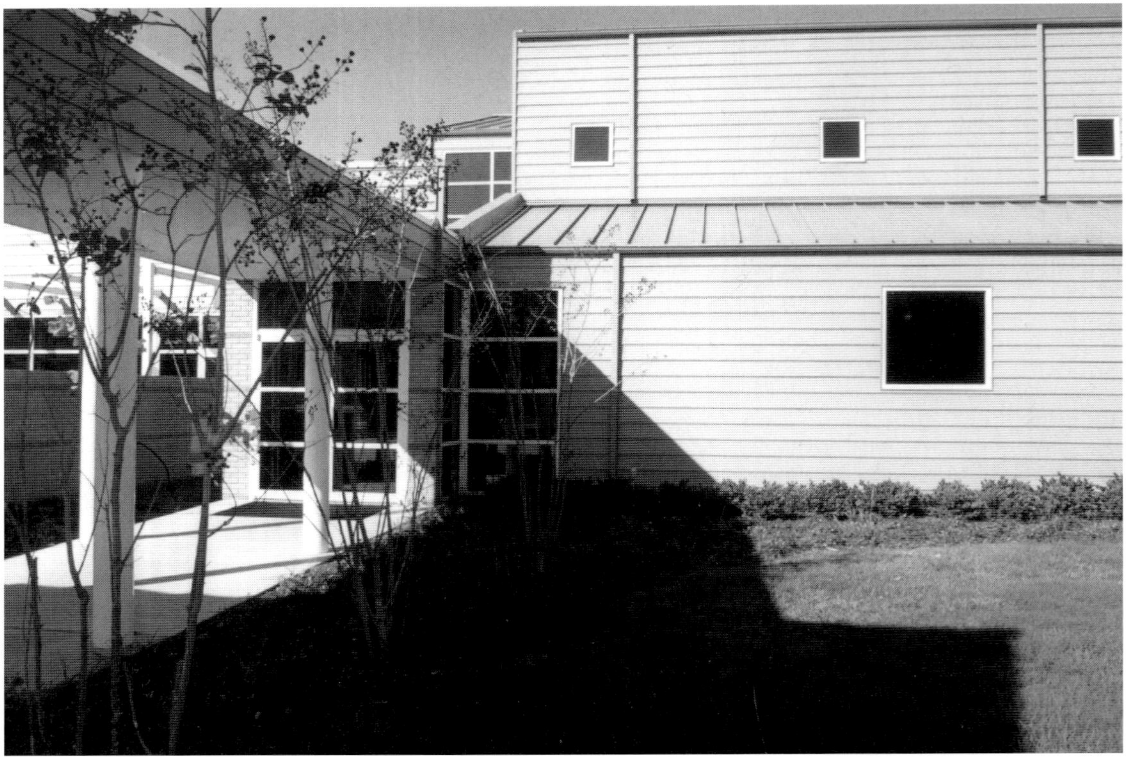

Fig. 5.2

building housed twenty-eight to thirty staff, and supported more than 1,100 patient visits per month. The architectural vocabulary and palette of materials referenced the eclectic mix of nearby residential and agricultural buildings, which are predominant throughout this region of Louisiana. Since children represent over 60 percent of all users at a typical health unit, emphasis was placed on the experience of the child. For the child, the intent of the design of all rooms, and the exam rooms in particular, was to create a health center as a welcoming environment—a health house. This intent is conveyed on the exterior as well as within.

The six exam rooms are correspondingly scaled and massed as embedded, yet flanked by quasi-autonomous elements. (Figs. 5.5 and 5.6) The subwaiting room is at the center of two banks of three exam rooms. The exterior wall plane is of masonry banded in red and beige brickwork. The roof is a standing seam steel roof, in blue. The entrance is protected by a porte cochère and a pedestrian

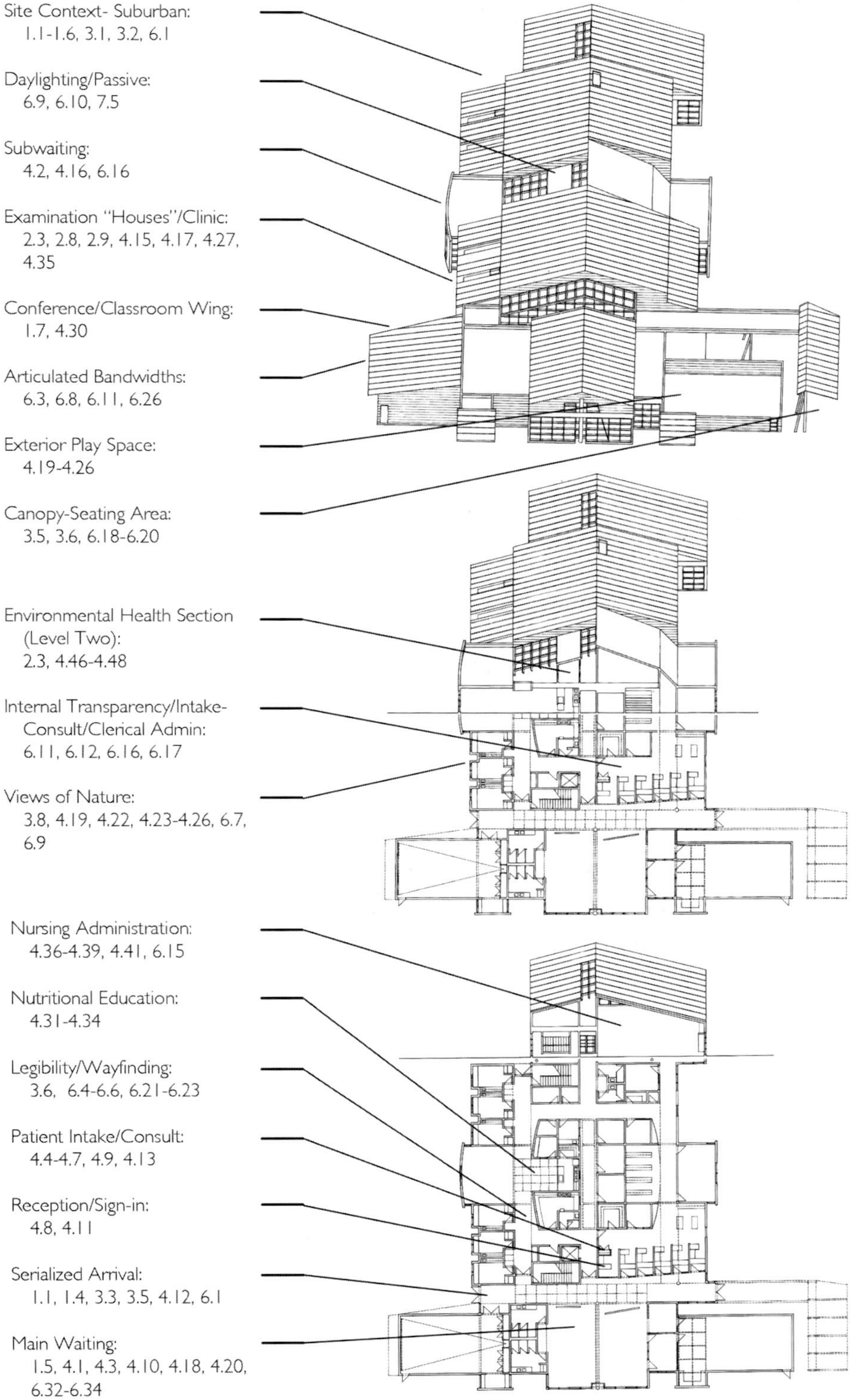

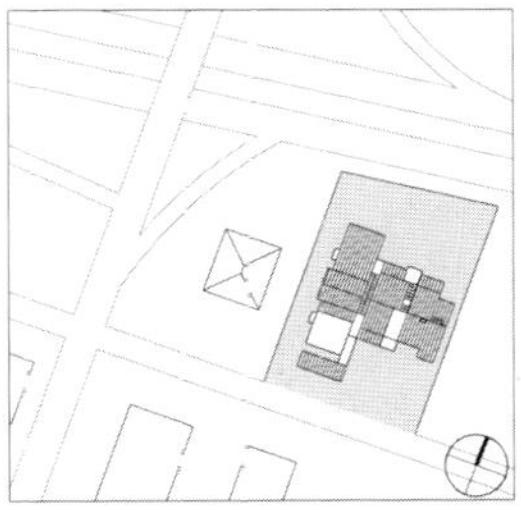

Fig. 5.3 a-c

Fig. 5.4

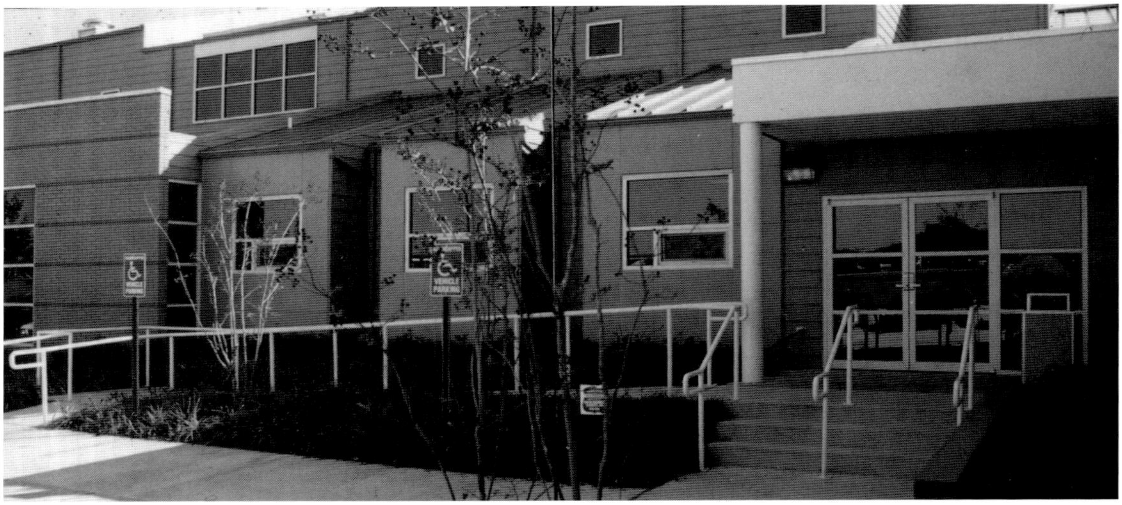

Fig. 5.5

canopy leading to the front door. The building's blue horizontal aluminum exterior siding reinforces its residential scale. The building's *T* partí is expandable, at a future date, into an *H* configuration on the adjacent undeveloped acre of land.

An access ramp adjacent to the entrance on the parking side of the site, next to the examination houses, circulates traffic and is partially screened by landscaping. The exam room "houses" were given individual expression, with exterior surfaces clad in the siding utilized throughout the exterior and, facing the north edge of the site, with aluminum panels in beige with a window set in a grid. Natural light is transmitted into the core areas of the building vis-a-vis skylights and clerestories (Fig. 5.7). Transparent connections exist along the main arrival axis (Fig. 5.8). A large skylight above this axis transmits daylight into the interior (Fig. 5.9). Transparent connections continue between the patient intake and the main waiting room, and between the waiting room and adjoining children's play yard (Fig. 5.10). The staff sought to eradicate physical and symbolic barriers, which have typically separated the patient from the caregiver in the past, as in the openness between the nutritional education demonstration

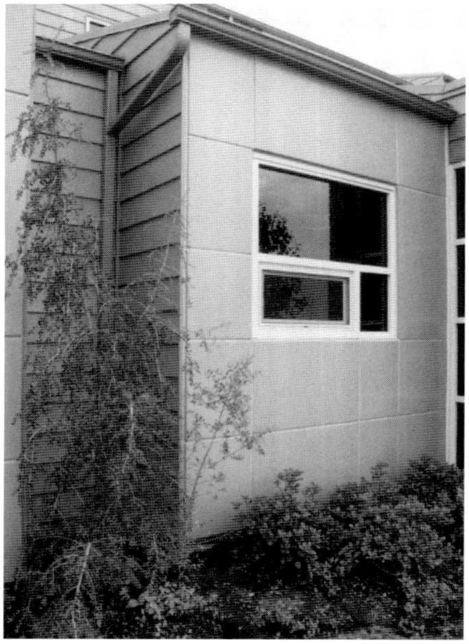

Fig. 5.6

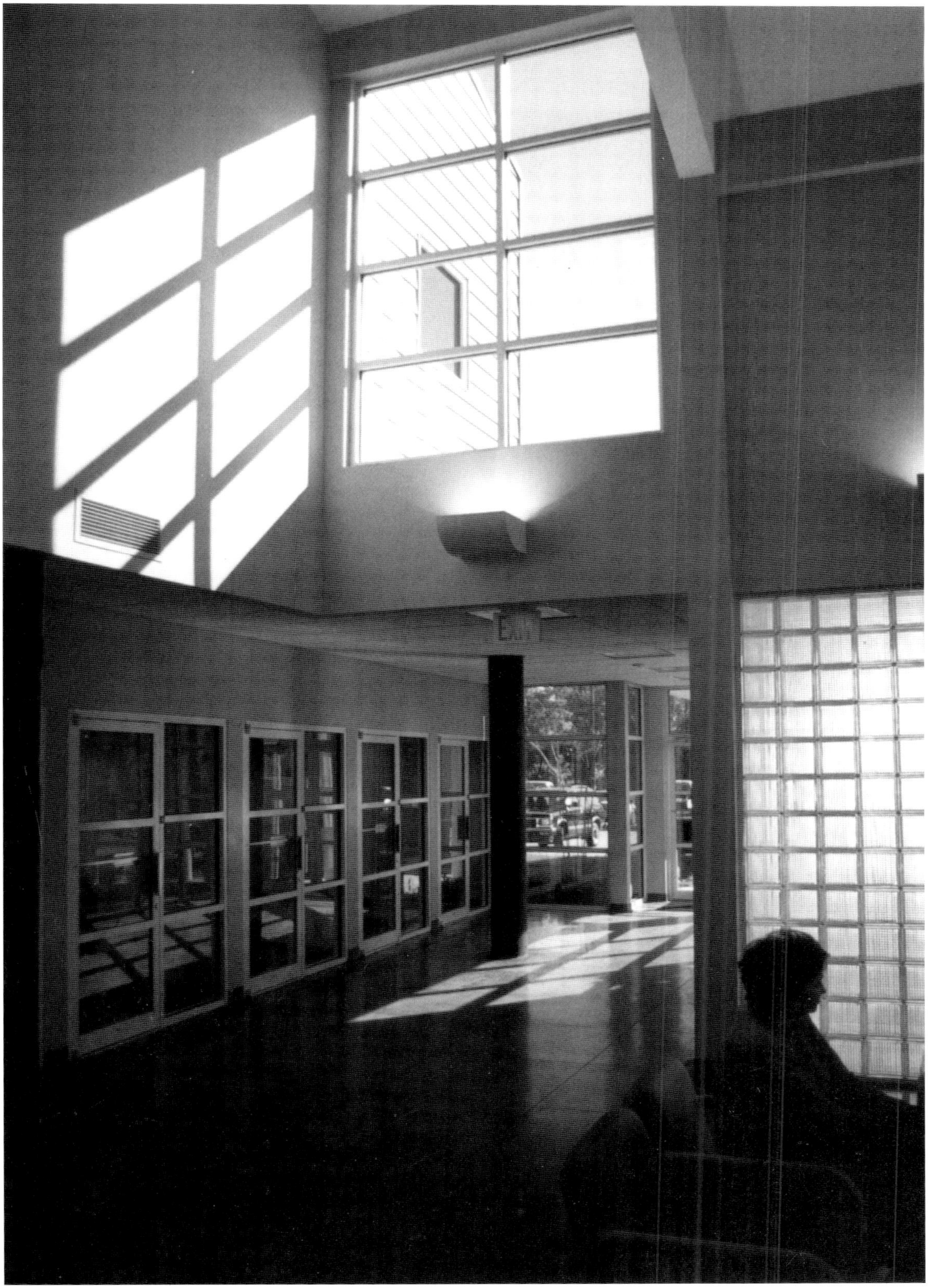

Fig. 5.7

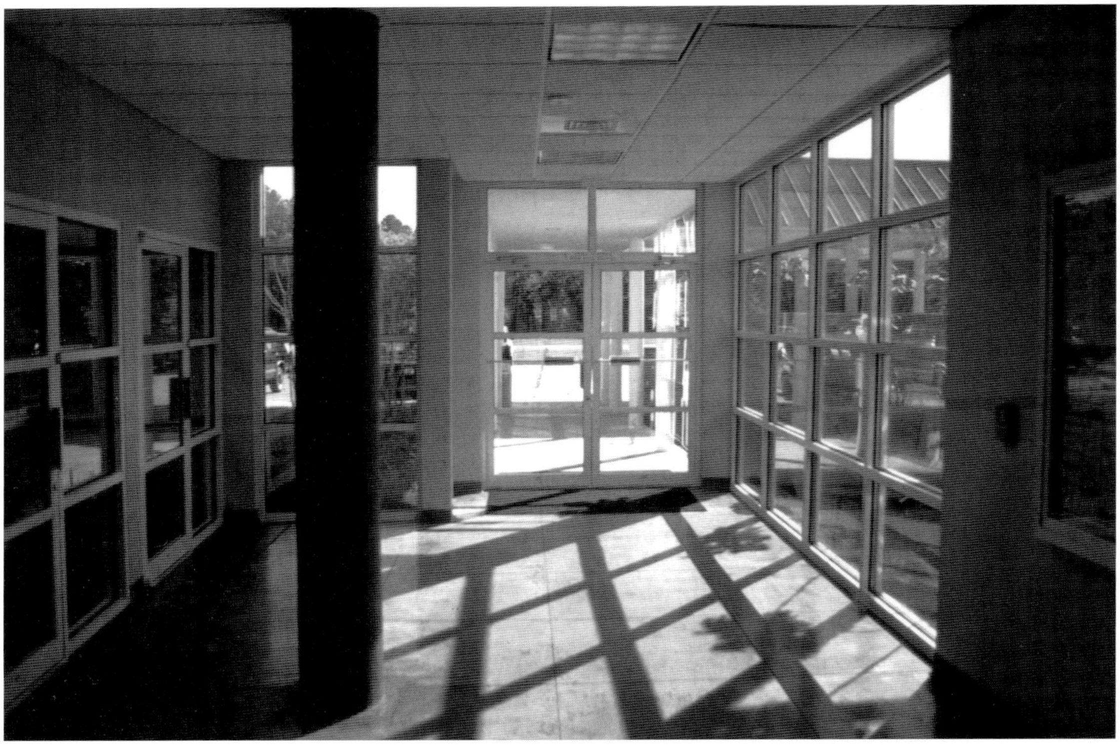

Fig. 5.8

kitchen and the subwaiting room (Fig. 5.11). The demonstration kitchen area can be shut off from the waiting area vis-a-vis a roll down aluminum open mesh screen.

Transparency is also achieved between the five patient intake/clerical offices. This was the first case study to demonstrate to the full extent the heightened level of patient confidentiality attainable by having the intake office glass walled on the public side, and open on the clerical work side. Staff involved in the planning of clinics in other parts of the state visited this facility to see firsthand an alternative to the old-school arrangement of the patient having to literally yell one's private information across an open counter, in full view of everyone. Strong visual connections between interior and exterior spaces throughout the buildings aid in the building's wayfinding amenity for its occupants (Fig. 5.12). The floors in the public realms are of scored stained concrete and carpeted in the clinic, staff work areas, and the environmental health pro-

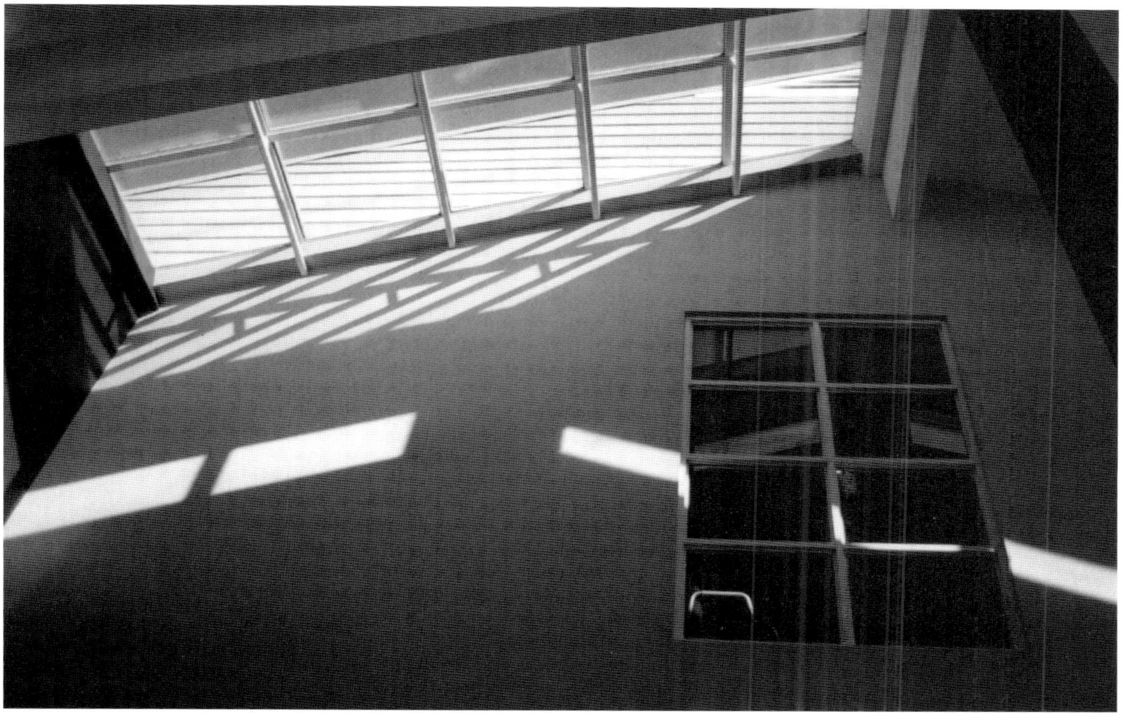

Fig. 5.9

Fig. 5.10

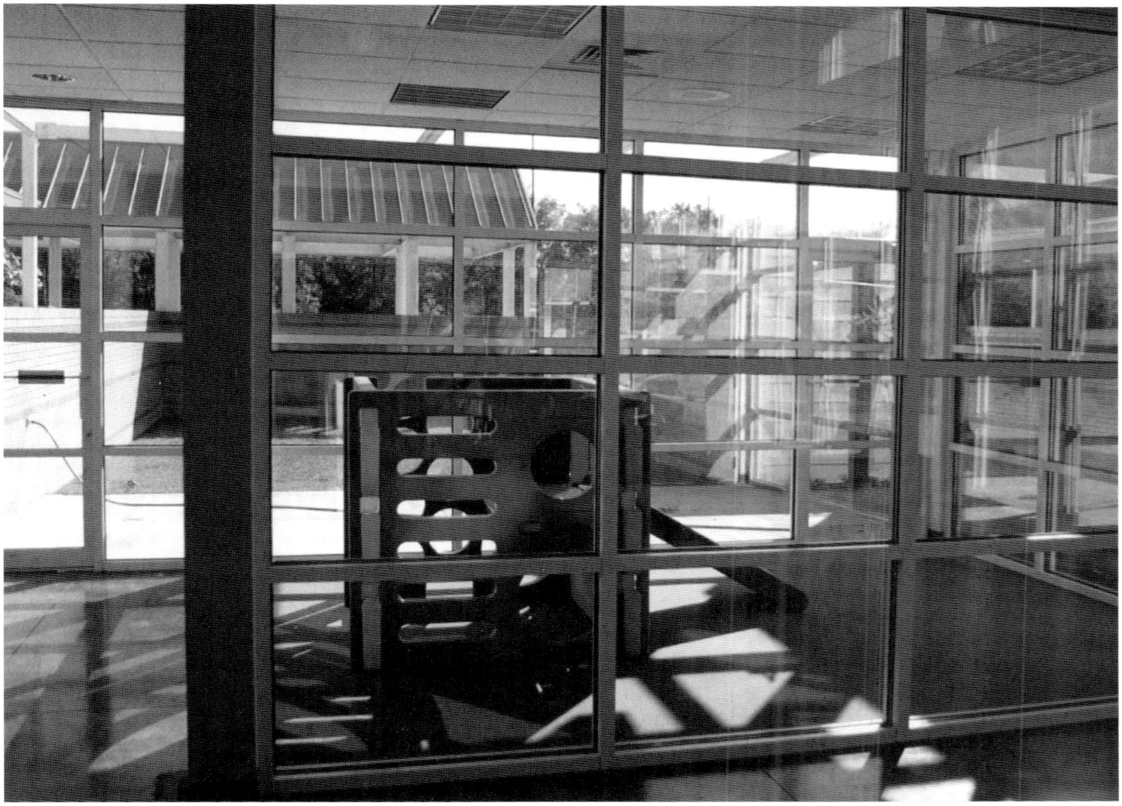

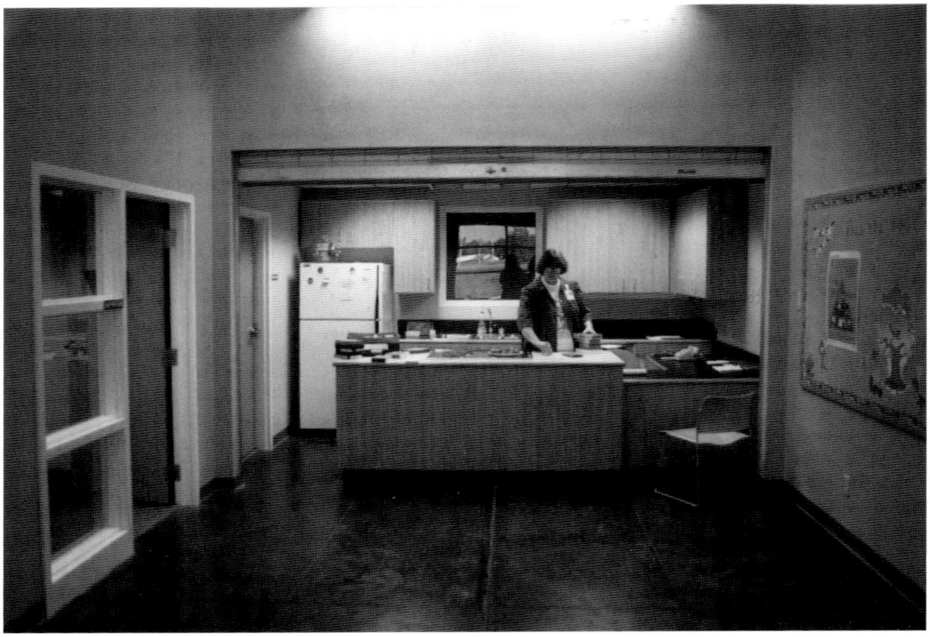

Fig. 5.11

gram area on the second level. These areas are accessed via an elevator across from the reception/sign-in counter on the main level, situated at the midsection of the arrival axis.

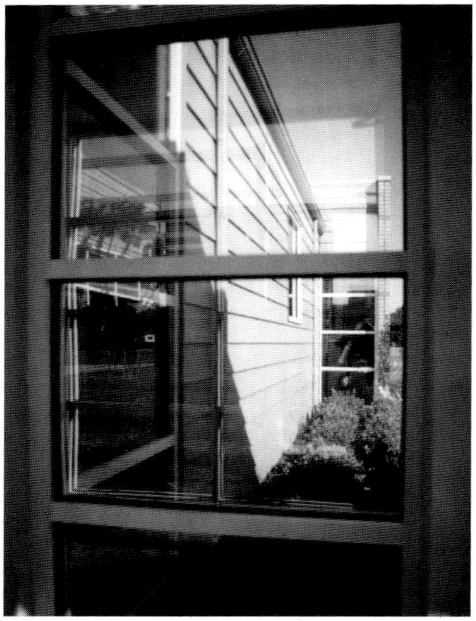

Fig. 5.12

This replacement facility opened in 1994. At the one-year interval the building was evaluated in terms of its overall performance. The entire staff completed a survey, as well as a group of patients and parish officials. Numerous interviews were also conducted. This stategy was subsequently applied to all SFI replacement facility assignments and is discussed in greater detail at the end of this chapter. Survey respondents cited its inviting exterior appearance and architectural imagery, a successful interior staff and patient flow pattern, the absence of noisy spaces within, the ambient spaces dedicated for children, the design of the nutritional education demonstration kitchen, the muted interior color scheme, the building's views from the windows to the outside, the natural daylight, and the building's interior circulation. Also cited as positive features were the flexivity of the waiting rooms, clerical workspaces, and nursing administrative areas, the residential scale of the building, and its landscaping. Negative assessments centered on a roof leak in the roof above one of the exam rooms (repaired soon thereafter).

Caldwell Parish, Columbia

Local elected officials in this parish were under pressure, on relatively short notice, to finance and build a new parish health unit because the health unit staff had been given notice they were being evicted from a building they shared with a DHH-operated mental health clinic, in a facility built on the edge of town in the 1970s. In Columbia, a town of 10,000 thirty miles south of Monroe, the health unit had had a handshake agreement to share space with the mental health clinic. This case study demonstrated how all parties could work together towards a common goal, when the need for rapid response is essential. The two programs had been sharing space and each had outgrown their respective quarters. The mental health facility, built with federal funds, was designed

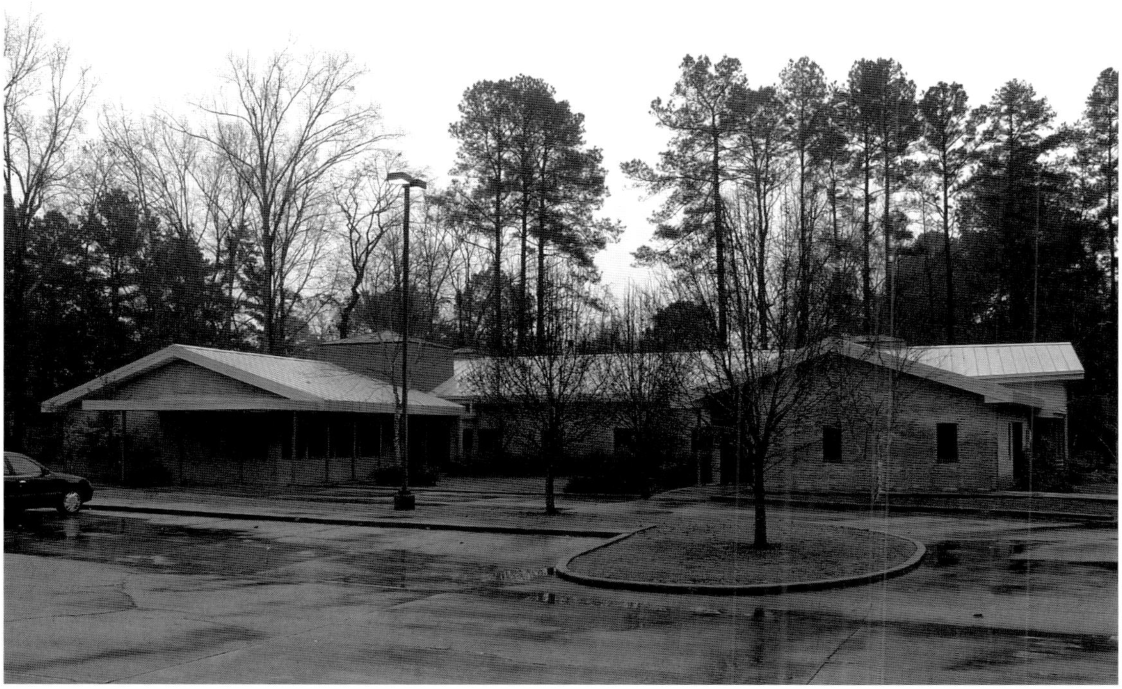

Fig. 5.13

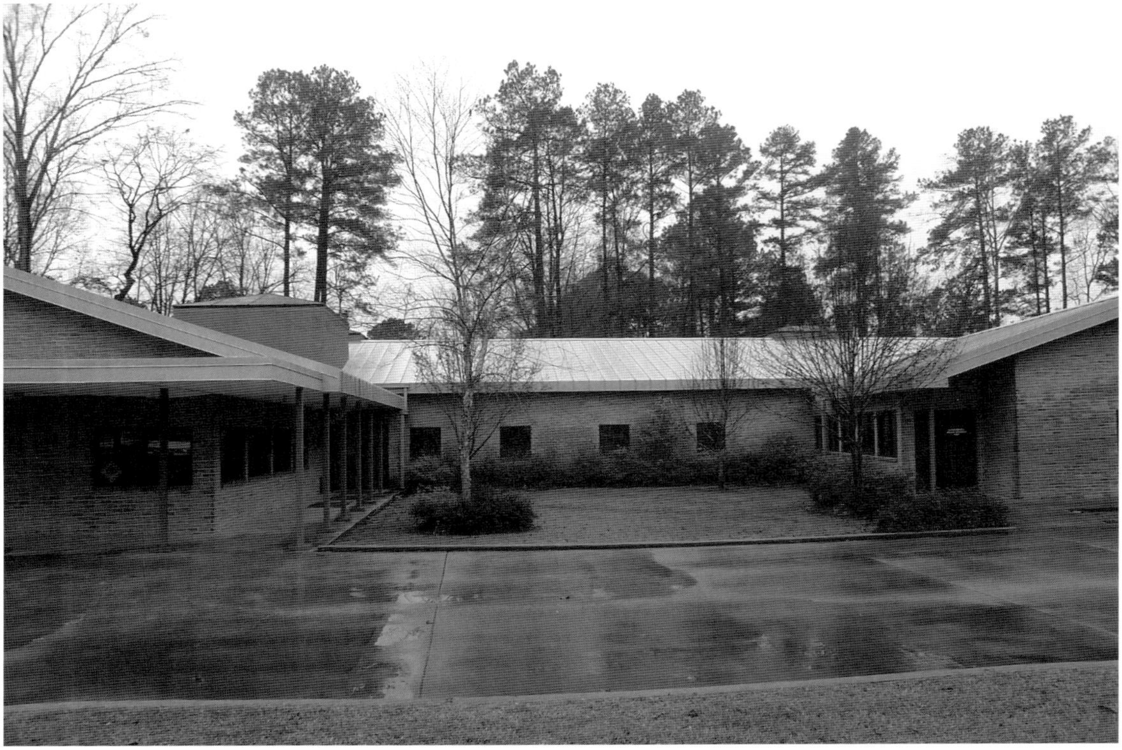

Fig. 5.14

with a four-sided courtyard at its center. It was an attractive, yet overburdened because it had not been designed to house a public health clinic.

For the new facility a wooded 2-acre site was selected across an access driveway leading to the parish's community hospital, situated across an access driveway. This site adjoined a residential neighborhood on the main road into town. This building, which opened in 1995, is a three-sided courtyard *U*, configured to preserved as much of the wooded setting as possible (Fig. 5.13). The building was 8,000 BGSF. Total construction cost was $900,000 (1995). This parish, as many had done, funded the project though a combination of a local millage tax and a local bank loan. This commission, similar to the clinic in West Monroe, was designed as a joint venture of R-2ARCH with Hugh Parker Architects of Monroe. The program called for a waiting and separate subwaiting room, clerical functions and four intake workstations for clerical staff, a clinic with four exam rooms, a nutritional education kitchen, multiple storage spaces,

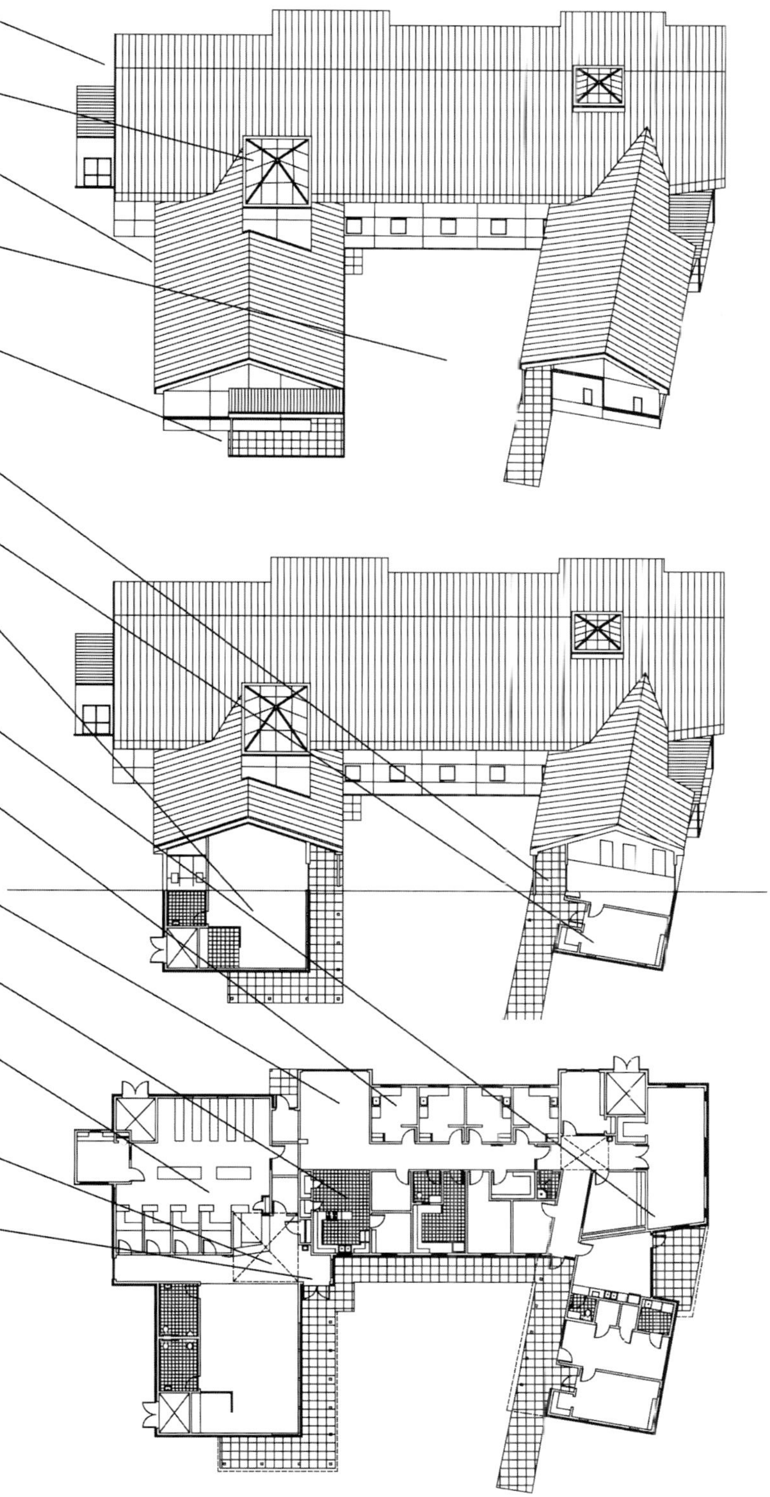

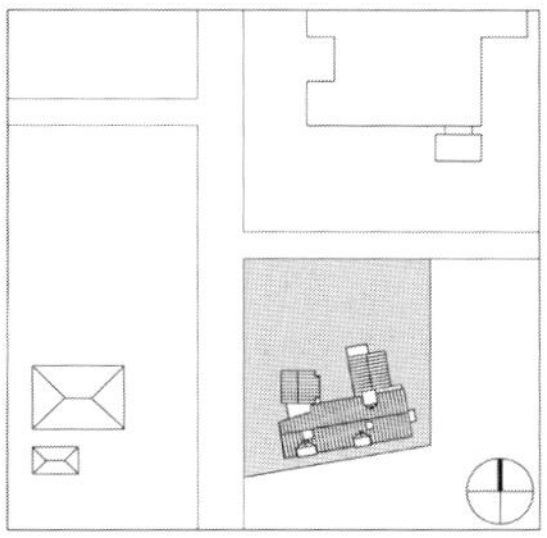

Fig. 5.15

Fig. 5.16 a-c

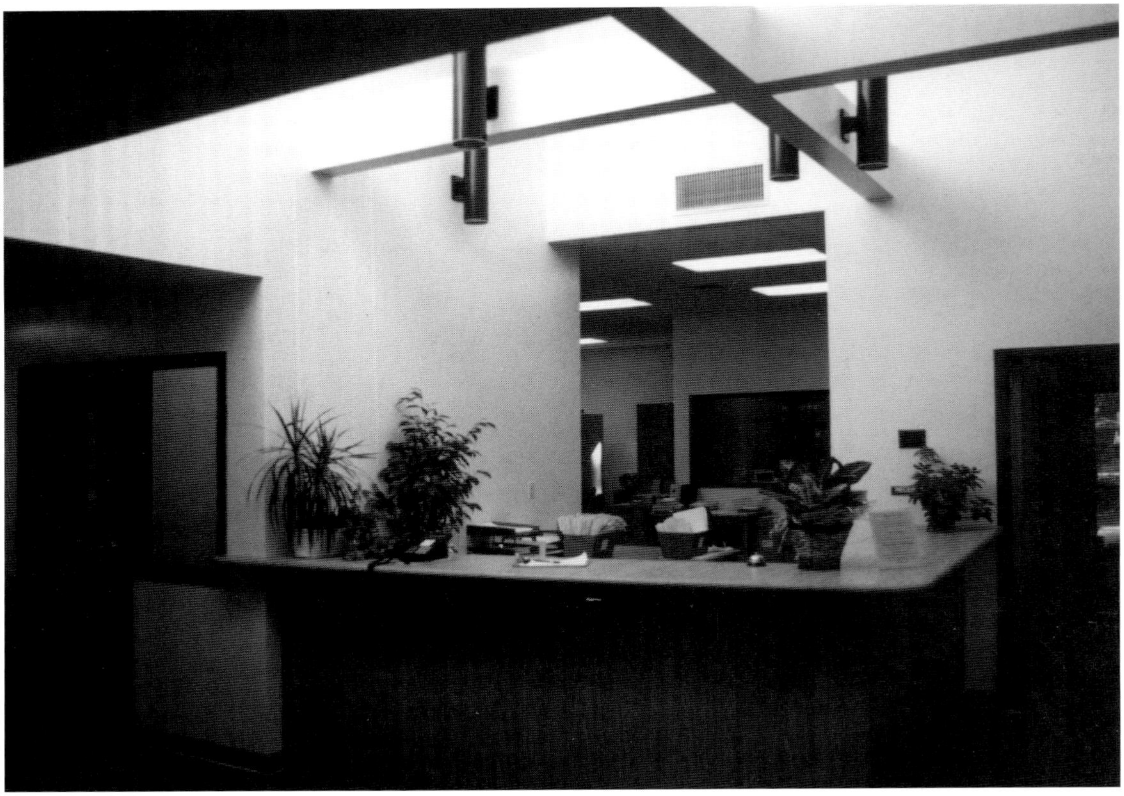

Fig. 5.17

a staff lounge-kitchen, and the environmental health program section. This replacement facility would nearly double the amount of space compared to the space occupied in the mental health clinic.

The partí was comprised as an articulated triad of the three principal realms inherent in the building type—the arrival/clerical realm, the clinic realm, and the environmental health realm. The courtyard facilitates wayfinding, as a means to access the clinic via its own dedicated entry, and, in turn, it affords direct access to the environmental health wing through a separate entry (Fig. 5.14). The building was sited to afford patients and staff therapeutic amenity insofar as facilitating visual contact with nature (Fig. 5.15 and Fig. 5.16). The main arrival wing houses the waiting room and patient restrooms and the mothers' alcove for breastfeeding infants. The appointment desk is clearly visible from the main entry and is adjacent to the patient intake area. The five patient-in-

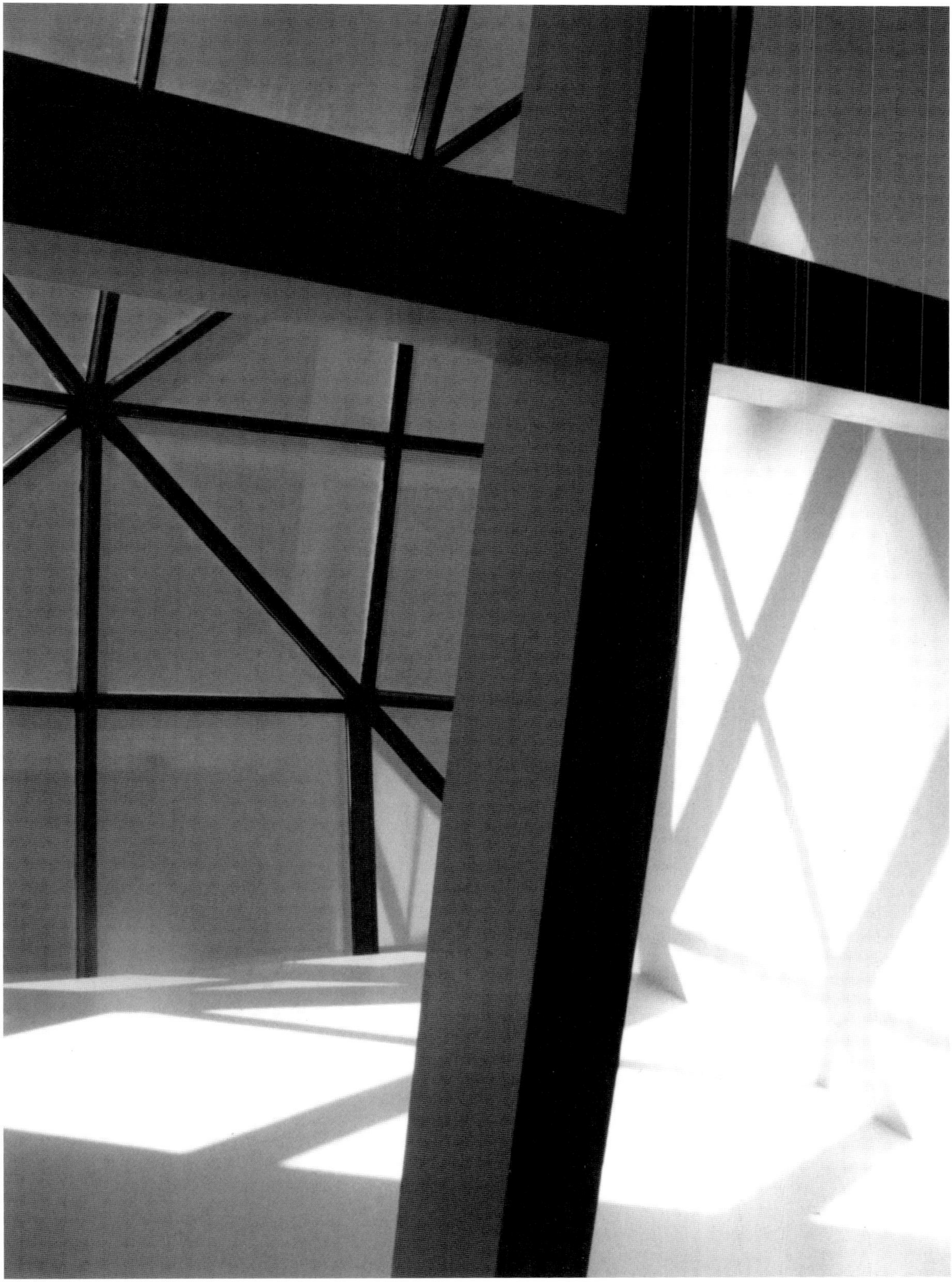

Fig. 5.18

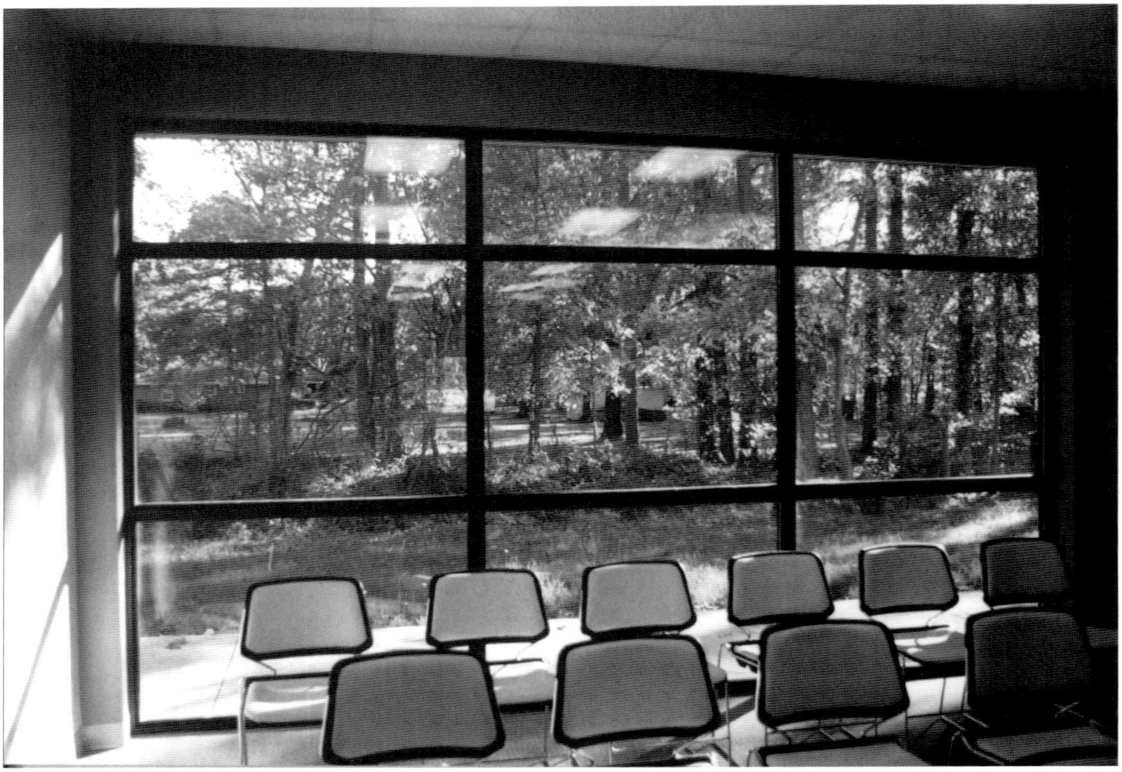

Fig. 5.19

take offices open up into the clerical workspace, containing a work island and the medical records storage area. The reception/sign-in counter is bathed in daylight from a skylight above (Fig. 5.17 and Fig. 5.18). Three skylights—at the appointment desk, the clerical-clinic threshold, and the clinic-nursing threshold—accentuated the transitional thresholds between these core realms, and also facilitated wayfinding.

Views to the wooded site from within activate the interior spaces in the clinic (Fig. 5.19). The clinic occupies the midsection of the building, with the exam rooms adjacent to subwaiting. On the courtyard side is the WIC kitchen, lab, patient specimen restroom, and staff offices. Nursing functions and clinic support spaces are housed in the zone between the clinic and the environmental health wing, with the staff lounge, semi-private patio, and staff conference/library situated between. The examination rooms were configured as autonomous entities, a variation of the concept previously incorporated at the West Monroe facility. Mock-ups were built of a typical exam room in order to arrive at the proper ergonomic relationship between patient, nurse, and setting (Fig. 5.20). This resulted in the creation of drop-down countertops, operable windows, and under-cabinet-mounted vertical file units. Both here and in the West Monroe facility, considerable attention was given to the scale and placement of the dressing alcove within each exam room. A full height wing wall with a seat was provided to function as a privacy screen; a pull curtain augmented this. Windows were operable in the exam rooms, as at West Monroe. The building's environmental health wing houses the parish sanitarians' offices, a second conference room, and environmental health support spaces. The aforementioned outdoor covered walkways leading from the parking areas to the main entrance of the clinic, and the entrance to the sanitarians' area, respectively, parallel the two wings.

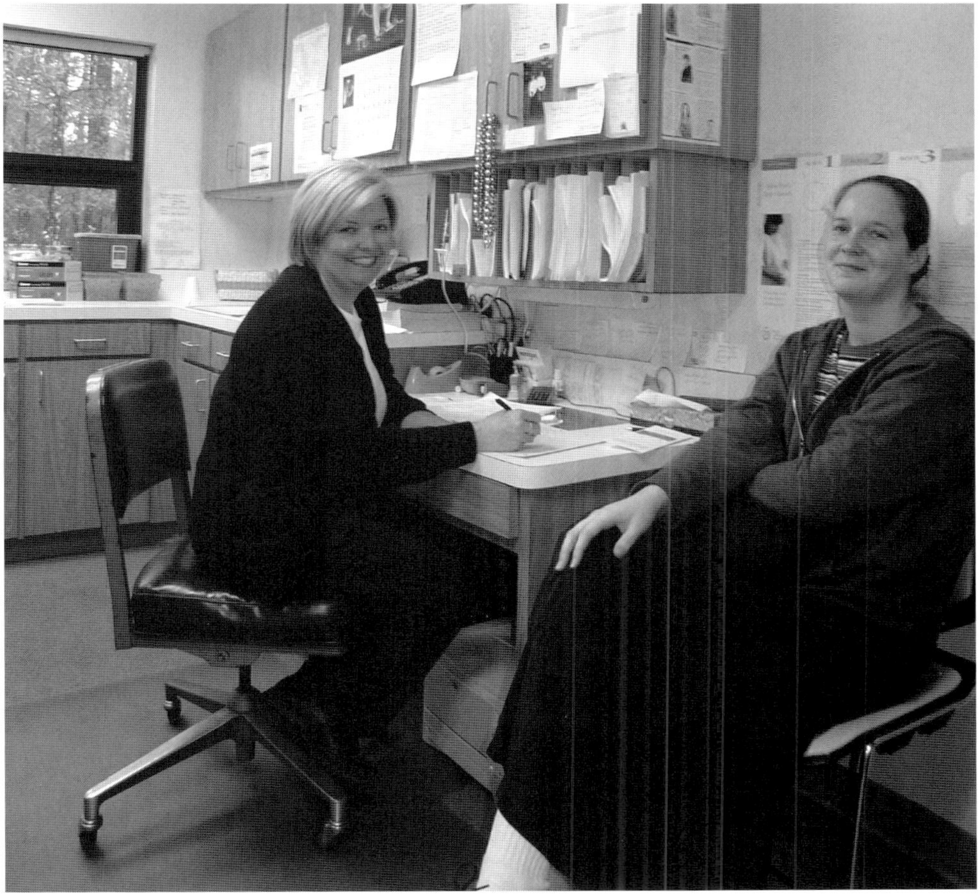

Fig. 5.20

The exterior colors, a sienna standing seam metal roof with red-toned face brick punctuated by black-framed fenestration, contributed to a residential aesthetic and scale. The post-occupancy assessment, one year later, reflected occupants' high level of satisfaction with the building, and principally with the staff and patient flow patterns, its overall quietness, residential scale, the colors of the exterior materials, the accessible relationship between parking and the arrival sequence, the views to nature, the natural daylight, the nutritional education demonstration kitchen, the sanitarians' work spaces, and the exam rooms. No specific architectural deficiencies were cited in the post-occupancy-assessment in terms of having any deleterious effects on the occupants, save for a roof that needed to be re-waterproofed above one of the exam rooms.

Tensas Parish, St. Joseph

St. Joseph, the parish seat of Tensas Parish, located on the west bank of the Mississippi River, about 120 miles upriver of Baton Rouge. It once was a thriving rural center of commerce for a multi-parish region. The parish has been losing population for decades, declining from a peak of nearly 30,000 in the 1950s to less than 6,000 in the 2000 census. The economy has traditionally been based on cotton farming, soy farming, and the lumber industry (see Chapter 3). The Mississippi Delta parishes, Tensas notwithstanding, continue to be among the poorest areas per capita in the United States. Agriculture, and the lumber industry, once had a major economic impact, but these industries were displaced because of technological advances and excessive deforestation. Nonetheless, this health unit had maintained a particularly strong civic presence in the community since its founding in the aftermath of the massive 1927 flood.

Since 1949 this health unit had occupied a plain storefront building on Main Street. Main Street, a two-block stretch, was once lined with bustling stores, saloons, and offices. Now only the historic parish library occupies a place of civic distinction along this street. Today the street is but a shadow of its former glory, with vacant lots the only remaining vestiges of long-vanished buildings. One restaurant remains, along with a few small shops, the mayor's office, and the aforementioned public library. Recent commercial development had consisted of the usual compliment of a Wal-Mart on the edge of town, fringe strip malls, and a few fast food outlets. A number of historic buildings remained, however, near the town center, serving as reminders of the town's rich past. This was one among a handful of health unit buildings not owned by the parish police jury (they leased it). As a result, maintenance and improvements had been minimal over the years. The owner of the building had enjoyed a comfortable long-term lease with the parish. In 1976, an addition was built at the rear. Although the parish's population diminished, the health unit endured as a civic anchor.

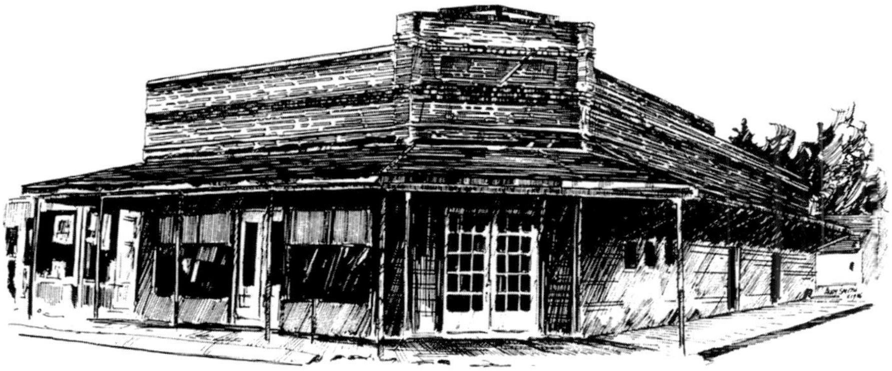

Fig. 5.21

The first proposal for a replacement facility grew out of an interest on the part of the police jury to relocate to a different site near the center of town. The structure they had in mind at the time, a one-story ranch house, was to be adapted to a healthcare facility. But with only 2,750 square feet and a program requiring three exam rooms, a lab, WIC demonstration kitchen, waiting room, a medical records and clerical area, two intake stations/offices, and an environmental health office, not to mention myriad code requirements making it impossible to pursue this strategy, the residence was soon judged to be inadequate. Soon thereafter, a capital outlay request to the state legislature yielded $250,000, with a local match in funds amounting to an additional $250,000 in 1995.

Henceforth, a larger clinic was designed compared to the house-cum-clinic strategy explored a year earlier, as local political leaders realized a new facility

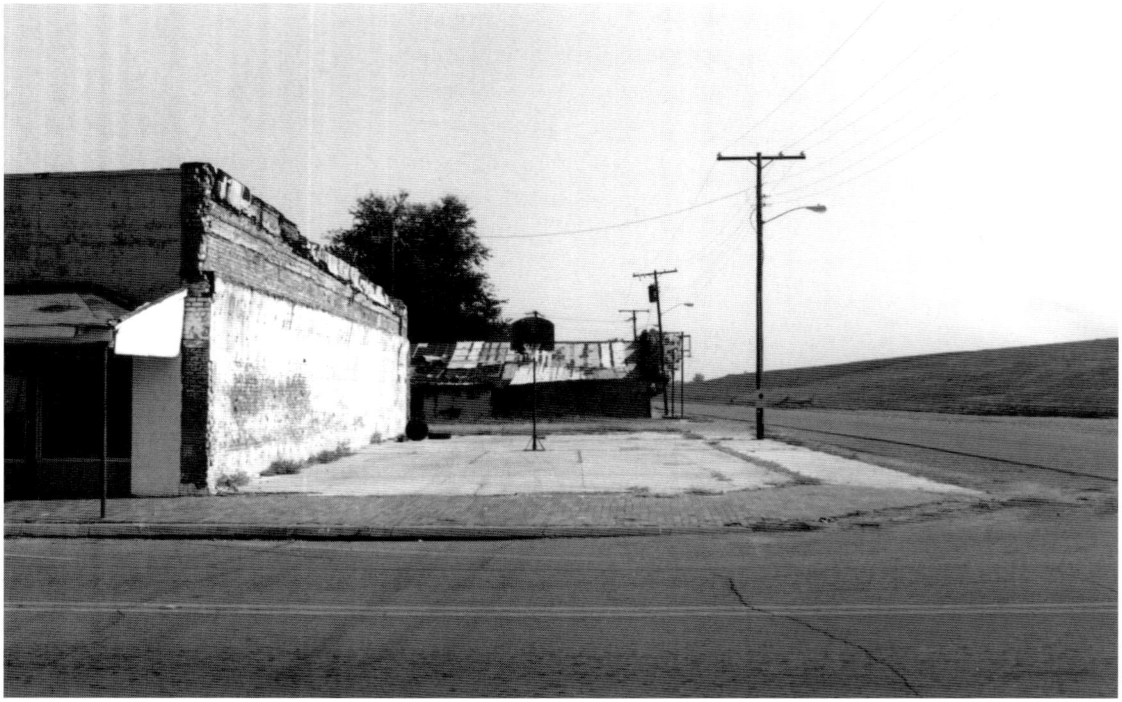

Fig. 5.22

might help spur the redevelopment of the once-vibrant Main Street. This renewed commitment to remaining in the town center was nearly short-circuited by heated squabbles among a handful of influential, wholly self-interested landowners, each lobbying for his parcel of land to be bought. This process bogged the project down for two more years. Eventually, it was agreed to purchase a site at the end of Main Street just across from the Mississippi River levee, on the former site of an infamous saloon that burned to the ground years before and had never been rebuilt. Everyone, it seemed, had a story to tell about it, as it concurrently operated as a "colored-only" and a "whites-only" bar side by side in the same building for at least three generations (see Chapter 3). Its local folklore made it all the more intriguing as a site because it held civic significance, as a symbol of the Jim Crow era, and belied the town's resilience through good economic times as well as bad (Fig. 5.21 and Fig. 5.22).

A second proposal, presented to the police jury in 2000 was for a 6,000 square foot, two-level clinic, necessitated due to the narrowness of the corner

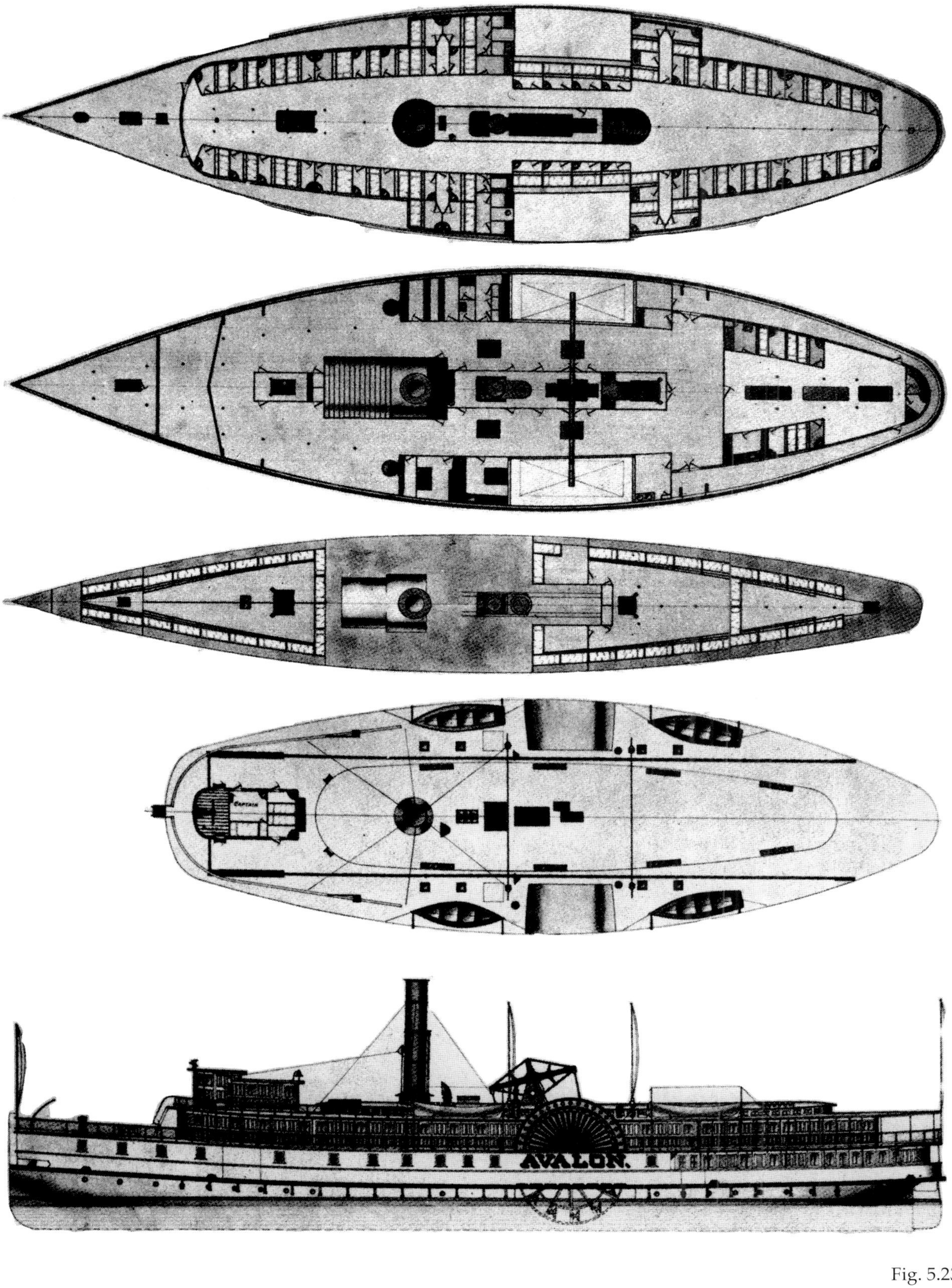

Fig. 5.23

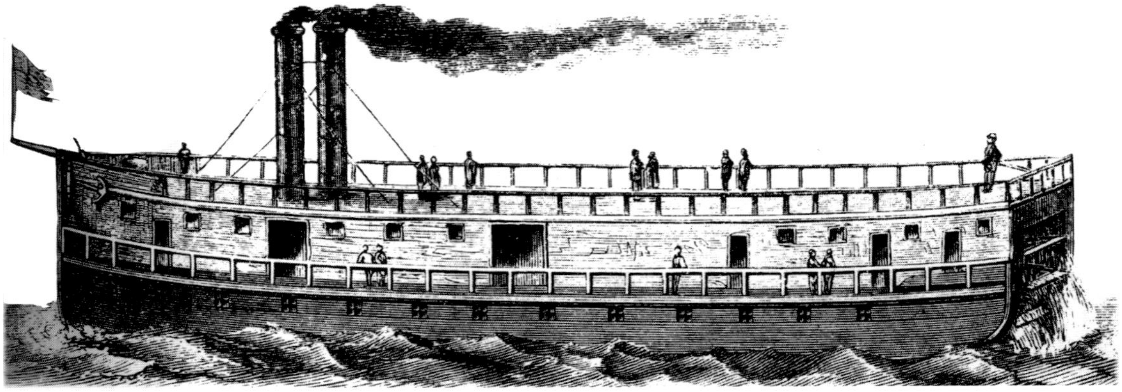

Fig. 5.24

site at the levee's edge. The first level's oversized masonry was to be reminiscent of a stone-sheathed bank, as was common in many rural banking institutions built across America in the late-nineteenth and early-twentieth centuries. The two-level partí was rooted at the base of Main Street, as a civic anchor. The site extended the entire block fronting the levee. Parking was located to the rear, as was an access drive and porte cochère. A second entrance, fronting Main Street, would provide access to a multipurpose/community room on the second level and the environmental health suite. Parking was readily available along Main Street. This second entrance was intended primarily for evening events in the community room. The main entrance to the clinic, beneath a porte cochère, led to the waiting room. A children's playroom and outdoor play space was situated to the right, and the intake stations/clerical offices to the front, with one doubling as a reception desk. Also included were four exam rooms, subwaiting, nutritional education kitchen, and support spaces.

The Mississippi River has had a colorful, fascinating history of its own. As a major highway for transportation of goods during the nineteenth century, it was unsurpassed in the amount of tonnage that passed along its waters. The principal port cities along this waterway were St. Louis, Memphis, Vicksburg, Baton Rouge, and of course, New Orleans, nearest the mouth of the river. Dozens of steamboats plied their trade along the river, stopping at various towns and former plantations along the way, including the town of St. Joseph, in order to pick up shipments of cotton. Many books have documented these ships, as they were in effect floating buildings. The architecture of the steamboats has

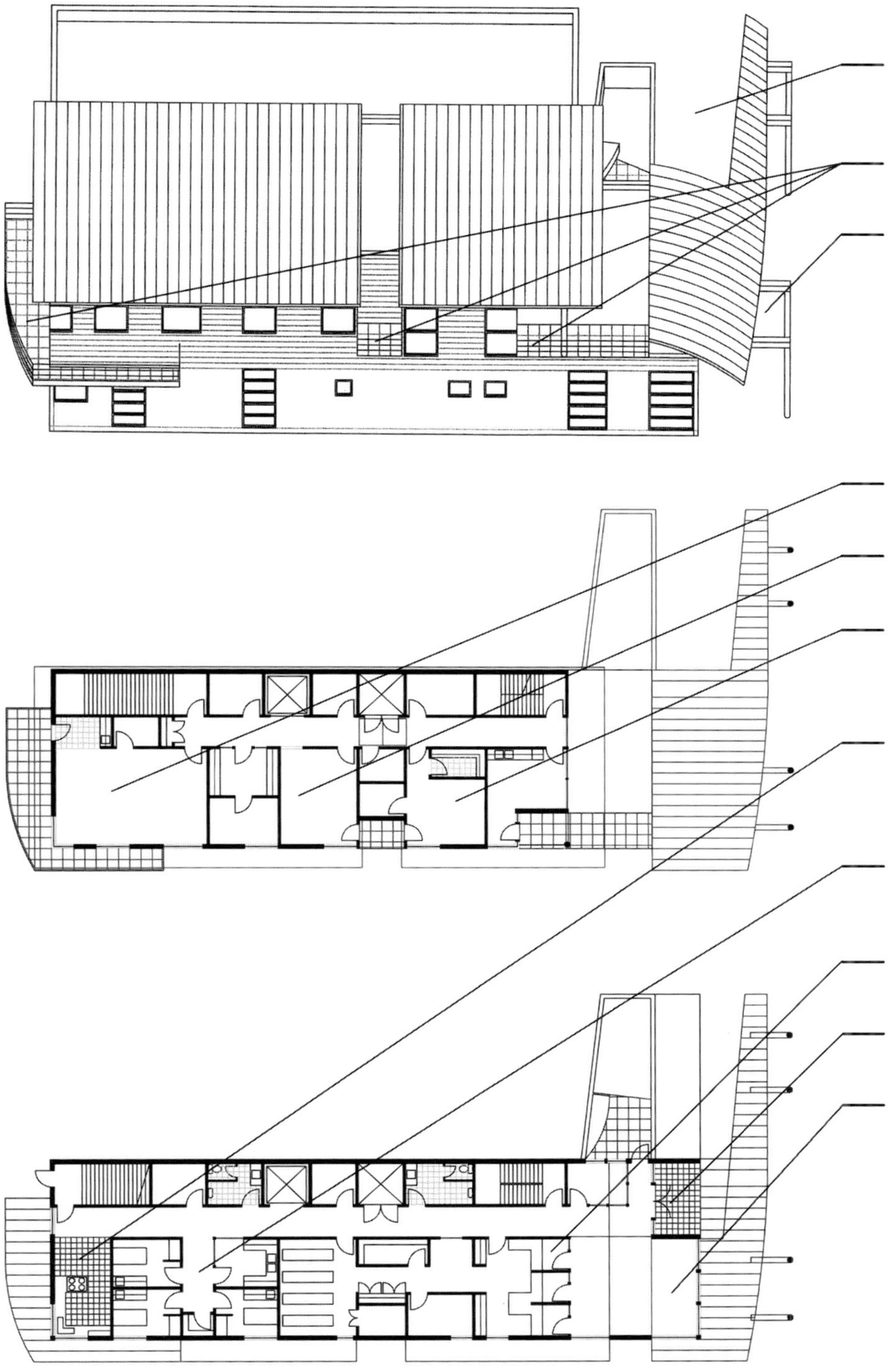

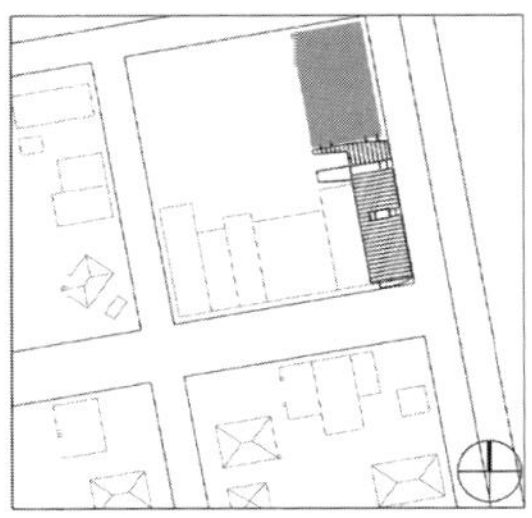

Fig. 5.25 a-c

Fig. 5.26

been the subject of numerous books documenting their many technological and spatial amenities. General plans of a proposed steamboat were submitted by the designers to the ship owners. These generally consisted of a profile and deck plan of each deck. Here are shown the plans for the steamer *Avalon*, built in 1888, with an iron hull, measuring 191′ x 31′ x 9′ (Fig. 5.23). The top deck of some of these river vessels afforded unobstructed views to the shoreline, as depicted in this engraving of the stern-wheeler *General Pike*, built in 1818 in Cincinnati (Fig. 5.24).[4]

The second level, not unlike the top deck of a nineteenth-century river steamer, was to house offices, the break room / kitchen, and an adjacent outdoor roof terrace for staff to take in views of the large ships passing by on the river on the other side of the levee (Fig. 5.25 and Fig. 5.26). All three viewing decks on the second level would afford dramatic views of passing ship traffic. The exterior red brick and the building's massing and setbacks complimented the adjacent historic buildings and Main Street's aesthetic vocabulary. Unfortunately, a clear ownership title to the preferred corner site could not be obtained. In 2003, after further political maneuvering, a replacement facility opened (not shown), built on a site at the far end of this same block, across from the levee.

Calcasieu Parish, Lake Charles

The 23,500 square-foot replacement facility for Lake Charles, completed in 2003, had been in the works for nearly ten years. The challenge was to reinvent this community care center on its present site without shutting down operations. Options to relocate to a new location proved unfeasible because the sites available would have been too far away from the neighborhoods where most of the patients resided far from public transportation. Its current location was excellent, adjacent to two bus stops at a major intersection. Second, the health unit, since its opening in 1962, had been part of an outpatient healthcare "campus." This campus housed a DHH-OPH region laboratory and the region administrative office relocated in 2002 to an existing building on the same block. The staff indicated in the post-occupancy survey in 1991 they were no longer able to fully implement the programs mandated by the agency, as the health unit building imposed too many limitations on a day-to-day basis. Besides the health unit, the site houses the aforementioned region laboratory (a replace-

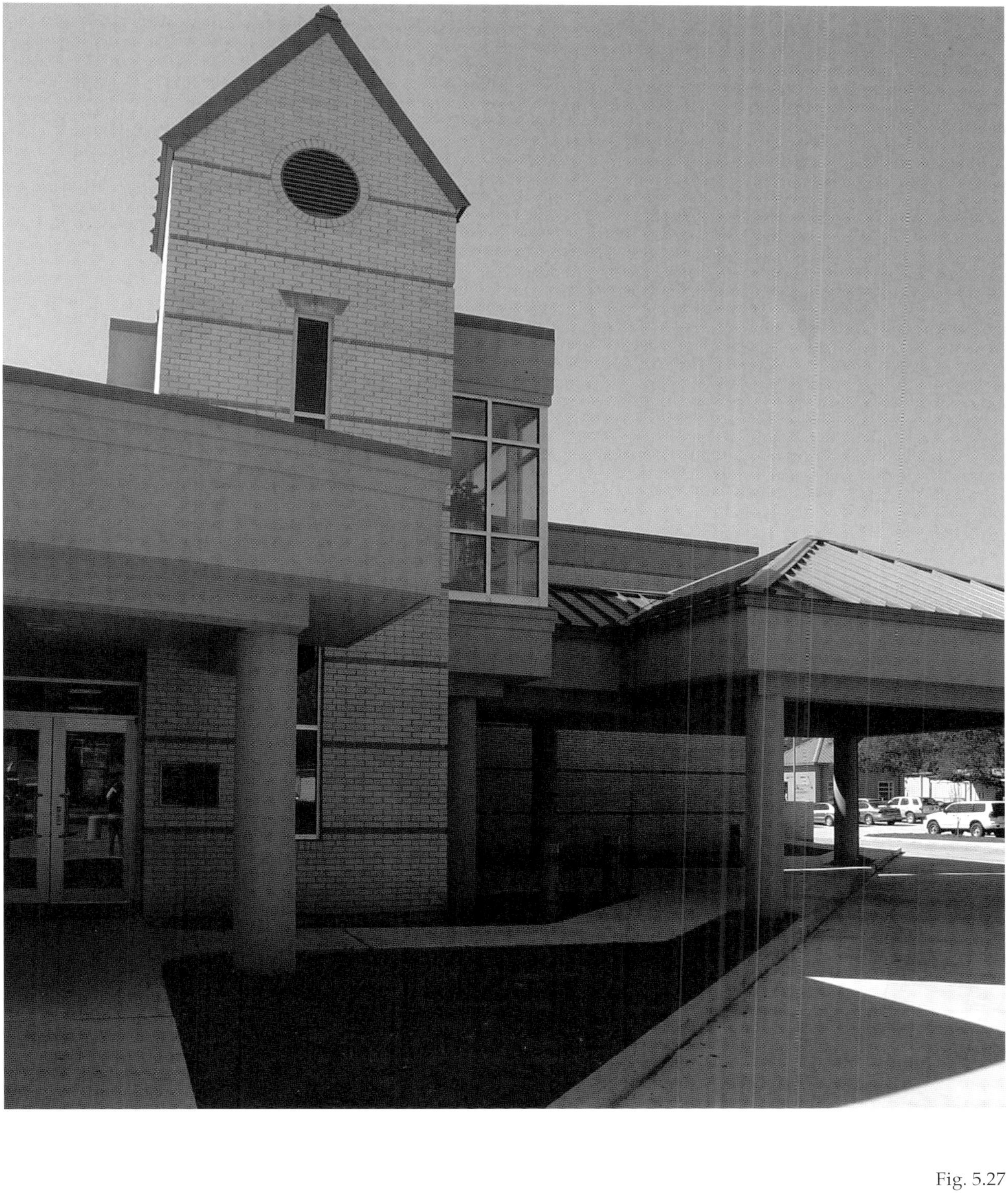

Fig. 5.27

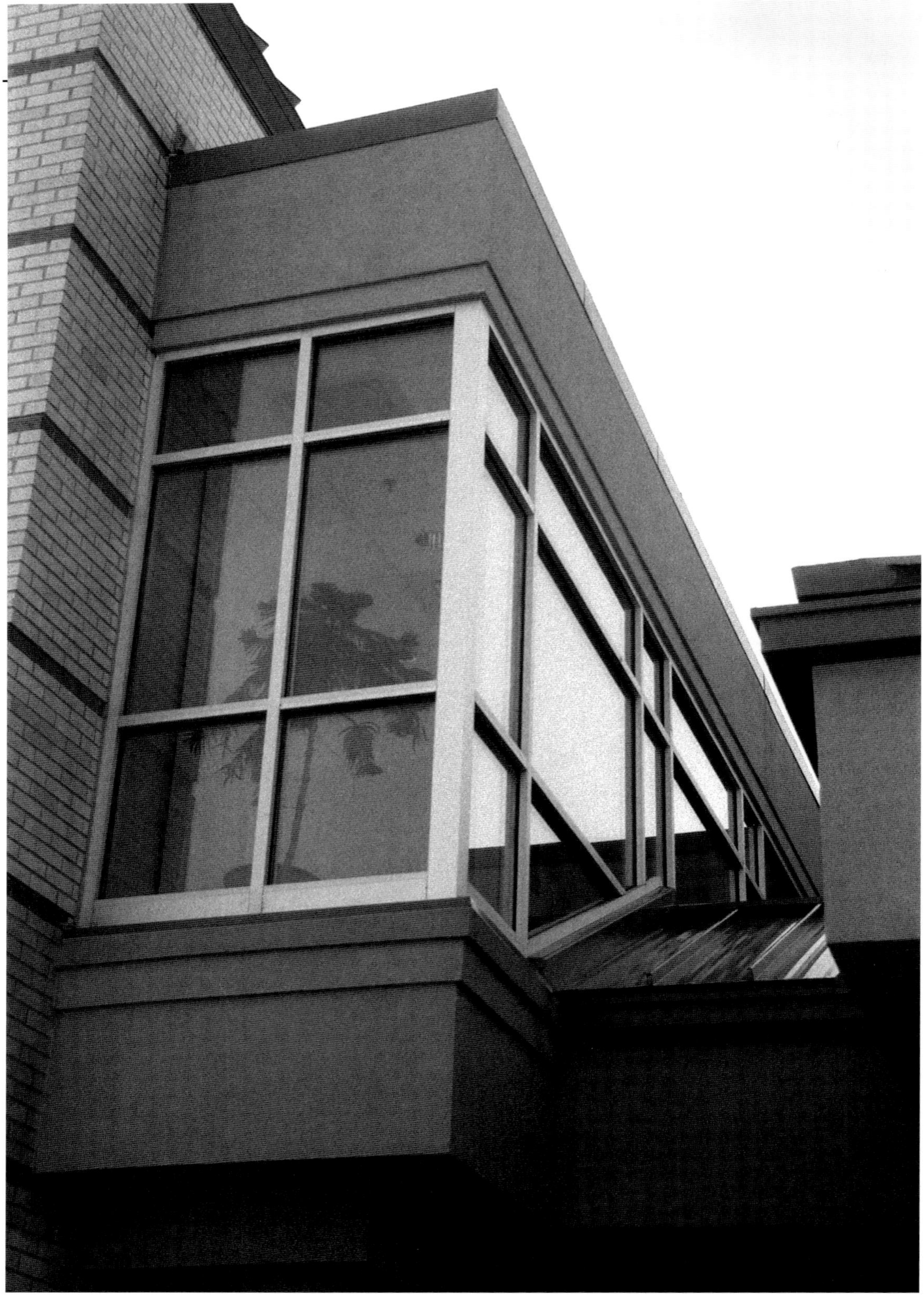

Fig. 5.28

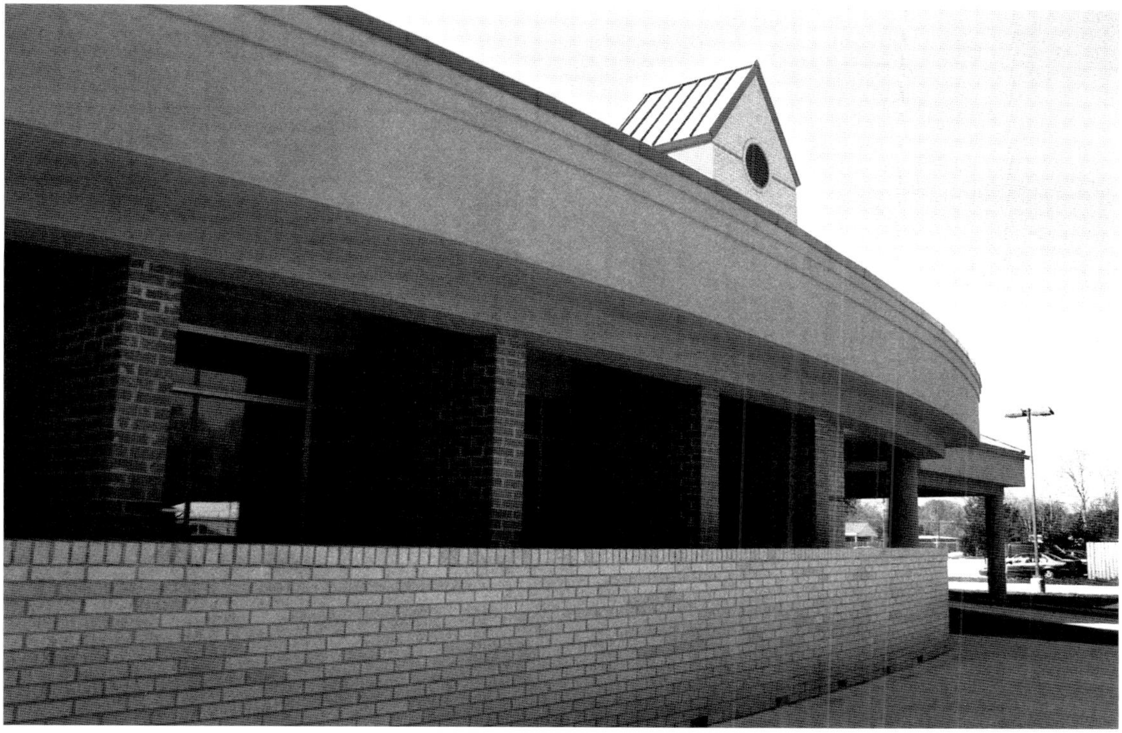

ment facility opened in 2000, replacing the original 1959 lab torn down to make way for the expansion of the health unit).

Fig. 5.29

The new facility, two levels in height, was built in eighteen months as a five-phase mix of demolition, renovation, and new construction (Fig. 5.27). Total project cost was $3.6 million. This stategy was worked out a priori with the staff in close collaboration with the architectural and engineering team. Meetings were attended by the directors of the various programs, the evidence-based SFI team, the local architect in Lake Charles, David Moss Architects (who served as the architect of record), and representatives from the state. In phase one the new lab facility was built. In phase two a two-level addition to the existing building was built. The first floor houses the clinic, and the second level houses the environmental health and vital records programs (Fig. 5.28). In phase three, the vacated lab wing and part of the old health unit space was demolished. Then, a new waiting room and intake space was built in its place. In phase four, the retained sections of the existing building were thoroughly renovated.

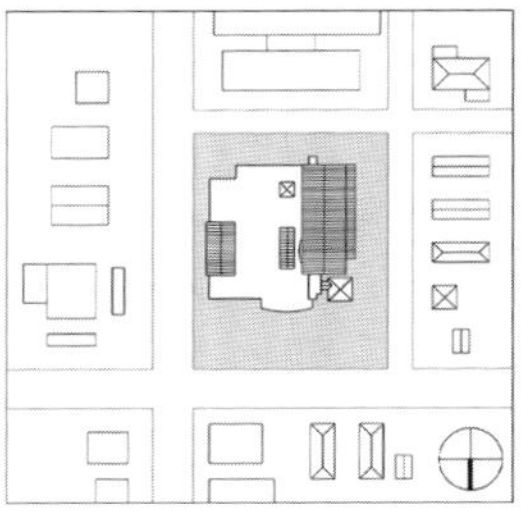

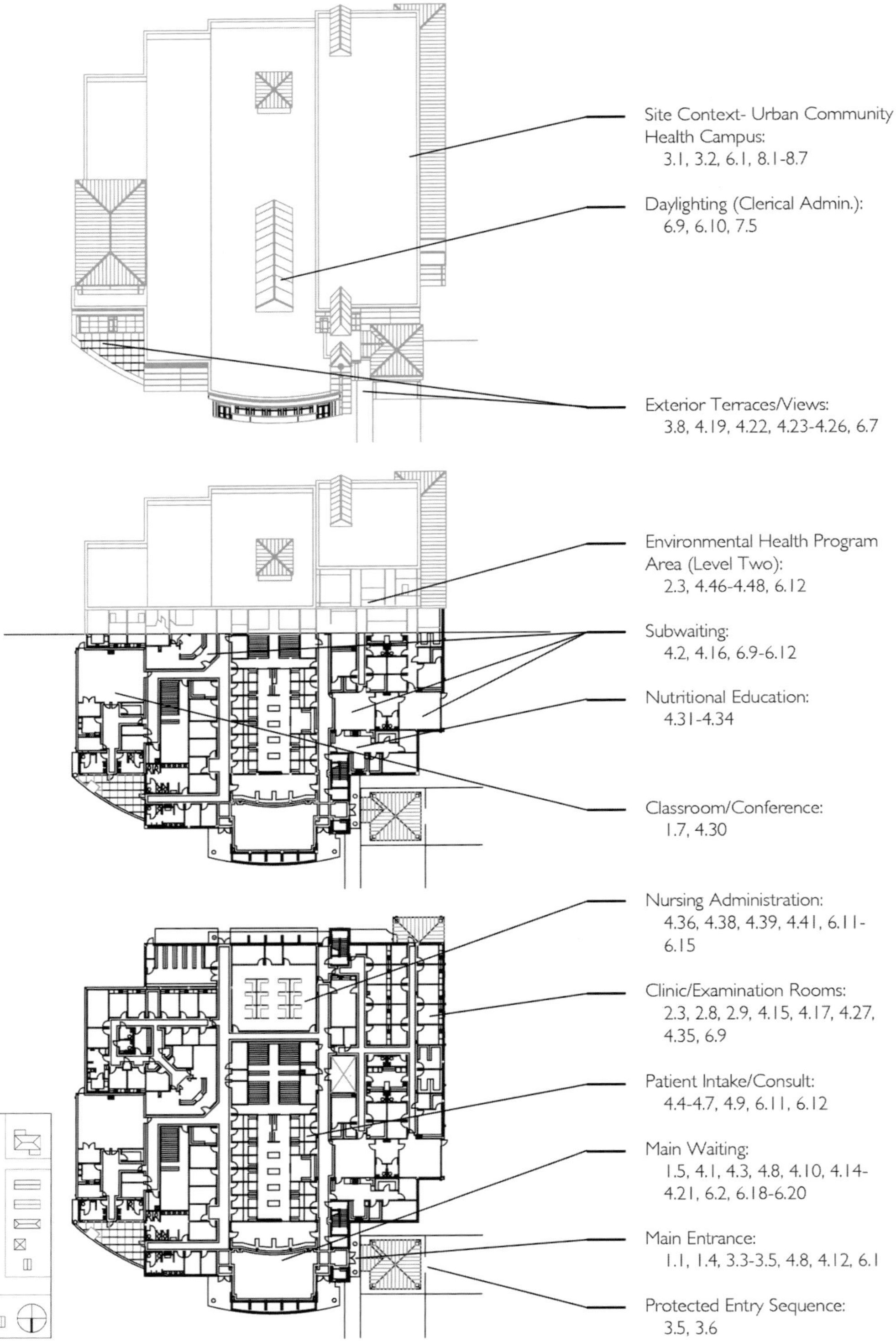

Fig. 5.30

Fig. 5.31 a-c

In the fifth and final phase, a new parking area was built on the site of the old lab. The program included environmental health, a comprehensive care clinic, a vital records program section, a clerical and administrative support section, and multipurpose rooms for health education and community outreach. The clinic contained fifteen examination rooms. The clerical intake stations/offices numbered sixteen.

A porte cochère is located at the main entrance. The second level houses the environmental health program and is accessed vis-a-vis an elevator and public stairway. A reception and waiting area functions as a lantern at night. The environmental health area houses fifteen full-time staff. The full-time staff housed numbers sixty. On the first level, the main entrance leads directly to the reception/sign-in counter. The main waiting room is configured along the front of the building, and an exterior wall screens direct views of cars in the adjacent parking area (Fig. 5.29). Two banks of six clerical stations each flank a reception desk and an open clerical core work zone. This space has clerestory windows. The main records room adjoins this clerical work zone, with a rolling "spacesaver" file system. The record room adjoins an open plan office for fifteen nursing staff. Core clinic functions adjoin this space. On one side are ten exam rooms, and on the other, five. One side houses the communicable diseases clinic and the Children's Special Health Services (CSHS) clinic. The clinic on the opposite side houses family planning and child and maternal health programs.

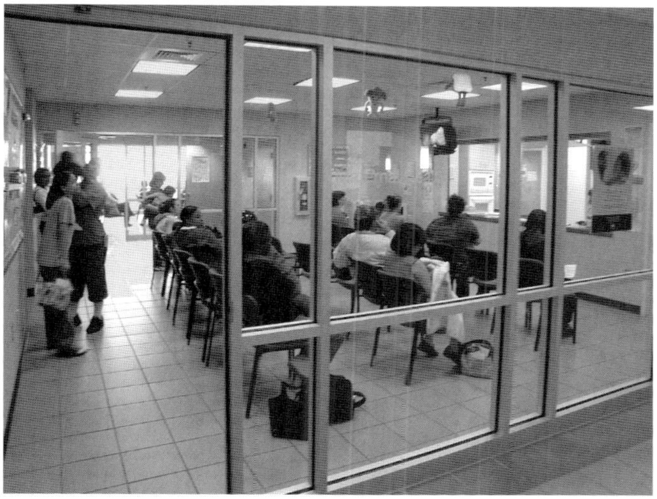

Fig. 5.32

The footprint was pre-determined by the aforementioned restrictions imposed by the site. The completed building is set back from the busy intersection. Parking for seventy-five vehicles is provided. Waiting rooms are decentralized to provide a safety valve, depressurizing occupancy demands on the main waiting room and the nutritional education kitchen (Fig. 5.30 and Fig. 5.31). This facility provides services to 175 patients per day.

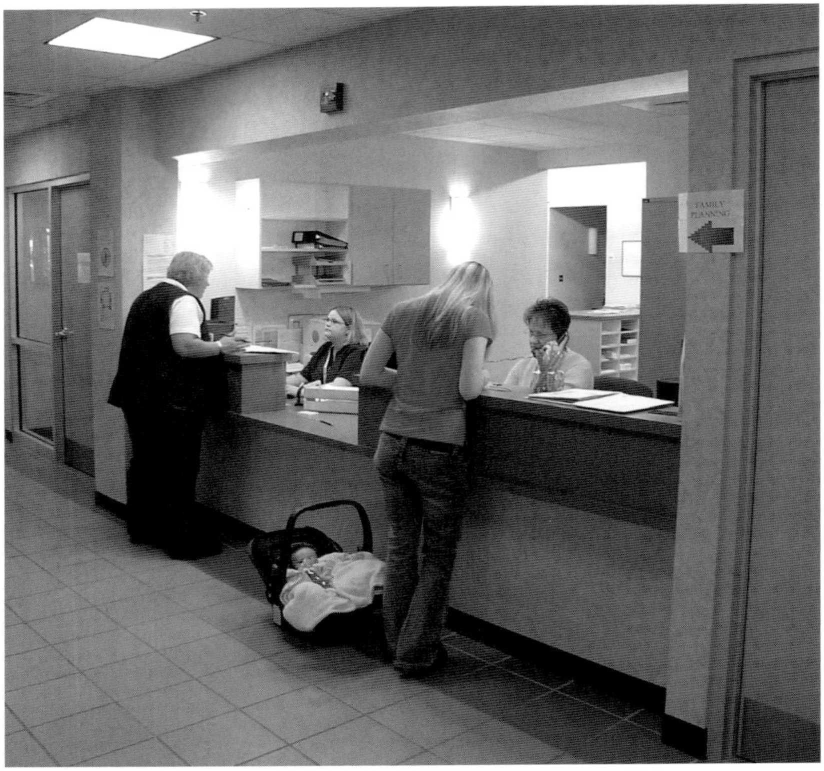

Fig. 5.33

The subwaiting areas are adjacent to the clinic areas and to the nutritional education demonstration kitchen (5.32). The sign-in counters for the clinics are decentralized (Fig. 5.33). This reduces potential overcrowding at the main reception counter at the front. The participation of the end-user occupants, and their collaboration with the A/E team and SFI team, and the various consultants, served as a precedent, demonstrating how a large urban community healthcare facility can be, in effect, completely rebuilt on its original site without relinquishing a centrally located prime land parcel. It also disproves the assumption that a new site is always the preferred option. The architectural assessment completed one year after occupancy indicated that the outcome has been a source of renewed pride and sense of accomplishment for all who were involved. This reinvented and significantly expanded care setting dramatically symbolized a renewed commitment to the future of public healthcare in the Lake Charles community.

Jefferson Parish, Metairie

This International style clinic, built in 1961, symbolized at once the best and the worst of the Hill-Burton era (Fig. 5.27). The site for this facility was problematic from the start. The patient must manage to navigate a labyrinth of small side streets and a bridge underpass with no direct feeder road. Upon arrival, one is rewarded for the effort. The Jefferson Parish East Bank Health Unit, regardless, remained one of the most elegant post-World War II modernist health clinics built in the American South. This building's clear organizational partí, its high level of architectural detailing, and the use of experimental building materials and assembly systems set it apart from its peer facilities built during his period. The owner, the Jefferson Parish Council, not realizing the clinic's architectural significance, had neglected to maintain the building over the years, and was on the verge of abandoning it in favor of a new building on an open suburban site some miles away. The evidenced-based SFI team set out to convince the parish council that this building was indeed worth saving and restoring to meet the community healthcare needs of the new millennium. Jefferson Parish, with a population of 650,000, is situated immediately next to Orleans Parish. The health unit is six miles from downtown New Orleans. Total project cost was $850,000. Renovation was completed in 2003.

Not unlike its International style precursor, the Finsbury Health Centre in London of the 1930s, the Metairie clinic was initially programmed and designed to articulate three main realms—a mental health center, a public health education auditorium, and a public preventive health clinic. As at Finsbury, the auditorium at the Metairie facility is situated at the center, flanked by two wings, with the public health clinic, a two-level volume, the larger of the two, to the east, and the mental health clinic a one-level volume to the west side of the auditorium. This configuration creates a semi-enclosed courtyard in the arrival area at the center, with entrances to each of the three realms. On the interior a corridor wraps around the courtyard, connecting all three (Fig. 5.34).

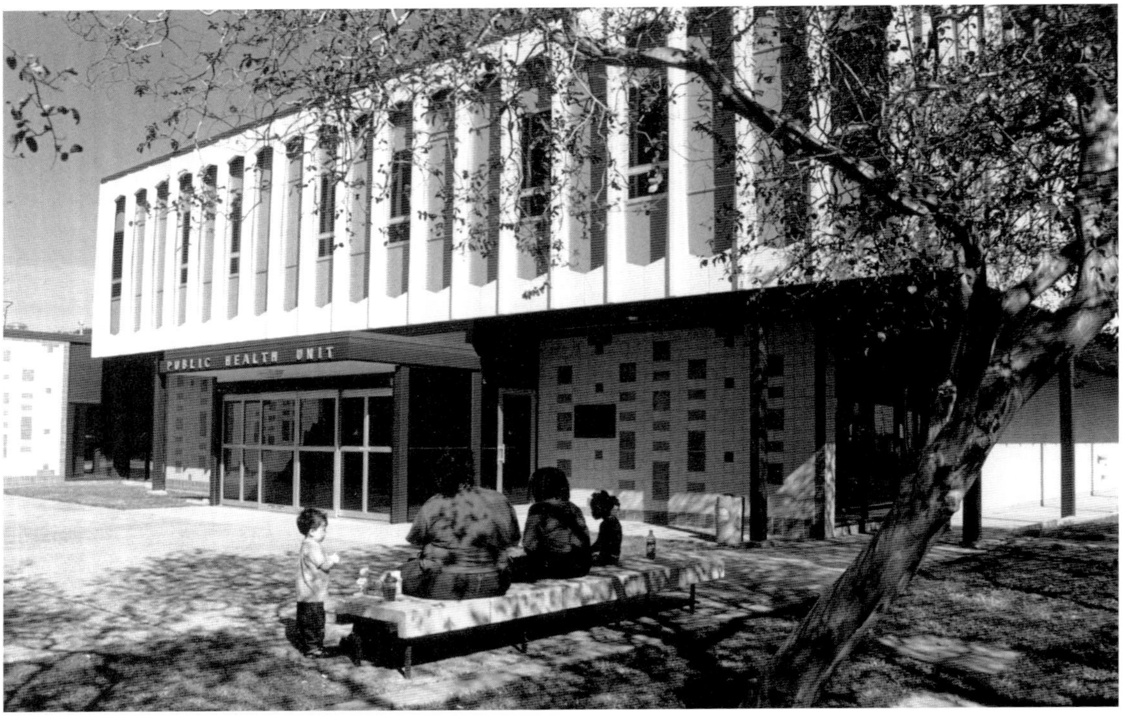

Fig. 5.34

While innovative in terms of its construction and tfunctional organization, the building had not been renovated since its opening. This fact is noteworthy in light of the exponential population growth in this community in the post-World War II era. It is now the second most populous parish in the state (behind Orleans Parish). This area emerged as a suburb of New Orleans in the post-World War II decades and the health unit experienced a ten-fold increase in use since its opening forty-five years ago. The Metairie facility was built as a suburban clinic but its high level of utilization now placed it firmly within the ranks of the urban clinics in the statewide network of parish health units. In the 1991 post-occupancy survey the staff remained firmly committed to its location in terms of its proximity to the patients most reliant on its services. The staff unanimously indicated extreme dissatisfaction with the obsolescent conditions within, however.

In 1998 the parish council voted to pursue improvements to the health unit, and at the same time explore possibilities for the construction of a replacement facility elsewhere. Cost feasibility studies were conducted, and it was concluded that it would be too expensive to purchase, or assemble, through eminent domain powers, a parcel of land large enough near to the existing location. Meanwhile, in 1991 a new health unit opened in the community of Marrero, on the west bank of the Mississippi River. At the urging of the staff, agency administrators, and the SFI team, a strategy of renovation and restoration was approved. The political decision to stay put at the present site, however, had not been based solely on the merits of the Metairie facility in and of itself. The unfortunate legacy of the parish's experience with the replacement facility across the river in Marrero weighed heavily. This pre-SFI facility (1990) had been plagued with costly retrofitting resulting from an inadequate HVAC system.

In this project, completed in 2003, the objective was to restore the exterior without making significant exterior architectural modifications. The one exception was the addition of a glass-enclosed entry vestibule, because, patients sitting nearest the main clinic entrance had been unbuffered from external weather conditions. The interior was gutted and rebuilt in a two-phase sequence while the clinic remained fully operational. The auditorium was renovated. An emergency shelter, recently mandated by the parish, was created together with a multipurpose classroom on the second floor. The space vacated by a mental health clinic temporarily served as the home of the health unit during a twelve month period. ADA-mandated handicapped access improvements were implemented throughout. No major modifications were made to parking areas or access drives.

The main waiting room was expanded, yet retained in its original location. Five intake workstations were incorporated. A new nutritional demonstration kitchen was constructed and adjoined the main waiting area. A subwaiting room was created to the rear, in the clinic, and the environmental health program was consolidated on the second floor. The SFI team provided the schematic design, the phasing schedule, and design review oversight, working with Cusack and Cusack Architects serving as the architect of record (Fig. 5.35 and Fig 5.36).

It is a well-known fact that New Orleans is acutely vulnerable to massive flooding in the aftermath of a Category 3 or greater hurricane. The site of the health unit in Metairie flooded repeatedly over the years due to heavy rain-

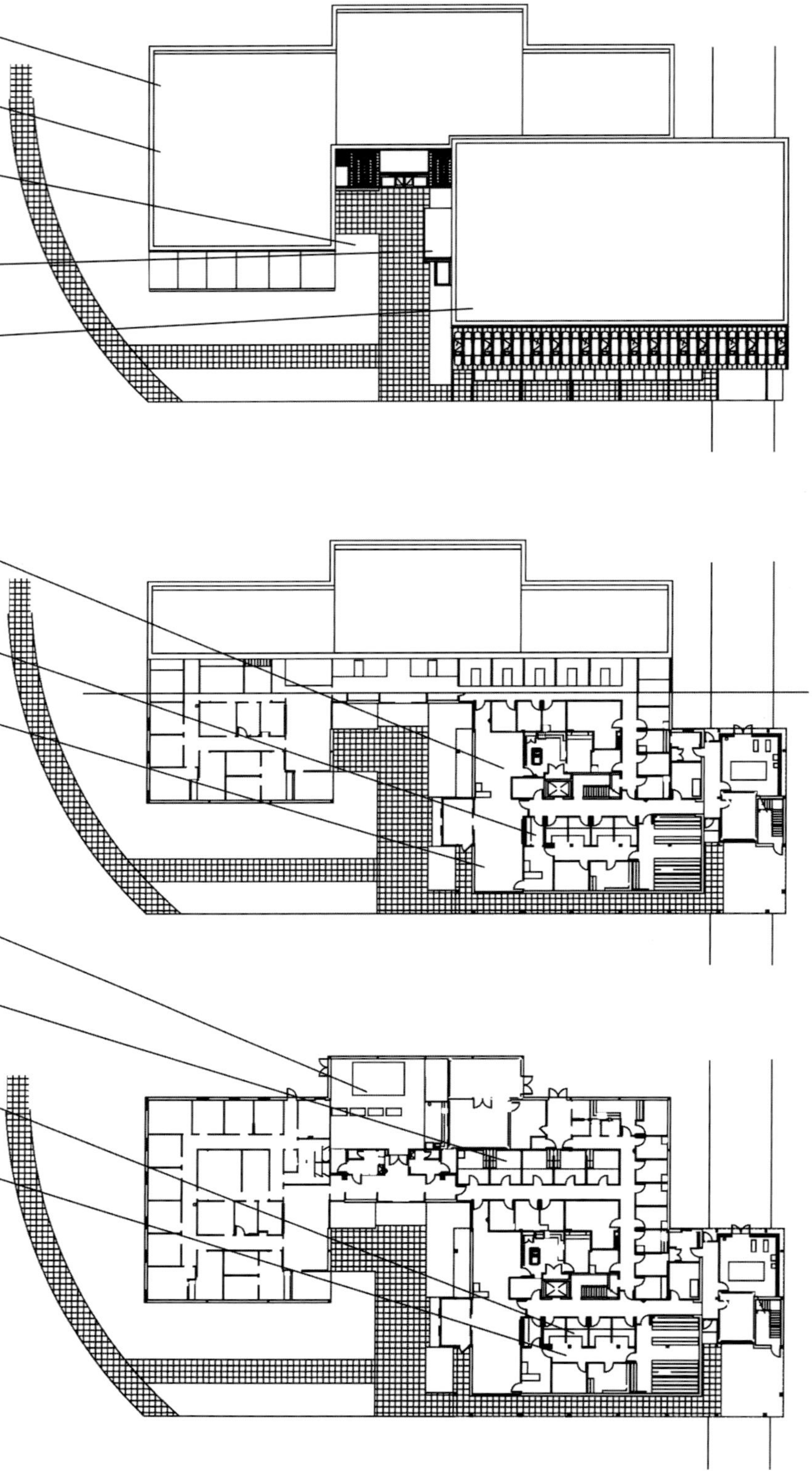

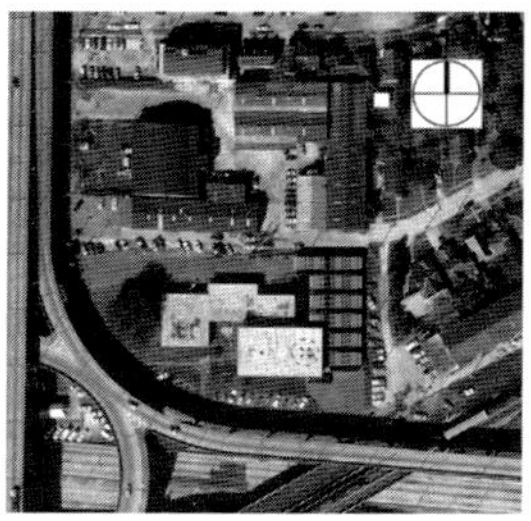

Fig. 5.35

Fig. 5.36 a-c

storms, and a few staff persons retain memories of the 1947 flood that put the area under four feet of water for many days. Due to the coastal erosion crisis in Louisiana, the New Orleans area is now more vulnerable than ever in its history to massive damage due to flooding, with the potential of hurricane-driven waves topping the eighteen-foot-high levee system which rings the city and portions of the outlying metropolitan area. The water would most likely enter over the tops of the levees which line the Lake Pontchartrain shoreline. September 2004's Hurricane Ivan, a Category 3 storm, threatened to take dead aim on the city. Miraculously, it veered to the east at the last minute. A direct hit would have put the first floor of the health unit under as much as ten feet of water for many weeks. The parish council, while prudent in allocating funds to create a special needs shelter in the scope of the renovation, soon realized it alone would be far too small to meet the needs of the community.

In response, immediately after the Ivan event, the Rapid Response Design Studio in the School of Architecture at Tulane University (under this author's direction) embarked on a project to expand the Metairie facility's capacity as a special needs shelter. Working collaboratively with the parish and with DHH-OPH officials, a 5,000-square-foot portable, temporary facility was programmed. It contained sleeping quarters for fifty medically fragile persons and their family caregivers, triage capabilities, emergency aid clinic, decontamination area, provisions for a medical staff, Red Cross personnel, emergency food services, and a communications command center. The resultant shelter is re-deployable—shipped to the site and erected on 24-36 hours notice. It would be owned, stored, and assembled by Jefferson Parish. The deployment scenario called for three such shelters, purchased by the parish, one for deployment in Metairie at the health unit, and two to be deployed elsewhere, including the West Bank, adjacent to the second levels of existing community hospitals. The inclusion of American Red Cross personnel is noteworthy, because at the present time this organization designates New Orleans as the only community in the United States it will not enter prior to a natural disaster, such as a hurricane event, to set up its emergency relief operations. In fact, to underscore the severity of this situation, the Red Cross estimates up to 100,000 deaths would occur in New Orleans in a worst-case scenario. This shelter is re-deployable prior to a natural disaster, and would be operational either before the event or able to open its doors in the immediate aftermath. Because the Metairie location would be the first American Red Cross emergency response station in the metropolitan area, the adjacent roadway overpass (Causeway Boulevard) would be designated as an emergency airlift zone (Fig. 5.35). Of the four two-student teams who produced designs for this emergency shelter, the work of the team of Julia Ford and Claudia Foronda is presented below.

This prototype can be transported to the site via existing roadways or via the rail tracks which border the site (Fig. 5.37 and Fig. 5.38). Ten (or more, depending on site configuration and size) premanufactured modules are delivered to the site. A steel frame undercarriage is erected, and this system is also transported to the site in containers. Once the undercarriage is in place, at a height of fourteen feet above the parking lot, the modules are placed atop the grid by two highboy lift vehicles working in tandem (Fig. 5.39 and Fig. 5.40). When fully deployed onsite, the shelter would connect to the existing second floor of the health unit, at this point functioning as the "mothership." The permanent component of the shelter houses a dining room and food services unit, flexible space to be used by staff or as overflow for shelter occupants, the central IT-computer server room, and general support (Fig. 5.41).

This re-deployable facility is accessed via roads, in the event surface roads are passable, via helicopter (Fig. 5.35), or via boat. The modules for habitation are constructed of stainless steel panels and steel frames. Conceptually, there are three core objectives: occupant safety and security, and a system that has the ability to extend and be re-deployable on other sites. Translucent panels with embedded objects and the curvature of the modules express nautical references. The arrangement of circulation spaces extends that of the mothership, thereby allowing for natural daylight to enter the lens aperatures of each module. These interlocking structural components slide into one another and interlock. Cross beams and columns secure firmly this system in all other directions, thus providing rigid stabilization in the face of a Category 5 hurricane's 155-mile-an-hour winds (Fig. 5.42).

New material innovations were researched for incorporation to enhance the experience of inhabitation and to enhance the structural qualities of the building system. Patterned resin panels afford many options of impregnated patterns and colors. The Struttura©™ panel line produced by 3-Form Corpo-

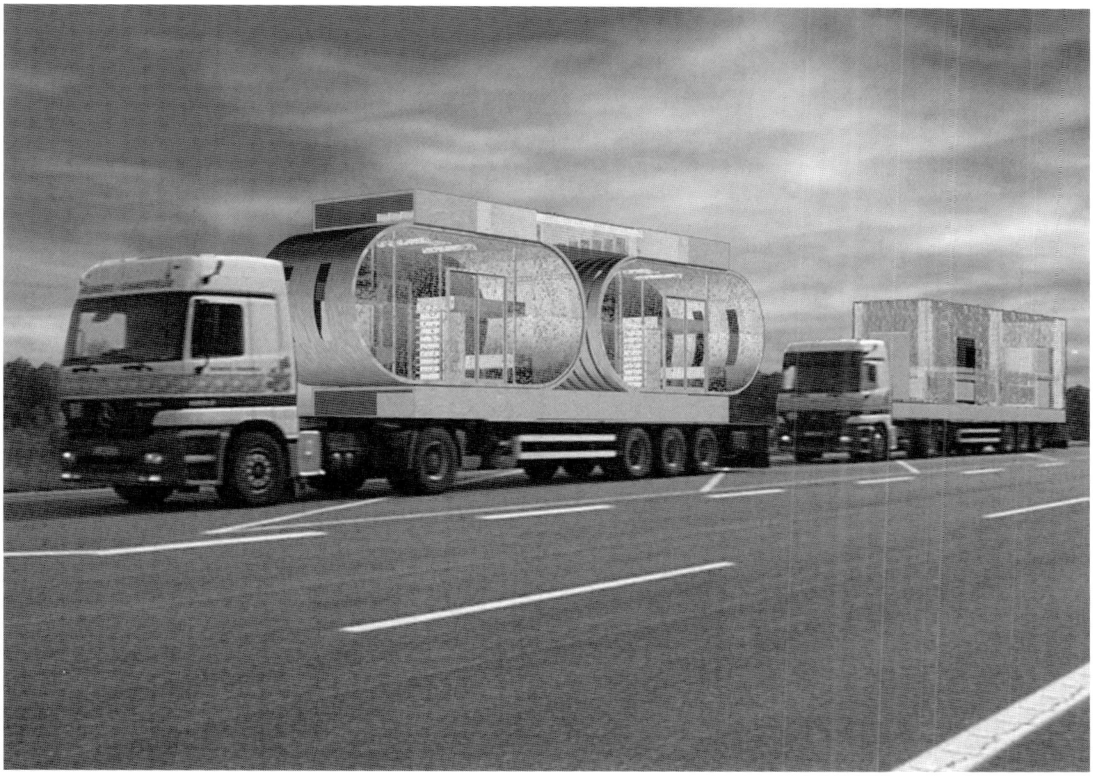

Fig. 5.37

Fig. 5.38

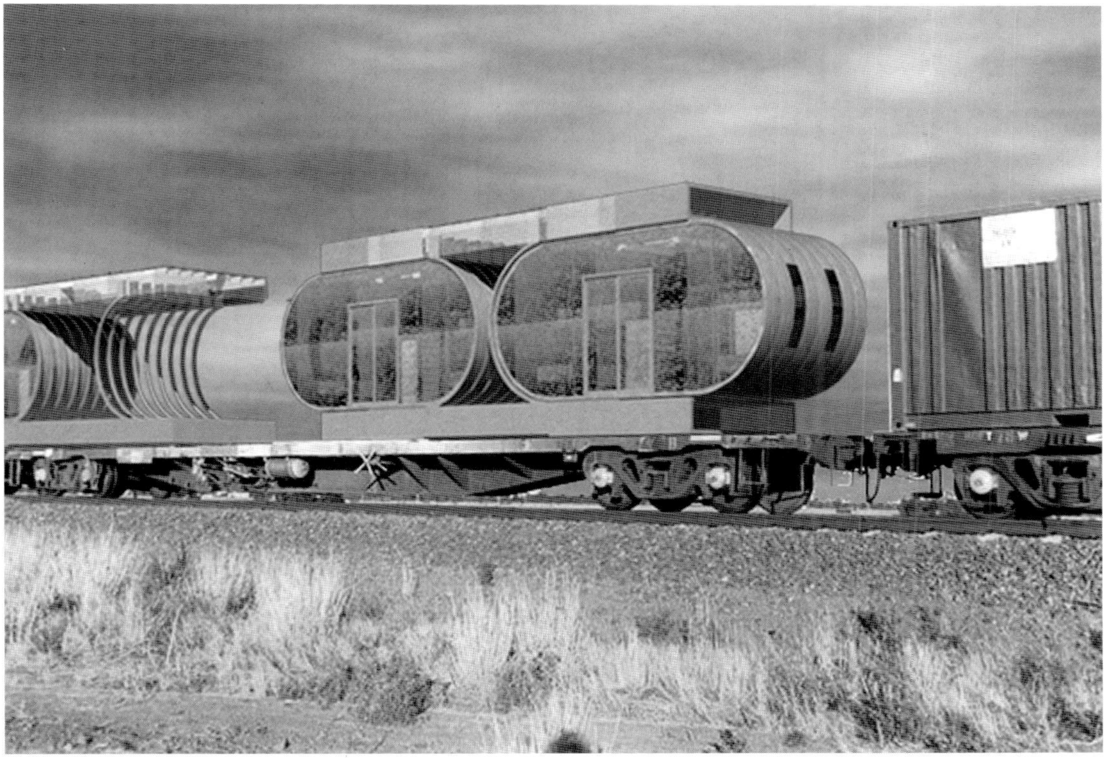

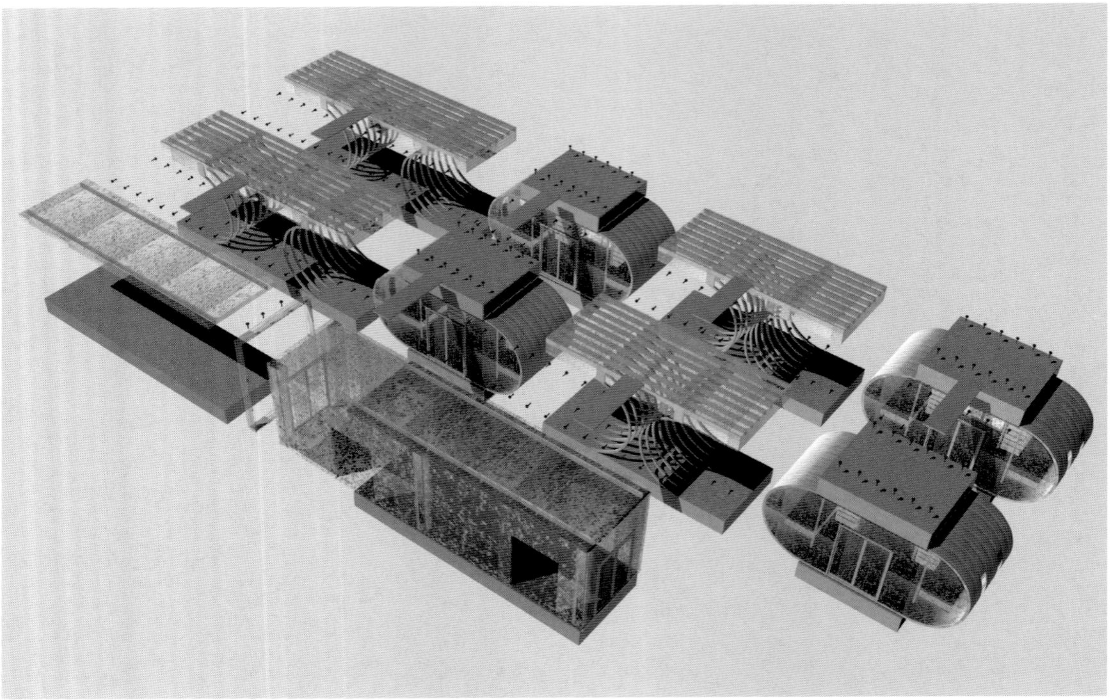

Fig. 5.39

Fig. 5.40

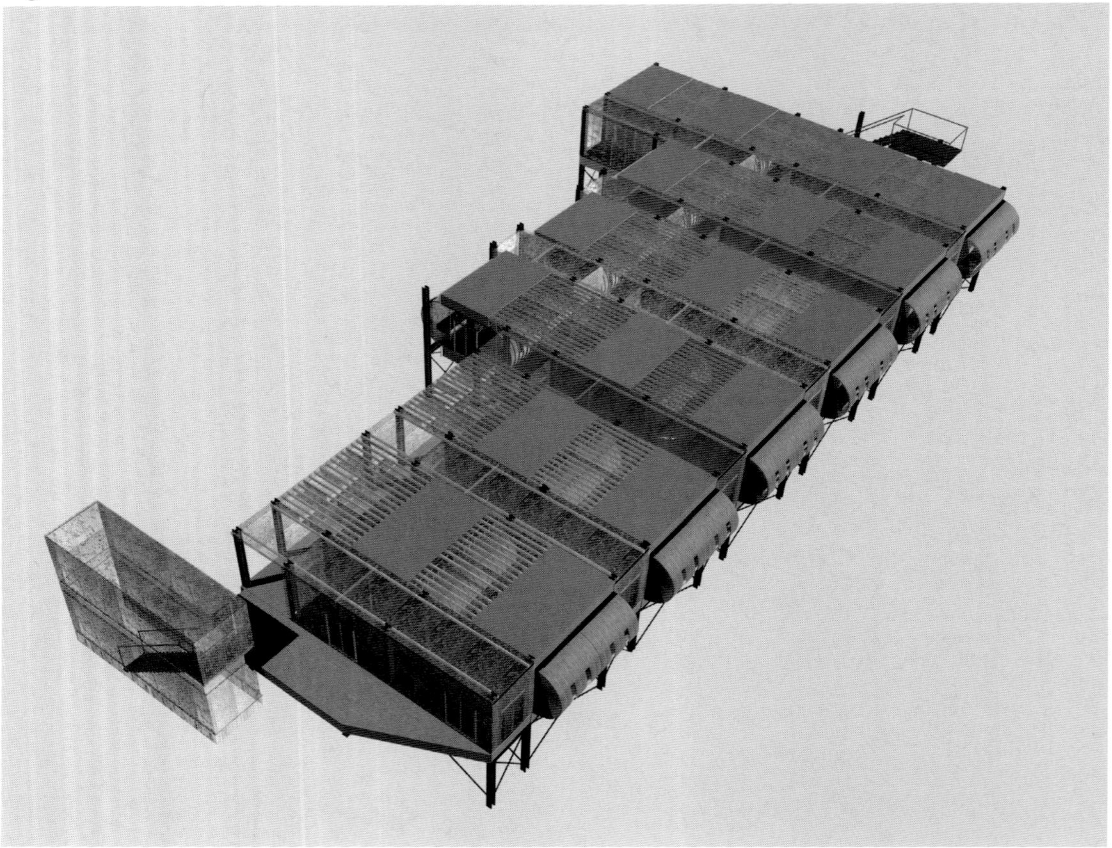

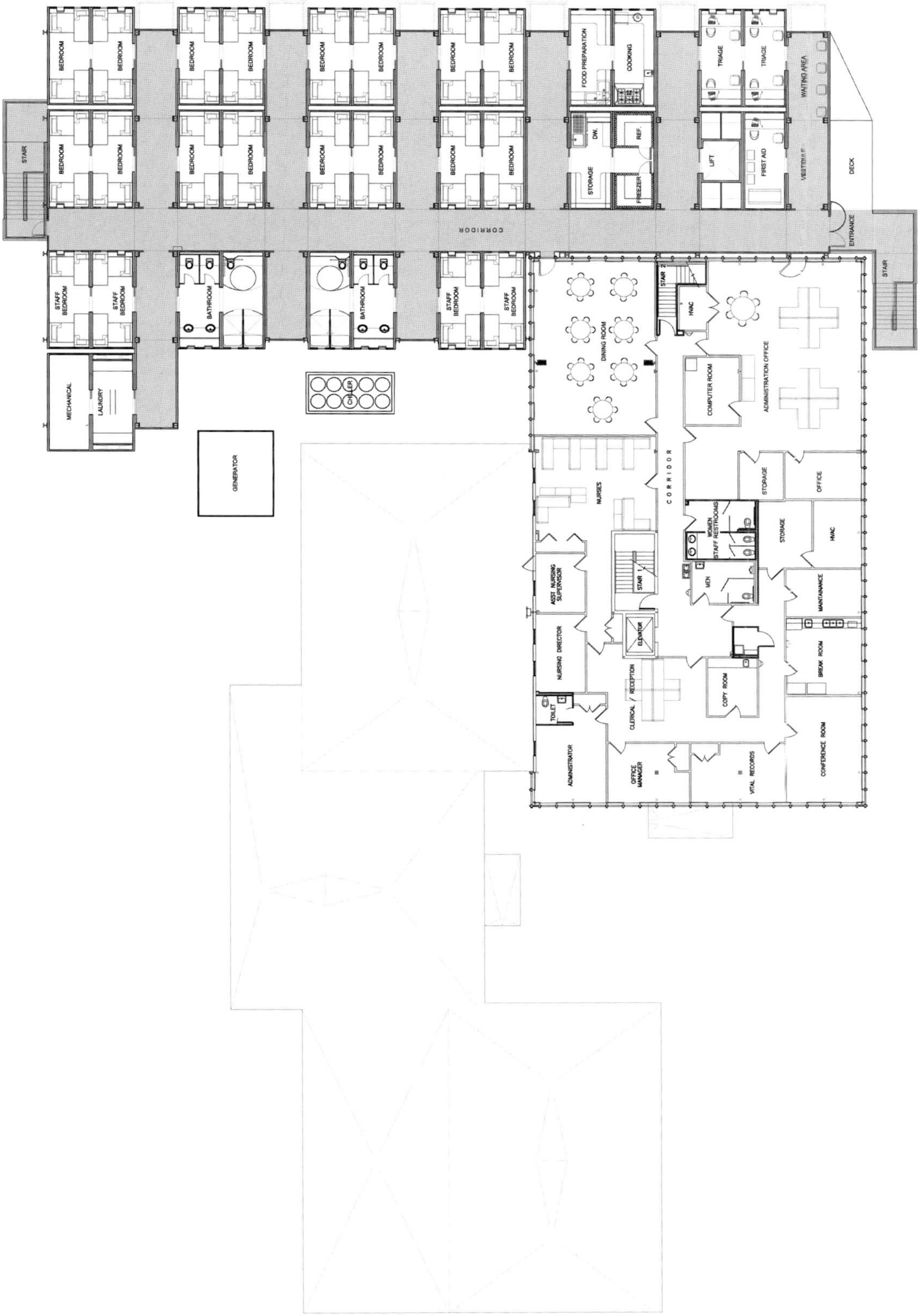

Fig. 5.41

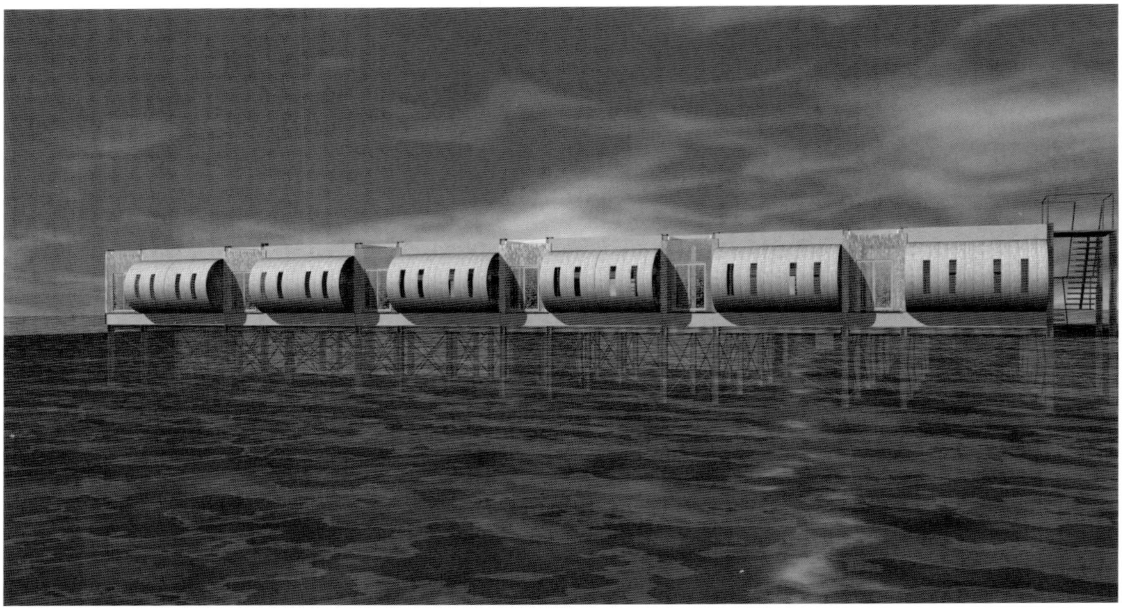

Fig. 5.42

ration is used, as is Nanogel©™, an insulation system produced by Kalwall. These components are lightweight, effective as insulating elements, and light transmissive. The typical module is composed of of a network of panels sheathing the primary and secondary structural systems. Panels can be sandwiched and injected with Nanogel to further increase stability. These panels are translucent, transmitting light while affording privacy. Bubbloy©™, a recent invention, is produced by Caltech. Made of palladium, copper, nickel, and phosphorous, it posses the "stiffness of metal but the springiness of a trampoline." It is an exceptionally lightweight material, thereby affording ease in transportation and erection atop the elevated structural platform. Each module, and the entire structural platform, is tethered to the site by stainless steel cables connected to pile driven anchors in the surface of the parking lot (Fig. 5.43 and Fig. 5.44).

The parish, in its decision to designate the second floor of the health unit in Metairie as a special needs shelter, funded the installation of a gas-powered emergency generator, to enable the clinic to remain open in the event of a natural disaster. This unit is situated on a nine-foot high steel platform, located on the north side of the two-level clinic component of the building. The special-needs shelter, as defined, is for use by non-hospitalized or persons recently

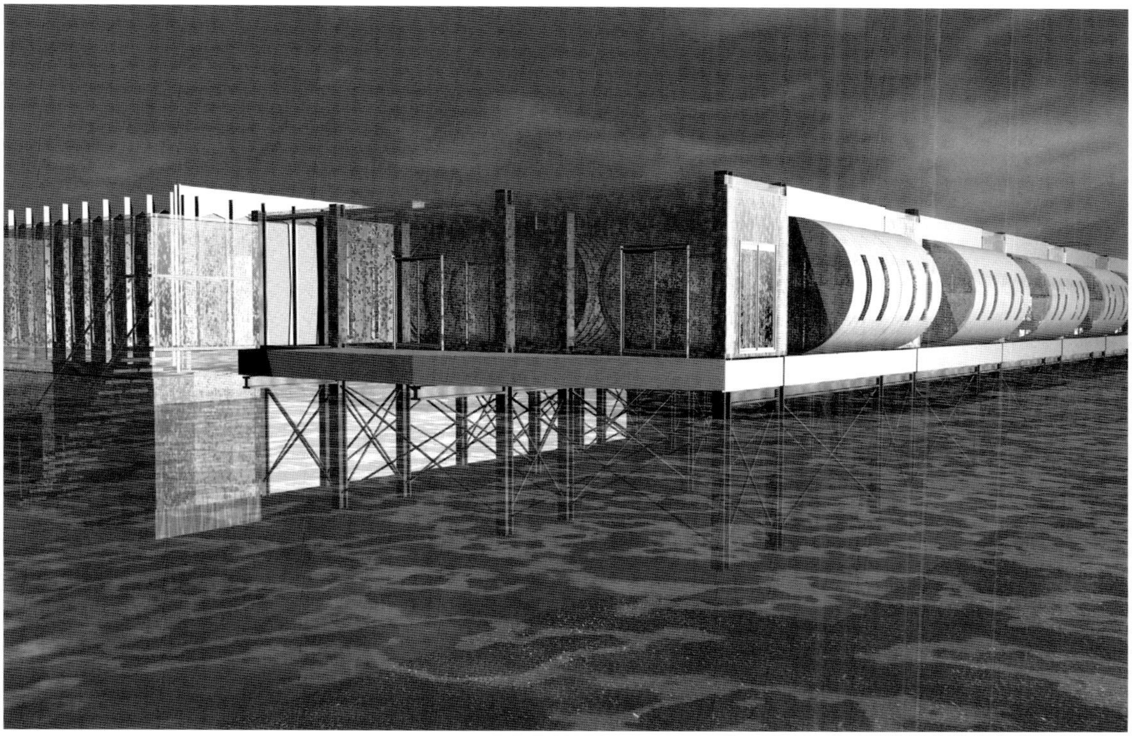

Fig. 5.43

Fig. 5.44

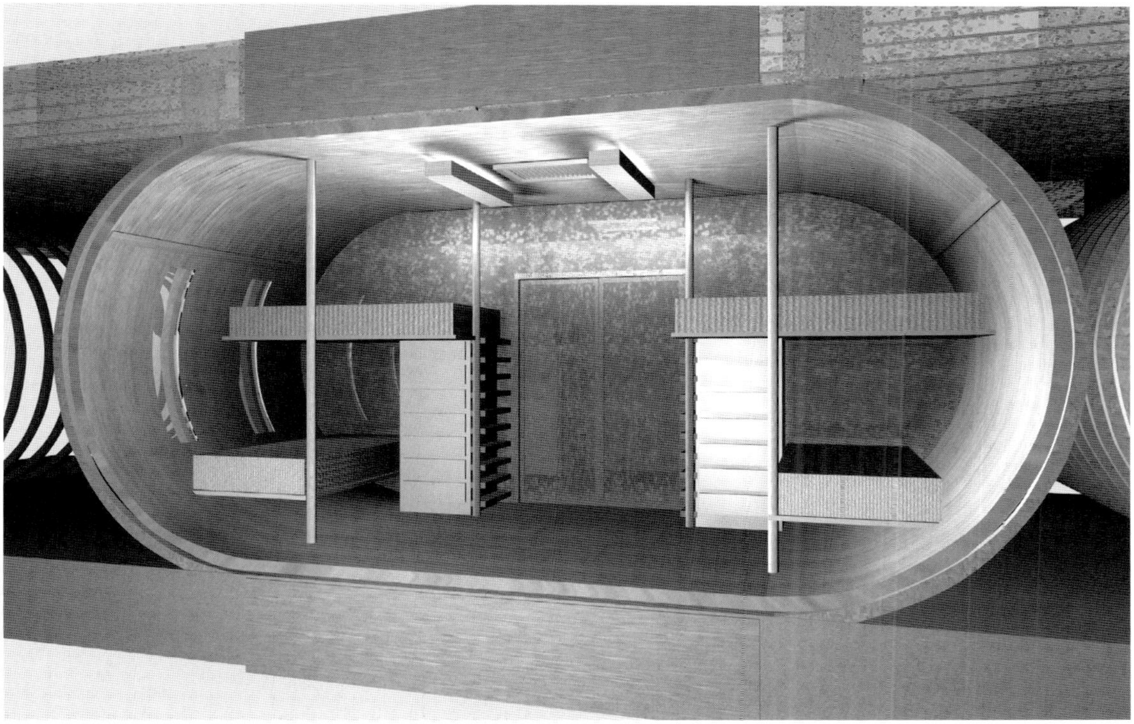

discharged from a hospital and in need of 24/7 home-based medical care by a family member. Elderly residents are generally the largest group to avail themselves of shelters of this type, followed by developmentally disabled persons of all ages. Metairie was therefore noteworthy for a number of reasons. The post-occupancy evaluation completed one year following the mothership building's renovation yielded very few problems or complaints on the part of staff or patients. This case study is an example of an historic modernist clinic having been restored to its former luster, and an example of the possibilities of opting to remain in the same location, a location that had evolved into a valuable asset over the years. Third, its updating reaffirmed the parish's and the agency's commitment to the health and well being of the community.

Avoyelles Parish, Bunkie

Since 1946, the health unit in Bunkie was housed in a small frame structure in a modest residential neighborhood. This one level, green frame building, situated alongside a two-lane parish road on the edge of town, was non-descript in nearly every respect. It had become rundown through years of use and neglect on the part of the local police jury. This small building was remarkable in many ways, for it symbolized both the highest aspirations of rural healthcare and its starkest realities. It was home-like, intimate, and accessible to its constituency although thoroughly dysfunctional in terms of its lack of architectural accommodation. The parish was prompted to replace the old facility as a preemptive measure when it learned of its eminent closure by the state agency. When the mayor complained to local politicians the momentum gradually built among residents to construct a replacement facility and to keep the program operational. The Bunkie facility had been used as a satellite clinic, open only two days per week, as the staff traveled from Alexandria or the main parish health unit in Marksville on clinic days. A handful of these satellite clinics remained statewide.

Various sites were assessed for feasibility. Things were going fairly smoothly until a police jury meeting one evening when a schematic design proposal by the SFI team was scheduled for presentation in Marksville, the parish seat. Unfortunately, on that evening, the vote to proceed was not to be. A simmering behind-the-scenes feud between a police juror and the parish sanitarian flared into an open confrontation, a shouting match in the council chamber, only moments prior to the formal presentation of the proposed design. The juror in question angrily stated, in front of the packed room, "Y'all will never get a vote worth a dime from me as long as that man is involved with this [proposal] in any way!" He stood up, pointing his finger directly at the red-faced sanitarian sitting in the rear of the room. Silence fell. At that moment, it would appear to be impossible to rebound from this spectacle. After the meeting adjourned, it was learned the sanitarian had denied a sewerage permit only a few days earlier toa relative of the angry elected official.

The Marksville area is steeped in the rich legacy of Native American civilization. The descendents of the most prominent branch of these indigenous settlers had become wealthy since opening a casino a few years earlier on tax-exempt reservation land in Marksville. Tribal leaders had stated the tribe would help pay for a new health unit if built near the reservation. The site chosen met that criterion. Additionally, it had been decided that as a tribute to the tribe's philanthropic patronage it would be appropriate to reference its rich architectural heritage in the architecture of the new health unit.

In describing on the area's historic past, Linda Treash writes:

> Back when Highway 1 was the main road in Louisiana, angling across the state from Grand Isle to Shreveport and beyond, Marksville, the largest town between Baton Rouge and Alexandria, saw plenty of visitors. With the advent of the Interstate system, Highway 1 lost its traffic, and so did Marksville That is, until the Grand Casino Avoyelles opened in the mid-'90s, an Indian reservation casino smack on Highway 1. The Tunica-Biloxi Indians brought visitors back to Marksville. But the Tunica-Biloxi are not the first Native Americans to stir up Marksville. In 1926, a Smithsonian archeological survey came to town and set up shop on a bluff overlooking Old River, a former bend in the Mississippi that's now a wide but shallow marsh just outside the town. What happened on that bluff in the 1920s and '30s, as well as in the years between 100 and 400 A.D., provides another reason to make the trek up Route 1. . . . The big attraction on the bluff was a conical mound, 20 feet high and 100 feet around. In the 1926 dig, Smithsonian scientist Gerald Gowke and his crew dug a 25-foot wide, 60-foot long trench into the mound, unearthing a remarkably complex Native American burial site that was further excavated by a second crew in 1933. . . . (and) a 1938-1939 Works Progress Administration excavation. Five mounds and a 3,300-foot earthwork border were mapped out on the bluff. Sur-

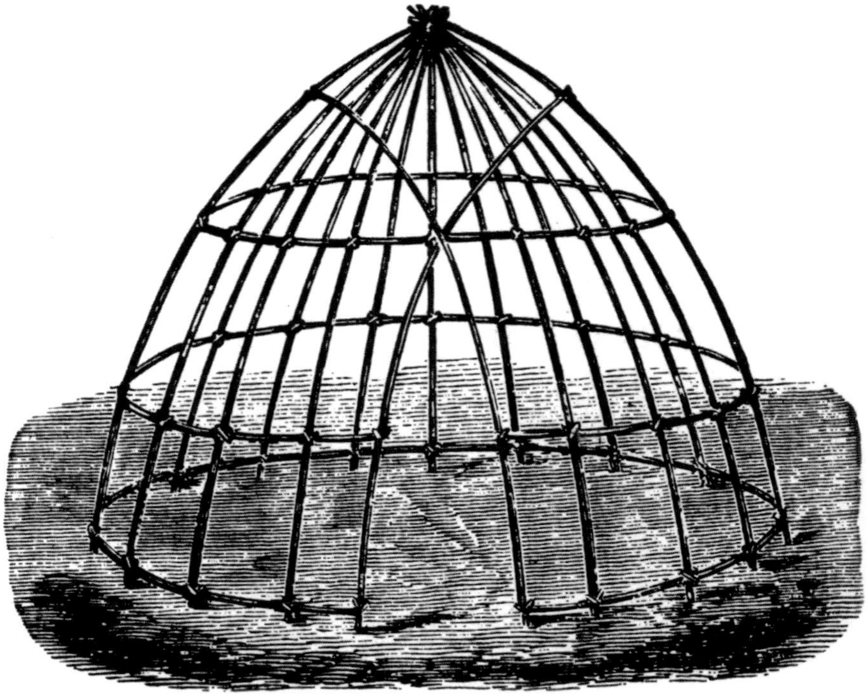

Fig. 5.45

prisingly, the mounds were not linked to the nearby Tunica-Biloxi tribe or any tribe then known to have inhabited Louisiana, but to the ancient Hopewell culture of Ohio and Illinois . . . without the serpentine motif (found on the pottery unearthed), archaeologists would have had trouble identifying the Marksville culture as part of the Hopewell. The original pots, which are among the oldest pieces of pottery found in Louisiana, are on display in the Smithsonian in Washington, D.C. . . . Thanks to the abundance of burial mounds in Louisiana, we know quite a bit about Native American religion, which centered on ancestor worship until 700 A.D. . . . relatives tended to be buried together in special houses, which were ultimately covered with earth, creating conical mounds. Later cultures added the worshipping of the sun and other deities to the continual practice of ancestor worship.[5]

All five of the original Hopewell tribal mounds remain, plus a later discovered mound, identified as "Mound X." These are located within a forty-two-acre state park and visitor's center. One ceremonial mound was used for civic functions; an aerial view, to the southeast, of the Marksville site in the mid-1930s depicted the elaborate layout of a community inhabited by perhaps two thousand tribal members at its peak. A vast earthwork spanning 3,330 feet surrounds the mounds. These were used as protective walls and as spatial markers for formal events. Members of the Marksville Hopewell community resided in a series of circular lodges outside the earthworks, along a bluff of the Mississippi River. The bluff is an old natural levee of the Mississippi, and this bluff is the highest point south of Natchez, Mississippi, some fifty miles to the north. The inhabitants of this ancient community were sophisticated, keepers of a fairly complex civilization. By the eighteenth century, tribal villages in the immediate area ranged in size from a few dwellings to dozens or more. Each major settlement centered on a temple and the house of the chief. These structures were situated across from each other, separated by a broad, open plaza. The plaza was used for ceremonial and athletic events. The dwellings of the local families were situated in close proximity to the fields, linked to the center of the village by an elaborate network of footpaths.[6]

Fig. 5.46

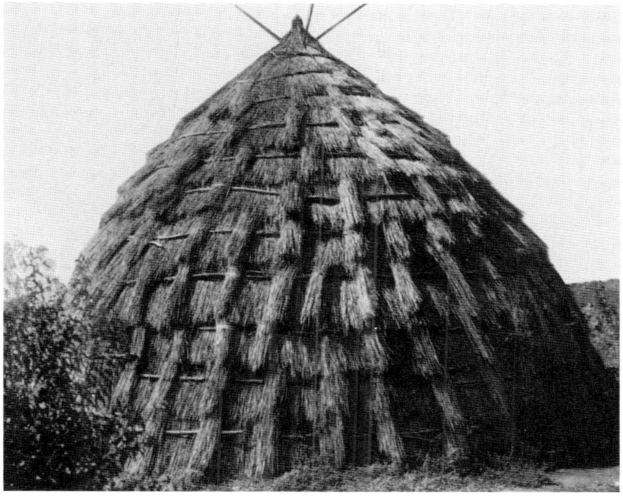

The wigwam remained a popular building type over the centuries. The bent sapling frame of a Winnebago house is covered with reed mats. Wigwams ranged in size from seven to twenty feet in diameter and were covered traditionally with reed mats and bark. Their separate frames and coverings rendered these structures transport-

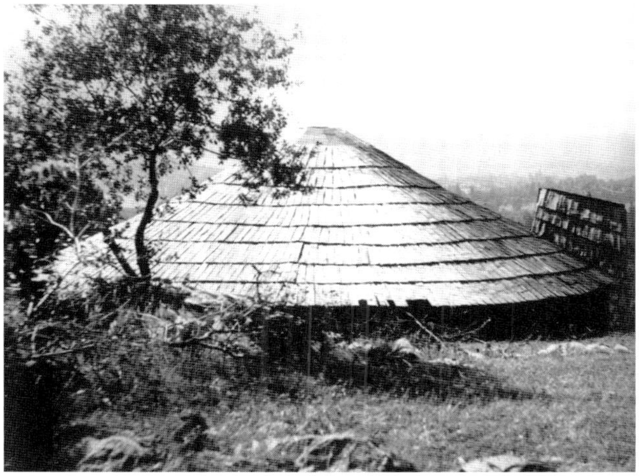

Fig. 5.47

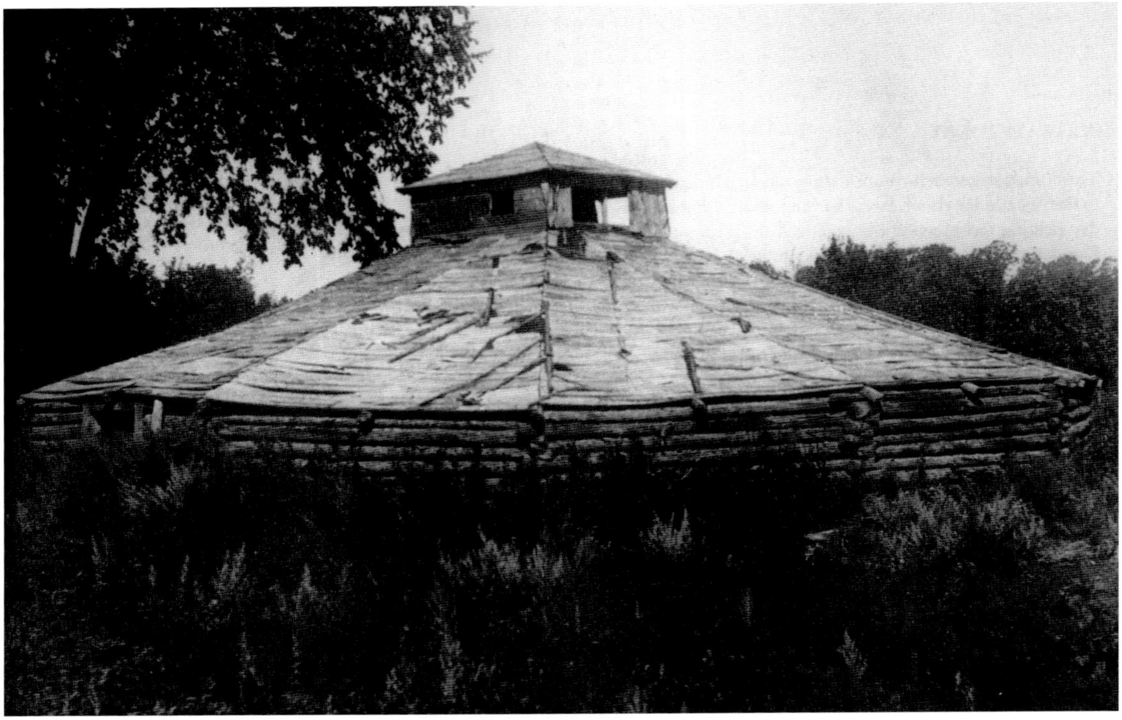

Fig. 5.48

able (Fig. 5.45). In 1691, an Algonquian told a Frenchman who was trying to persuade him to adopt a European house, "we can always say, more truly than thou, that we are at home everywhere because we set up our wigwams with ease wherever we go and without asking permission of anybody."[7] Another variation on the dwelling became referred to as the grass house. This example, photographed in 1927, was also framed of poles bent over an interior ring of posts and beams and bound together at the top. Horizontal sampling stringers strengthened the frame, which could be as wide as sixty feet across at the base. The thatch was anchored in tightly drawn together bunches, and exterior rows of stringers held it fast (Fig. 5.46).[8]

A building type known as the roundhouse appeared in the late nineteenth century. Ceremonial earth lodges, many of which were subterranean, were replaced by these round wooden structures. Roundhouses were built entirely at grade. They had pole frames and were roofed and sheathed with split planks or shakes. By this time, metal nails and split shingles had replaced the earthen

Site Context-Rural- Native American Community:
3.1, 3.2

Industrial Vernacular Expression:
6.1, 6.3, 6.8, 6.11, 6.26

Daylighting:
6.9, 6.10, 7.5

Identifiable Entrance:
1.1, 1.4, 3.3, 3.5, 3.6, 4.12, 6.1, 6.11, 6.26

Transparency/Views of Landscape:
6.12

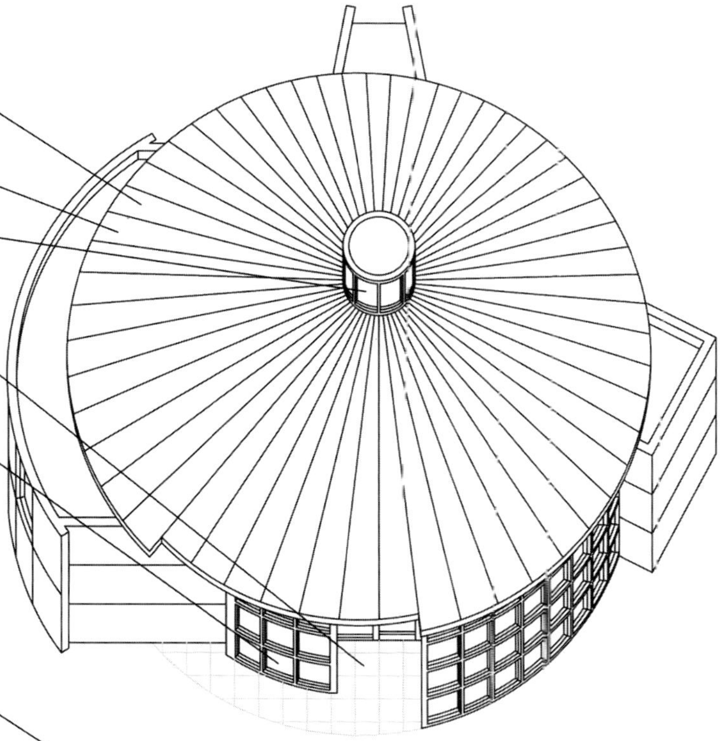

Patient Intake/Consult:
4.4-4.7, 4.9, 4.13, 6.11, 6.12

Reception/Sign-in:
4.3, 4.8, 4.11

Main Waiting (Flexive):
1.5, 4.1, 4.3, 4.16, 4.18, 4.20, 6.2

Environmental Health/ Classroom/Nutritional Education (Flexive):
2.3, 2.8, 2.9, 4.15, 4.17, 4.46-4.48, 6.16, 6.17

Entry Sequence:
6.4-6.6, 6.21-6.23, 6.25

Exam Rooms/Nursing Administration (Flexive):
2.3, 2.8, 2.9, 4.15, 4.17, 6.16, 6.17

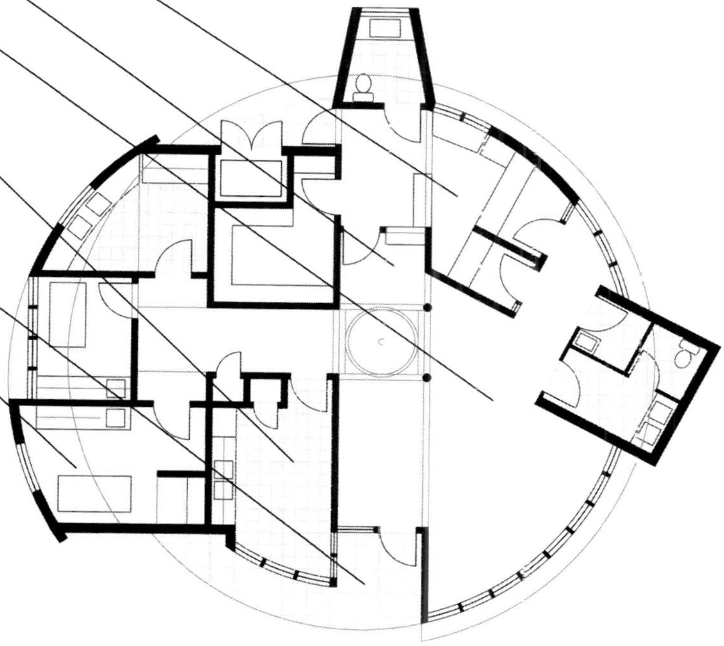

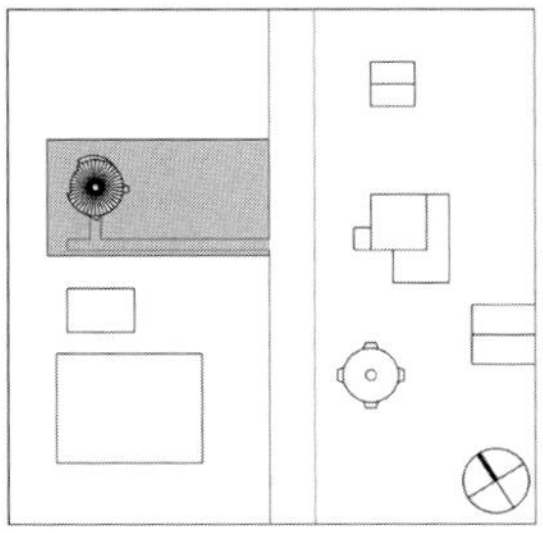

Fig. 5.49

Fig. 5.50 a-c

roofs of most traditional assembly halls. This Miwok roundhouse was photographed at the Bald Rock Rancheria, near Mooretown in Butte County, California, in 1924 (Fig. 5.47). A widely adopted type of civic structure was the community lodge, such as the Chippewa Drum Dance Lodge at Mille Lac, Wisconsin, circa 1910 (Fig. 5.48). These structures, which could hold gatherings of entire communities in private, symbolize the struggle of Native Americans during the early reservation period to preserve their religions and cultural traditions. Similar to the evolution of healthcare settings among Native American tribes, the Drum Dance was for centuries performed in an open circular area ringed with loges, signifying the universe. In the center, a large decorated feather drum was hung from four feathered staffs representing the cardinal directions. Over the decades, these open spaces were replaced with roofed halls, whose form most likely derived from the Plains Indian log-or-lumber dance enclosures that had become popular during the reservation period for housing the Grass Dance. These buildings were generally four- or six-sided, with turrets in the middle of their pitched, wood-shingled roofs. Wooden benches lined the walls, and the preferred floor was earth, beaten hard from dancing feet.[9]

In response to these indigenous vernacular civic building types, a 2,100-square-foot circular partí was developed for the Avoyelles Parish facility with a turret at the center of the roof peak (Fig. 5.49 and Fig. 5.50). This configuration was based upon the precedent of the traditional tribal meeting hall. This, and particularly the precursor of the local ancient tribal mounds built by the Hopewell at Marksville and elsewhere in the region, was acknowledged. Three elements push out at oblique angles from a radial core. A circulation axis is established through placement of the main entrance at one endpoint and the staff work zone at the opposing endpoint. Two exam rooms spin off radially. The core is resolved at the roof level with a skylight at the center, clearly visible from a distance at night. The building's perforated metal roof and its corrugated metal exterior walls are of earth tones. A sheltered outdoor area is adjacent to the main entrance. Views of the surrounding prairie landscape are afforded vis-a-vis floor to ceiling windows in the waiting and classroom areas. Storage, and clinic support spaces are provided. Two restrooms, one for patients and one for staff, spin off from the center core, freeing space in the core itself. Rooms are flexive: the laboratory doubles as the WIC demonstration kitchen, an exam room doubles as the nurse's office, and the waiting room transforms into the health education classroom.

Much more research is needed to document, preserve, and communicate the rich architectural legacy of Native American tribal culture and its role in the prehistory of Louisiana. This architectural proposal would, at the very least, have functioned as a strong civic symbol of the tribe's role with regards to the region's past, present and future—particularly in the wake of the tribe's newfound prosperity acquired through its 1990s entrepreneurial foray into the gaming industry, although this unbuilt proposal died, unfortunately, that night, in the parish courthouse in Marksville, only a few short miles from the remains of the ancient tribal villages. Eventually, the police jury abandoned altogether the prospect of a freestanding replacement. Two years later, a small storefront building on Main Street was purchased and renovated on a shoestring budget. Regardless, the unbuilt proposal's historical references, unbeknownst to the politicians that evening and overshadowed by other preoccupations were salient.

Lafayette Parish, Lafayette

A new parish health unit for Lafayette Parish had been in the works for nearly a decade by the time ground was broken in 1999. The health unit was housed in a building built in 1959 in an industrial neighborhood a mile and a half south of downtown. This facility, known as the "War Memorial" building, was simply unable to keep up with the pace of advancements in community public healthcare. This had become an acute issue during the previous ten years, as Office of Public Health programs evolved and expanded. The War Memorial site housed the Region IV Laboratory, also operated by the Office of Public Health. A Children's Special Health Services (CSHS) clinic was housed in a separate wing connected to the health unit by a covered walkway. By the 1990s the building had become dysfunctional, plagued with overcrowding, poor internal flow, and electrical and mechanical problems. Patients were seated in corridors, file cabinets were in open areas accessible to anyone, and parking was a chronic problem. During the 1990s—a decade of considerable stress for the staff—deferred maintenance was the norm.

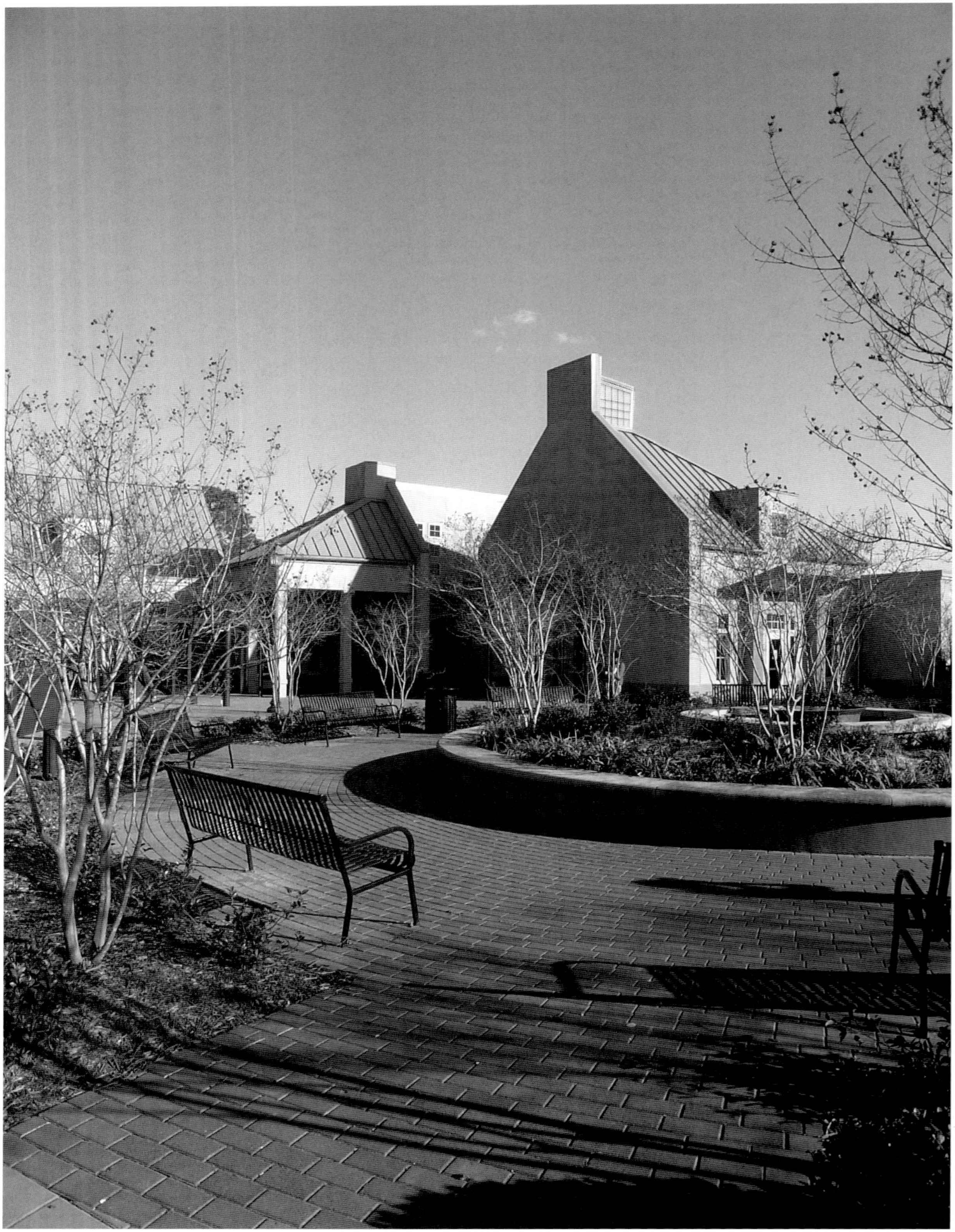

Fig. 5.51

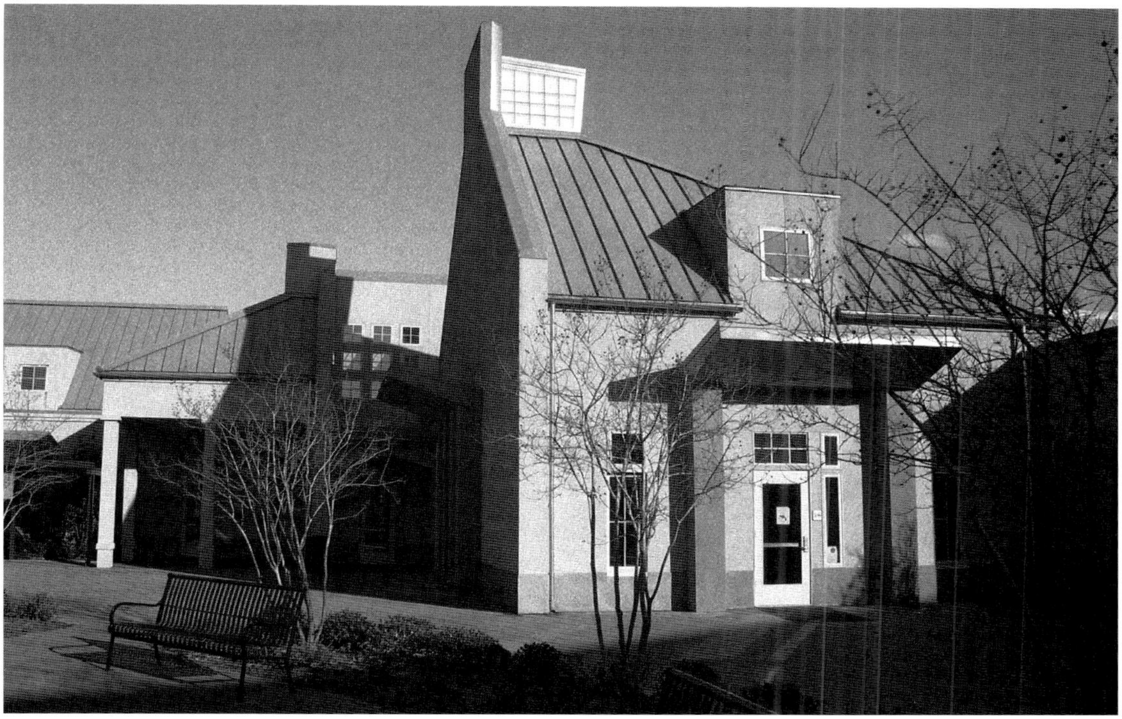

Fig. 5.52

A functional brief was developed and the SFI team evaluated multiple sites for a new facility. A debate over various lease-build options between the state and parish simmered, with little progress. Meanwhile, as for the nine CSHS regional clinics in operation statewide, all but one (New Orleans) was consolidated into the nearest (usually urban) health unit. In Lafayette, this would prove problematic, because the contract documents for the new facility were well underway at the time the consolidation policy was implemented. The architects, Architects Southwest of Lafayette, were instructed to accommodate the CSHS clinic and staff, and did so admirably. The new facility, which opened in 2002, was built on the northern edge of Lafayette near the older, established neighborhoods where many patients reside. A twelve-acre "civic services" campus was created. This campus consists of the health unit, a town hall facility, driver's license bureau office, and a police substation. It is located on a public transit line, and the various buildings, with the health unit at the center, create a pedestrian-scaled village streetscape ambiance, not unlike that of a college campus (Fig. 5.51).

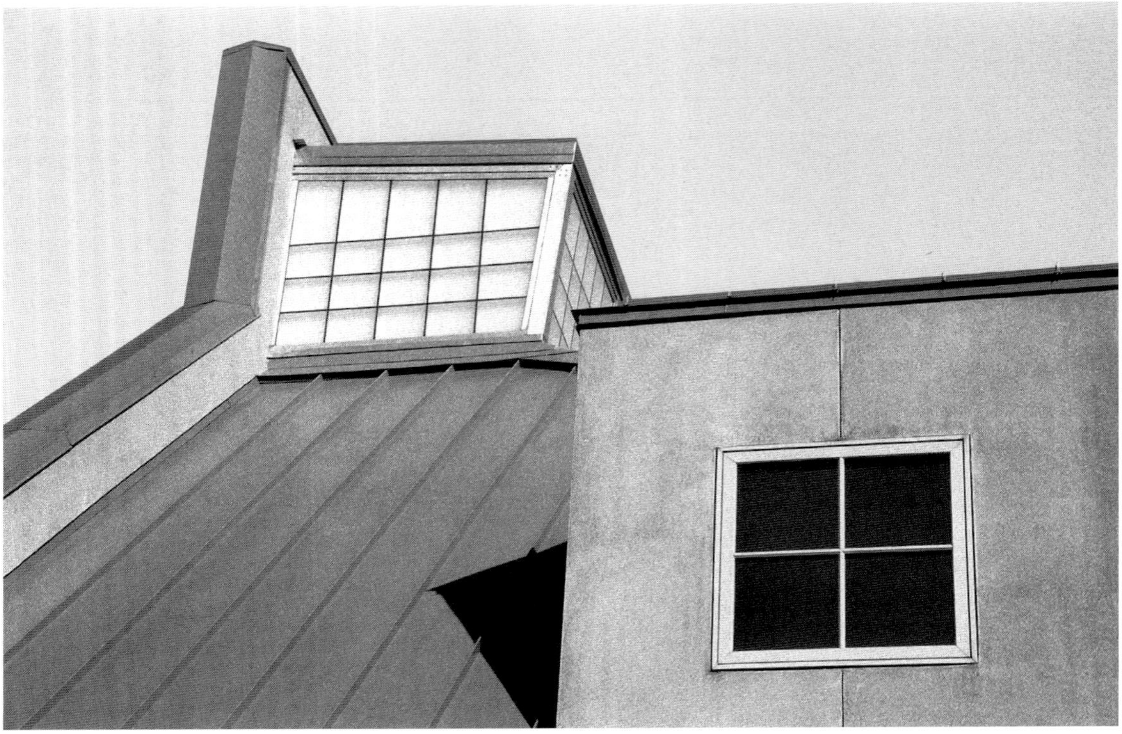

Fig. 5.53

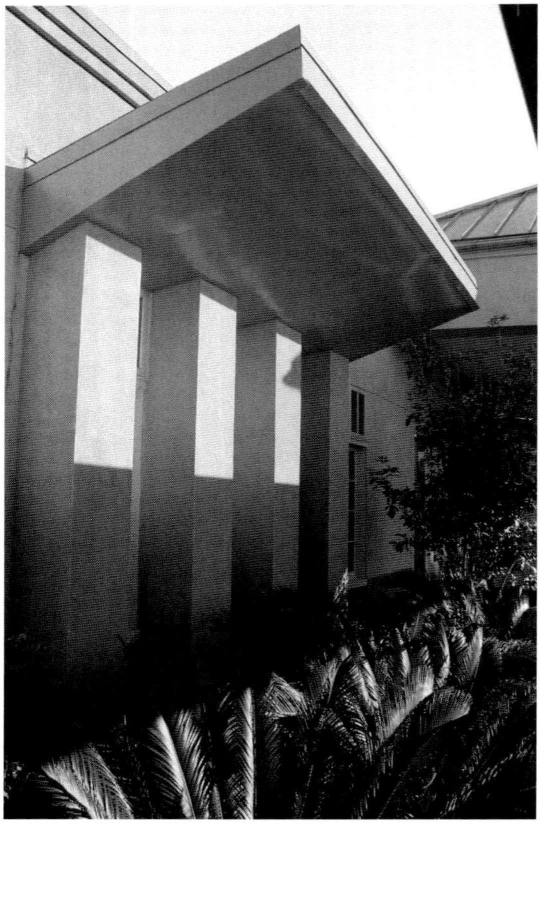

Fig. 5.54

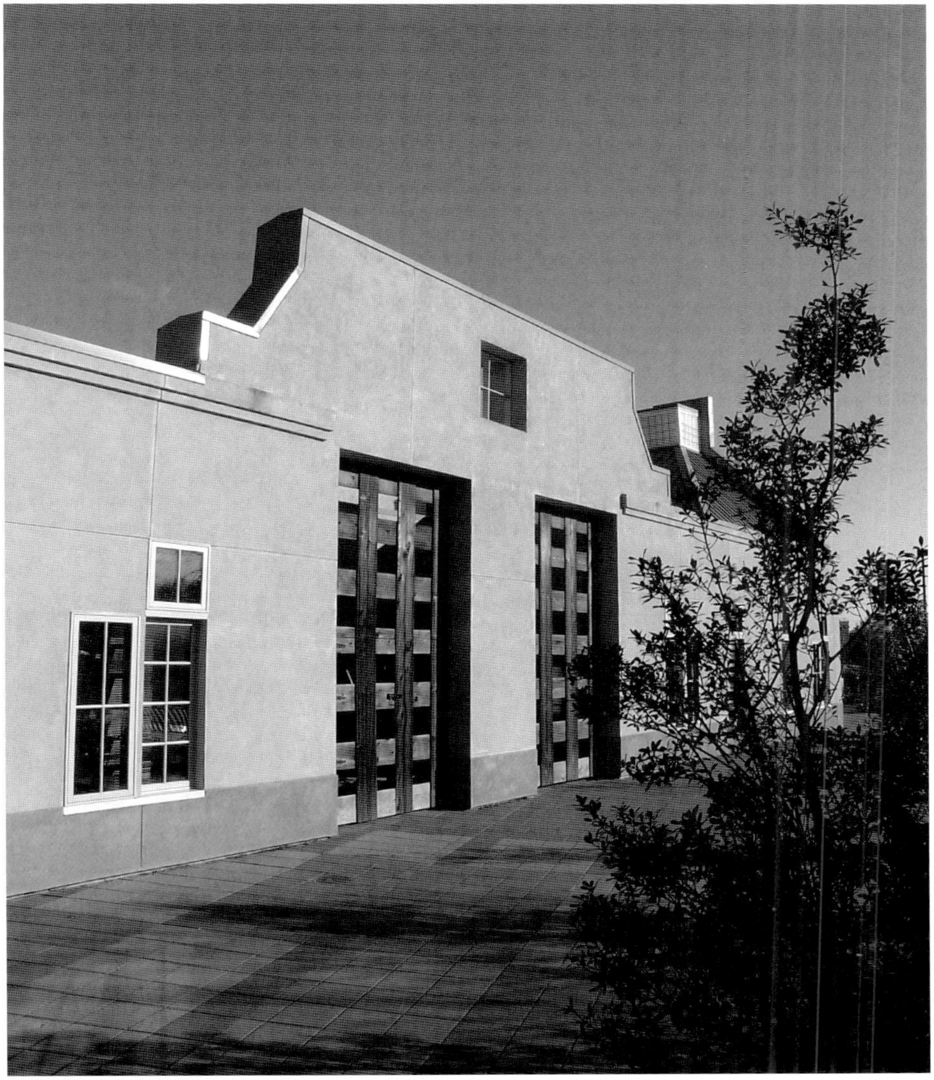

Fig. 5.55

A 24,500-square-foot building was configured on one level. Total project cost was $2.7 million. A linear footprint was necessitated due to the narrowness of the site and the limited frontage along the sole site edge, which fronted a roadway. On one side is the community town hall and parish services build-

Site Context- Community Services Campus:
3.1, 3.2, 6.1

Protected Entry Sequence:
1.1, 1.4, 3.3, 3.5, 4.12, 6.1

Indigenous Vernacular/ Expression:
2.7, 3.1, 3.10

Views to Nature/Seating/ Gardens:
3.5-3.8

Autonomous Environmental Health Section:
2.3, 2.9, 4.46-4.48

Patient Intake/Consult/Clerical Admin:
4.4-4.7, 4.9, 4.13, 6.11, 6.12

Reception/Sign-in/ Analogical Reference:
4.3, 4.8, 4.11

Serialized Arrival:
3.3, 3.5, 3.6

Main Waiting:
1.5, 4.1, 4.3, 4.10, 4.14, 4.18, 4.20, 6.2, 6.32-6.34

Examination Rooms/Clinic:
2.3, 2.8, 2.9, 4.15, 4.17, 4.27, 4.35

Subwaiting Area:
4.2, 4.16

Nutritional Education:
2.9, 4.31-4.34

Wayfinding/Pedestrian Street:
3.6, 6.3-6.5, 6.21-6.23, 6.25

Nursing Administration:
4.36, 4.38, 4.39, 4.41

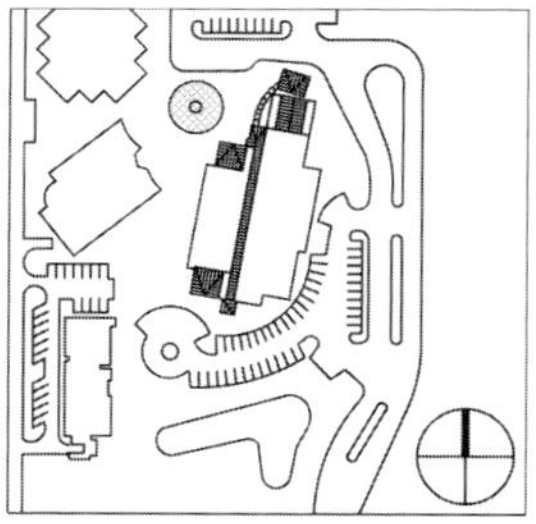

Fig. 5.56

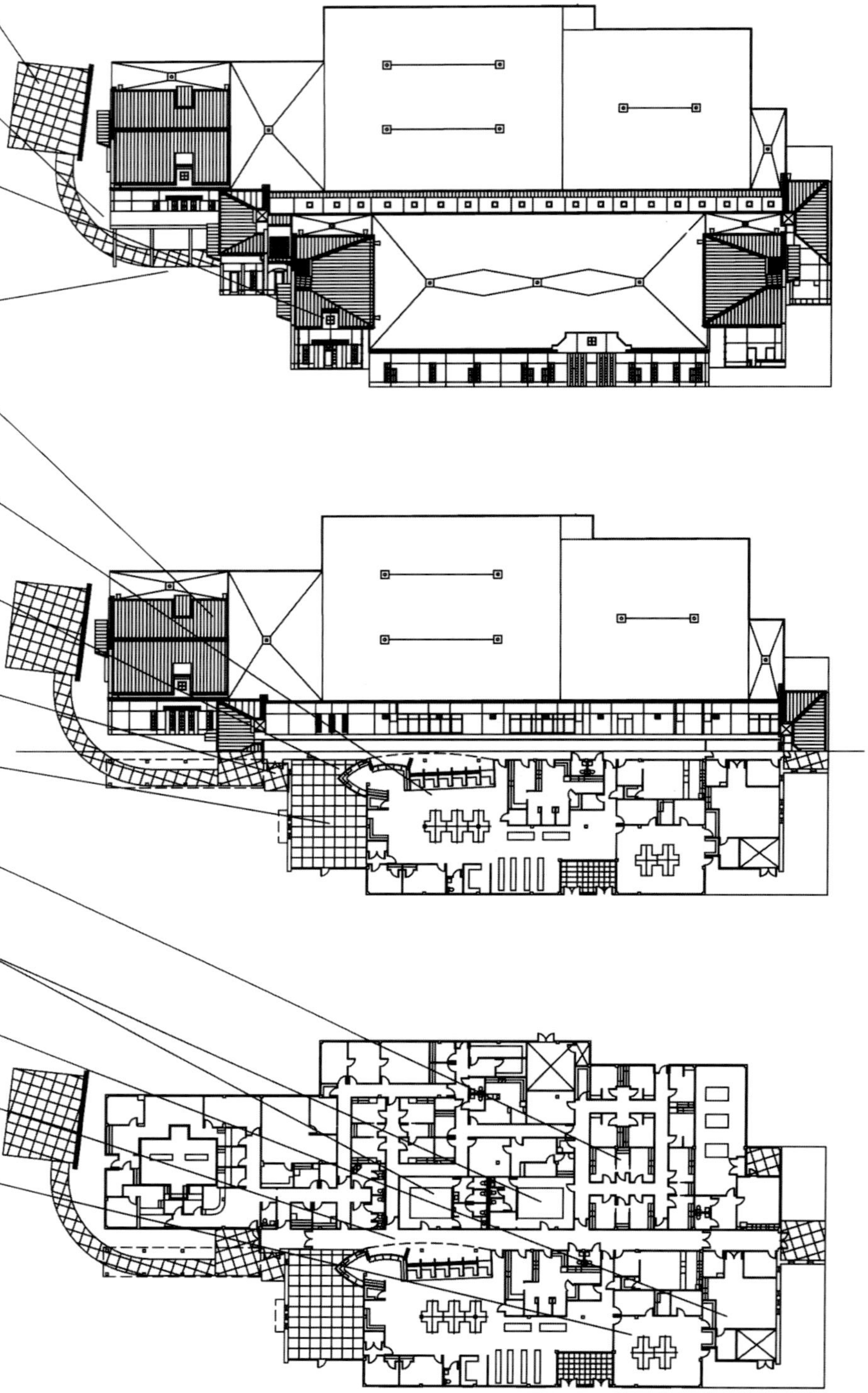

Fig. 5.57 a-c

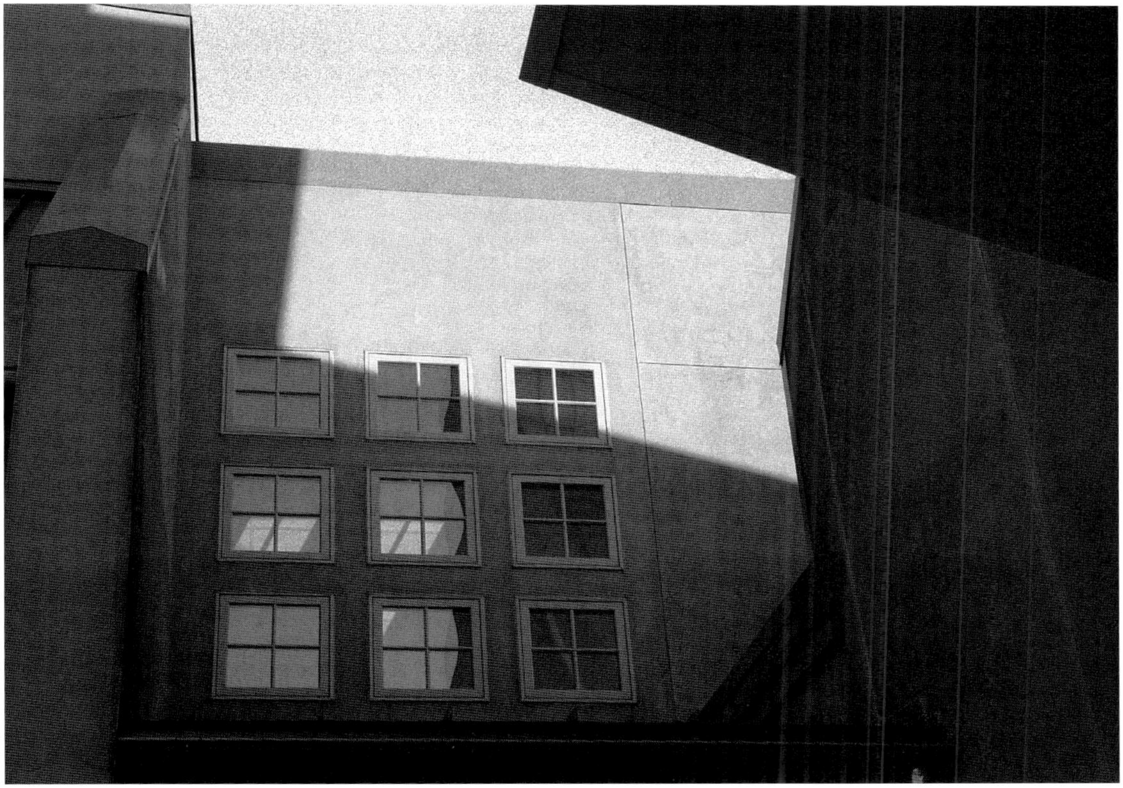

Fig. 5.58

ing; on the other are the main access drives. A circular fountain was built in the center to function as a focal point and key orienting element. The building is residentialist in its composition and aesthetic vocabulary. The endpoints of an interior pedestrian street are articulated, and the partí is distinguished as three residentially scaled elements. This concept of clinic-as-village is expressed in the environmental health wing, which appears from the exterior as a separate "house," independent from the clinic realm. This larger, linear element accommodates the clinics and support spaces, at the endpoints a pair of individual "houses," with gabled roofs, dormer windows, and two raised skylight-lanterns provide light to the spaces within (Fig. 5.52 and Fig. 5.53). The expression of indigenous vernacular architectural traditions in Acadiana, such as in the small courtyard on the administrative side of the building and the fenestration, are effective (Fig. 5.54 and Fig. 5.55).

The central circulation axis functions as a line of demarcation between the clinical, environmental health, and administrative realms. This linear "street" spans the entire length, from the covered canopy drop-off and main entry to the staff entrance at the opposing end of the building (Fig. 5.56 and Fig. 5.57). Clerestory windows transmit daylight into this pedestrian spine (Fig. 5.58 and Fig. 5.59). Patients sign in at the main counter, whose form evokes a small wooden shrimping vessel (Fig. 5.60). Subwaiting rooms are situated along the clinical side of the pedestrian street. On the opposing side are the intake stations for patients to consult with clerical staff and administration. The WIC demonstration kitchen and nutritional education classroom is also located along this "street." The clinic contains sixteen examination rooms, consult rooms, and support functions. Exam rooms are sized to be flexive—for treatment or consultation. Earth tones, maroons, and mauves are predominant throughout the building.

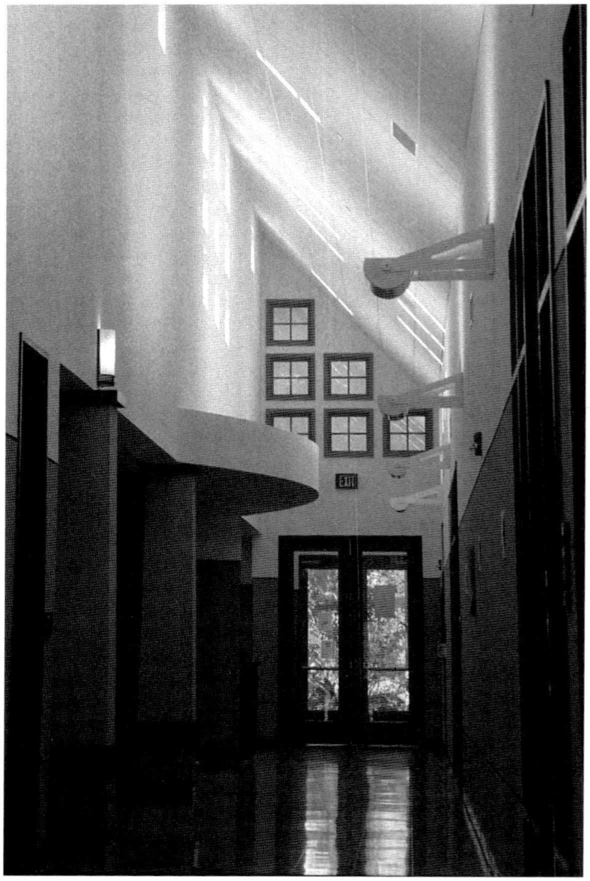

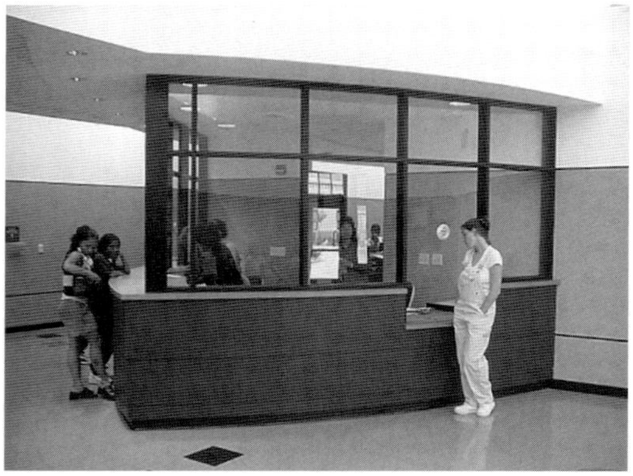

Fig. 5.60

Fig. 5.59

One year after completion, its occupants were most satisfied with the facility's access to public transportation, location within the community, imagery and aesthetic appearance, attractiveness of the grounds and the campus setting, and walking distances from parking areas. The post-occupancy evaluation also identified occupant satisfaction with the color scheme, interior daylighting, the sense of safety and security within, and views to the outside from the waiting rooms and the numerous room-to-room interior windows providing views onto the pedestrian street. Staff occupants were found to be most satisfied with the interior color scheme and the amount of natural daylight throughout. With respect to the exterior, staff occupants also cited the attractive landscaping, parking availability, attractive campus context, and, once again, the colors of the building.

Richland Parish, Rayville

For thirty years, the health unit in Rayville was housed near the center of town in a prefab metal structure shared with a branch of the state's Office of Social Services. In recent years the occupants endured the stench of a broken sewer line running beneath the clinic. This, compounded by the windowless conditions, was simply too much for occupants, especially during the long summer

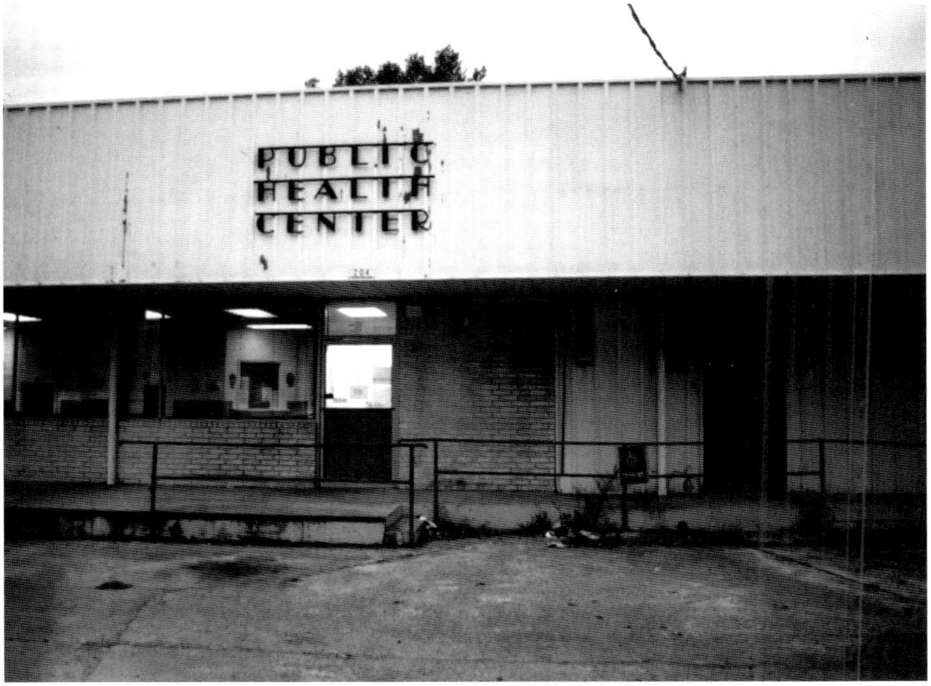

Fig. 5.61

months. Staff often complained of headaches, muscle aches, and nausea (Fig. 5.61). In 1998, the police jury, lacking a dedicated millage tax, approached the state for a capital outlay grant of $1.2 million for a replacement facility. Poor working conditions, combined with an absence of patient confidentiality, poor staff and patient flow, and inadequate parking, had been identified and documented by the SFI team in a post-occupancy evaluation conducted in 1994.

Only five parish health unit replacement facilities built during the 1990s were funded in Louisiana through capital outlay, with only two built with this source of state funds between 1985-90. Against the odds, the parish police jury pushed forward with its legislative delegation lined up in support, using the argument that the northern part of the state had been long neglected, and was overdue its fair share. Meanwhile, the parish had donated a seven-acre tract of open farmland at the edge of town near the Interstate 20. Without success the SFI team made the case for a site at the center of the community, only to be told, in the end, "Take it or leave it." It was remote, almost invisible from a civic infrastructural perspective, and yet, on the other hand, its openness and close geographic proximity to the lower Mississippi Delta flood plain were attributes. Historical precedent, once again, as in the case of Avoyelles Parish, allowed for a design response fusing the everyday cultural landscape of the present, with that of the past. Such a strategy would be achievable through the cross-referencing of predominant land use development patterns during the eighteenth and nineteenth centuries along the Mississippi River.

Fig. 5.62

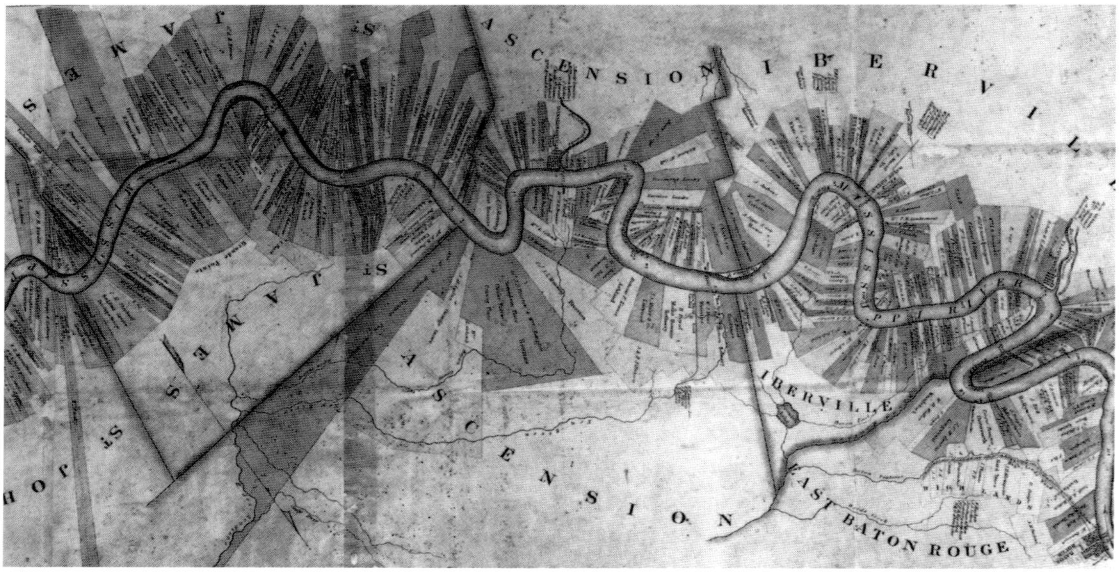

By the mid-nineteenth century, the subdivision of land along the river over two centuries had resulted in contiguous, irregularly shaped land parcels. Each parcel represented an autonomous plantation, each owned by a wealthy family. It was essential for each plantation to front the river, as the river was the main artery for commerce. An architect and engineer living in New Orleans, Marie Adrien Persac, developed a map of the region of the river from New Orleans to north of Baton Rouge, for the purpose of documenting the pattern of land distribution. This map, published in 1858, depicted land use based on the French colonial arpent system of land subdivision (Fig. 5.62). This map would have a lasting impact on continued land use and development patterns along the lower Mississippi River Valley. A section of this plat map, *Norman's Chart of the Lower Mississippi River*, illustrated the plantation parcels between New Orleans and Baton Rouge, identifying each landowner by family name.[10] Today's pattern of asymmetrical plat boundaries endures as much as a fascinating tapestry of bisecting, interdependent geometries, as a testament to the Old South era.

Form-generative computer software algorithms exist, where time is indexed, or imprinted, upon three-dimensional architectural space. In this way, animate as well as inanimate representations are able to be generated. Superimposed snapshots of motion demark time as the phenomenal movement between serialized frames and moments. This process yields kinetic, anthropomorphic, fluid spatial compositions. Tracing denotes the graphical notation of time, motion, and its visual and spatial corrolaries.[11] In the cultural landscape—the history of land subdivisions along the Mississippi, in this case—form, nature, space, and time become analogous with one another.[12] Geomorphologic and biomorphic tracings of time and human use upon the physical landscape become discernable. In a modification of this approach, landscape imprints were digitally transcribed into an array of landscape vectors representing the various paths the river had taken over hundreds of years and the resultant undulating shifts in the flow of the Mississippi River bed. As such, Persac's map was transcribed into a series of successive, undulating frames. These tracings were then transcribed into architectural terms in the proposed replacement facility in Rayville, where this author's transcriptions subsequently became the basis for the generation of an entire building. Of course, computer software algorithms such as this alone cannot be relied upon, as human experience must be central to any meaningful design process. This unbuilt proposal's (2002) biomorphic,

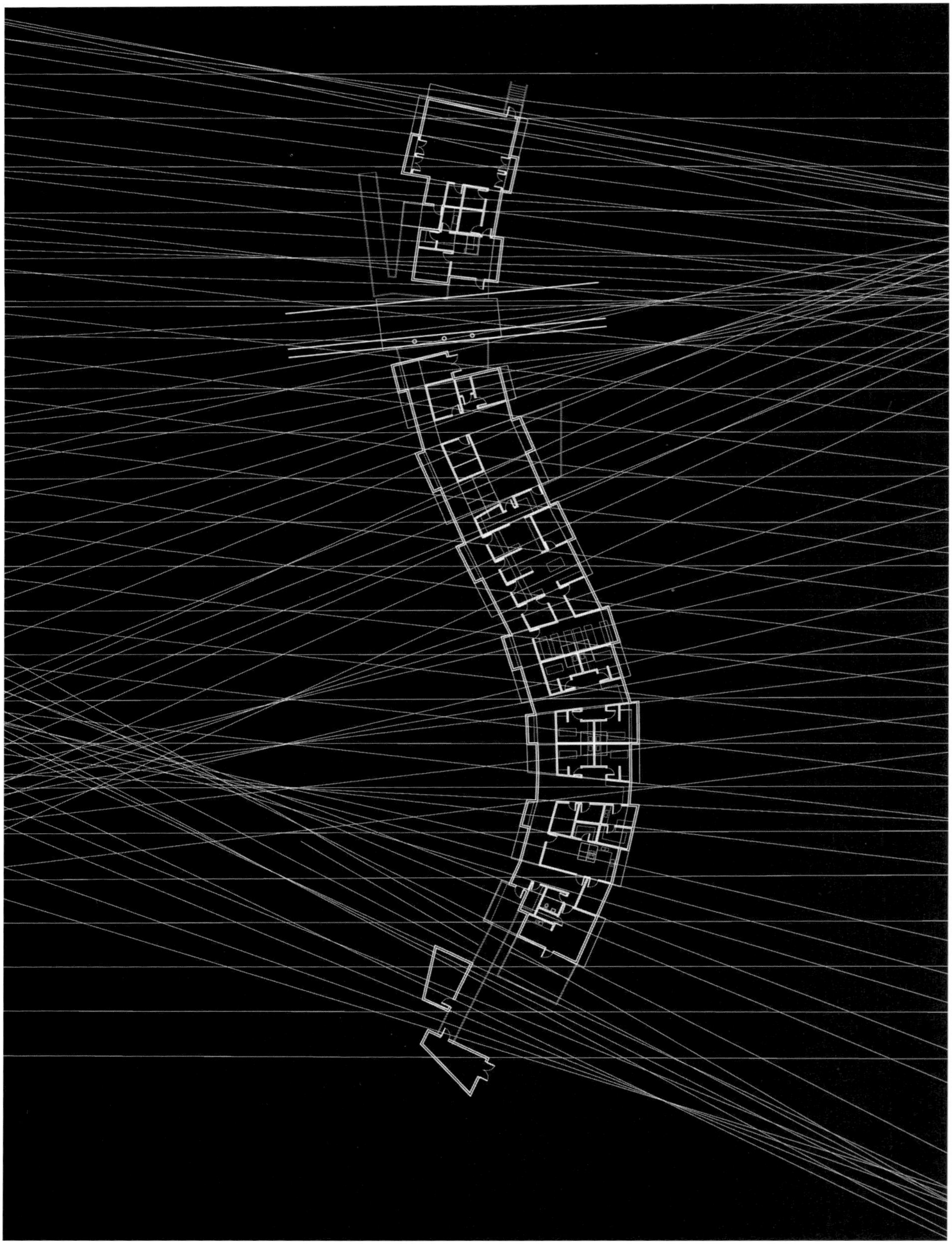

Fig. 5.63

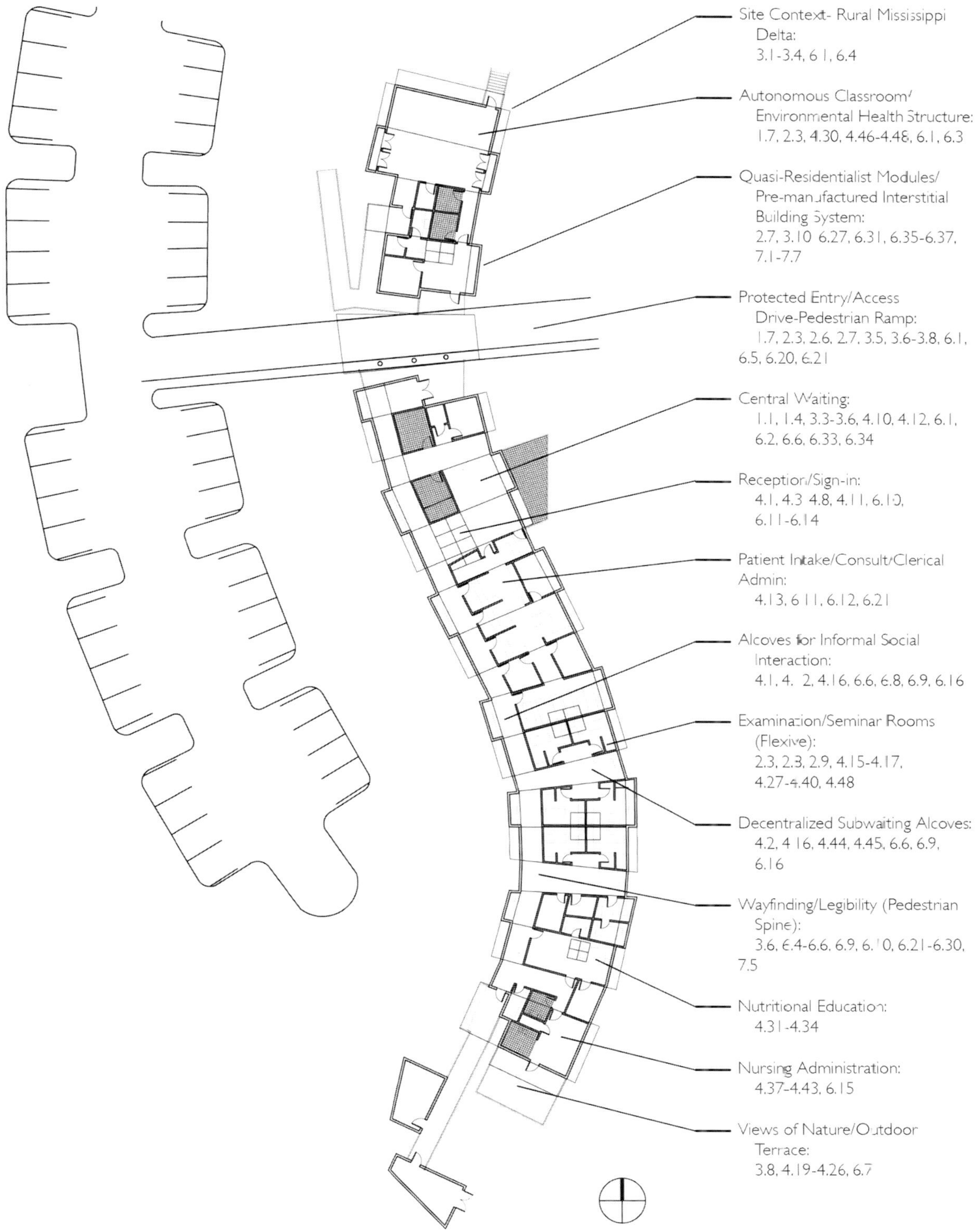
Site Context- Rural Mississippi Delta:
3.1-3.4, 6.1, 6.4
Autonomous Classroom/ Environmental Health Structure:
1.7, 2.3, 4.30, 4.46-4.48, 6.1, 6.3
Quasi-Residentialist Modules/ Pre-manufactured Interstitial Building System:
2.7, 3.10 6.27, 6.31, 6.35-6.37, 7.1-7.7
Protected Entry/Access Drive-Pedestrian Ramp:
1.7, 2.3, 2.6, 2.7, 3.5, 3.6-3.8, 6.1, 6.5, 6.20, 6.21
Central Waiting:
1.1, 1.4, 3.3-3.6, 4.10, 4.12, 6.1, 6.2, 6.6, 6.33, 6.34
Reception/Sign-in:
4.1, 4.3 4.8, 4.11, 6.10, 6.11-6.14
Patient Intake/Consult/Clerical Admin:
4.13, 6.11, 6.12, 6.21
Alcoves for Informal Social Interaction:
4.1, 4. 2, 4.16, 6.6, 6.8, 6.9, 6.16
Examination/Seminar Rooms (Flexive):
2.3, 2.3, 2.9, 4.15-4.17, 4.27-4.40, 4.48
Decentralized Subwaiting Alcoves:
4.2, 4.16, 4.44, 4.45, 6.6, 6.9, 6.16
Wayfinding/Legibility (Pedestrian Spine):
3.6, 6.4-6.6, 6.9, 6.10, 6.21-6.30, 7.5
Nutritional Education:
4.31-4.34
Nursing Administration:
4.37-4.43, 6.15
Views of Nature/Outdoor Terrace:
3.8, 4.19-4.26, 6.7

Fig. 5.64

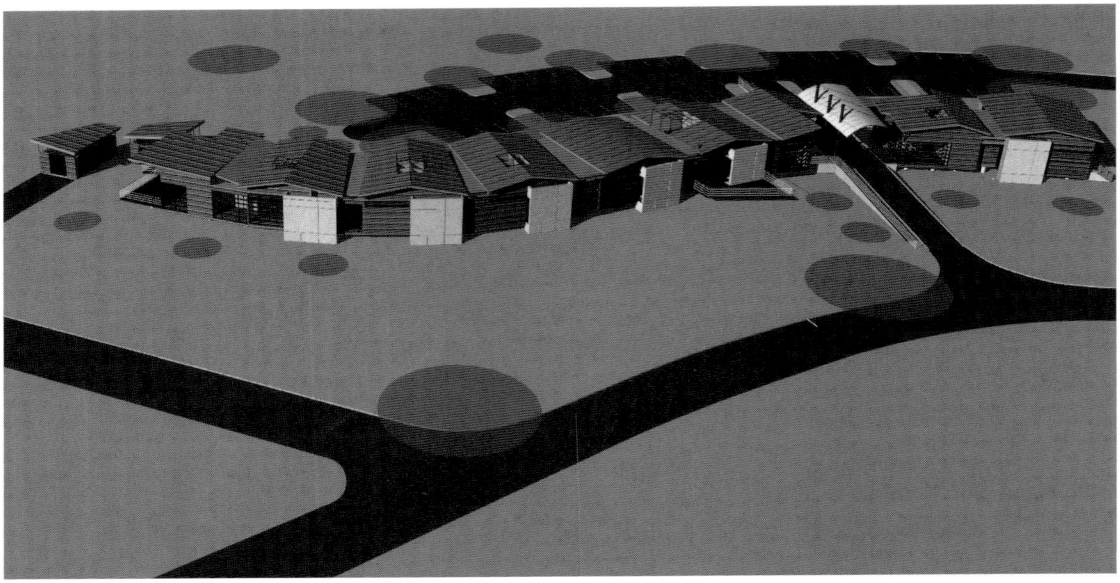

Fig. 5.65

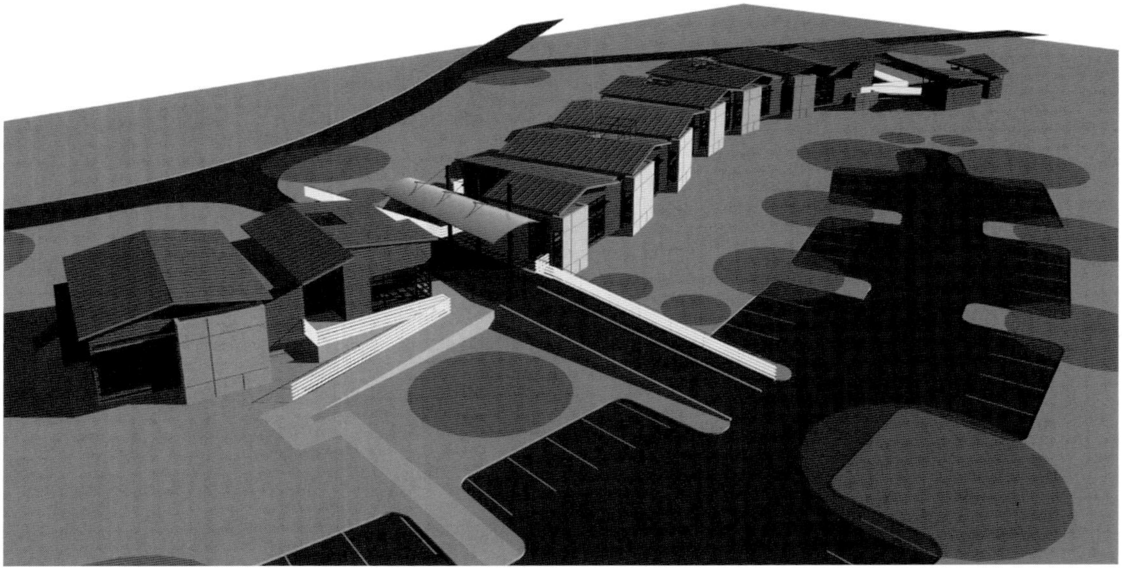

Fig. 5.66

undulating spine is therefore rooted equally in the day-to-day realities of human occupancy as in the serpentine tracings of the river delta and its various permutations through the centuries (Fig. 5.63).

The building houses an environmental health program, a clinical realm comprising six trans-programmatic exam rooms, and a clerical and administrative realm with a set of five combined intake-staff offices. Square footage totals 10,150, the building is elevated four feet above the delta flood plain (Fig. 5.64 and Fig. 5.65). The building's "legs" provide structural support for this to occur, and HVAC systems are supplied from beneath the main floor via an 18-inch depth interstitial two-way truss floor system. Its attributes include:

Decentralization—the main vehicular and pedestrian access point to the building near midsection. This allows for direct access to either an autonomous environmental health module, to one side, or the clinic, to the other (Fig. 5.66).

Flexivity—The partí is transformable, able to take on any number of alternative shapes, from linear to curvilinear, re-configurably. The premanufactured modular pods are similarly capable of horizontal accordion-like or variable expansion.

Parking/Site Access—the decentralized deployment of the environmental health program section apart from the clinic realm allows for options in the placement of parking areas, access drives, and pedestrian walkways.

Sustainability—a relatively thin, linear footprint allows for the retention of the maximum amount of existing natural vegetation on the site, and affords transmission of natural daylight into the building's modules (Fig. 5.67).

Fig. 5.67

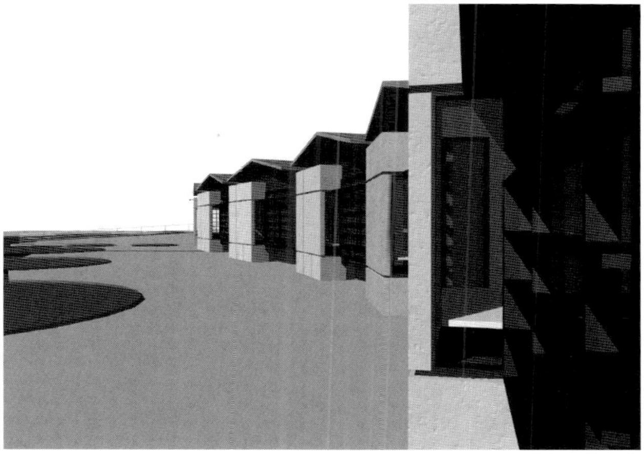

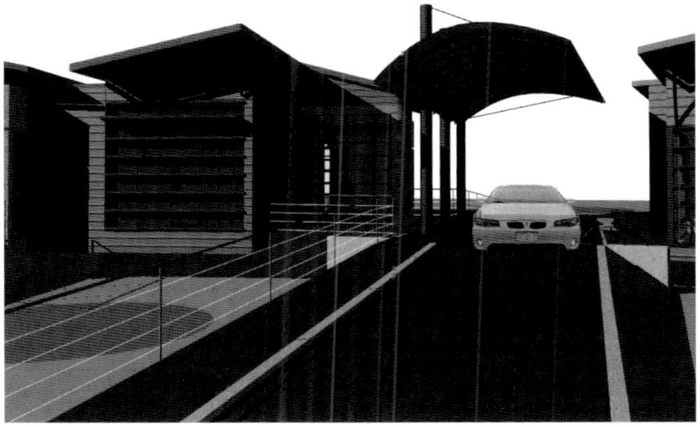

Fig. 5.68

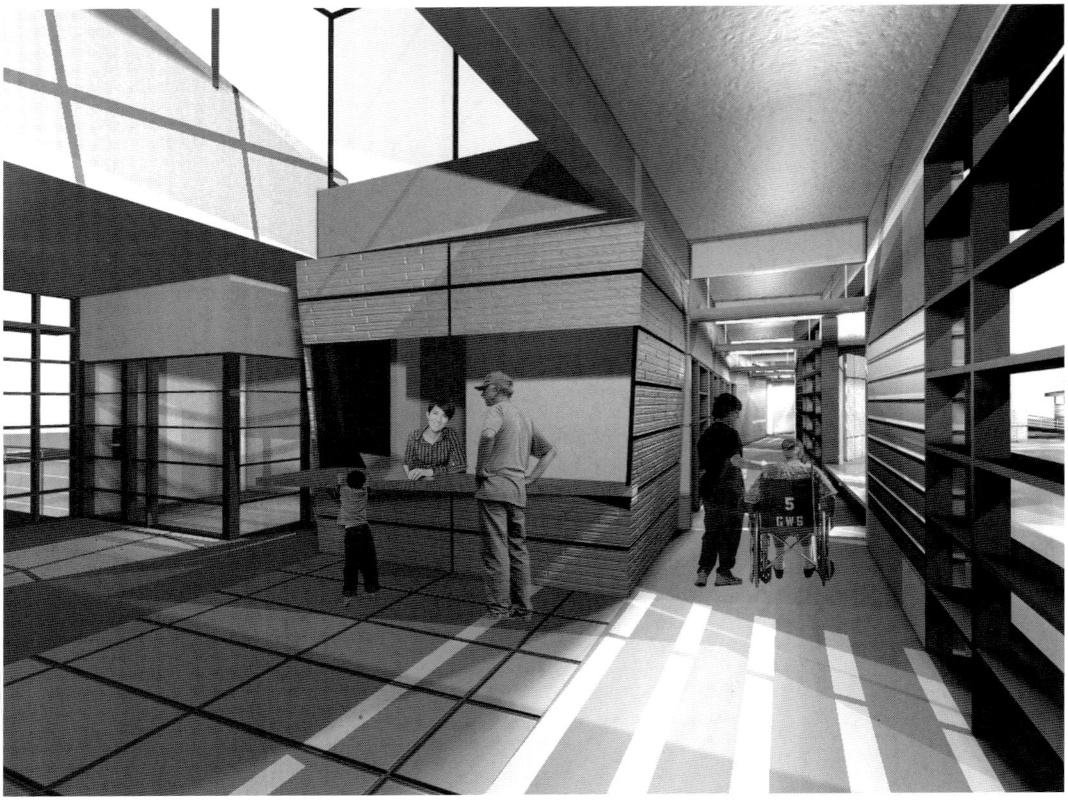

Fig. 5.69

Fig. 5.70

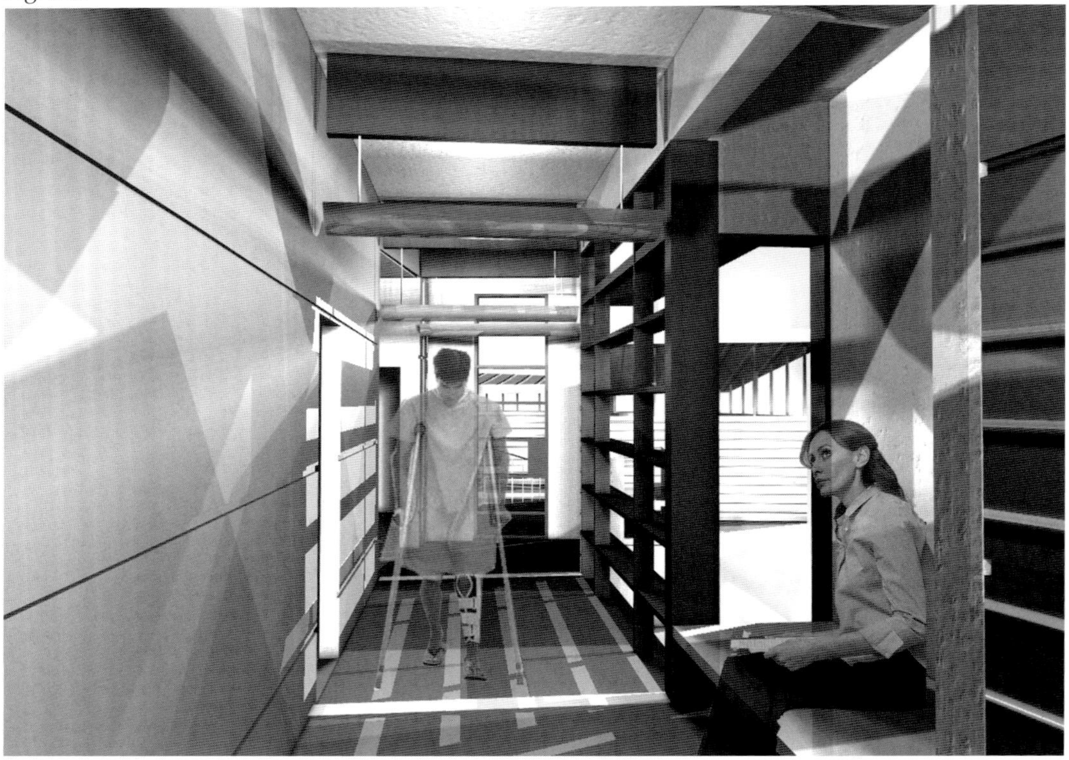

The fenestration in turn affords full views to the exterior landscape. At the porte cochère, one enters the environmental health offices to the left, or the main door to the clinic to the right (Fig. 5.68). On the clinic side, an arrival vestibule receives the patient leading to the appointment desk. The waiting room is to the left (Fig. 5.69). The patient is directed to one of the intake offices, subwaiting room, or to one of the seating niches arrayed along the circulation spine (Fig. 5.70). The patient proceeds to one's examination, returning to subwaiting to await word of a test. The nutritional education/WIC kitchen is located at the tail. For staff, an entrance is provided to the rear of the clinic near the staff parking area. The staff lounge and kitchen is located in the tail, with an adjoining outdoor terrace. The circulation spine allows for informal interaction in window seating nodes. The built-in seating dispersed along this spine functions as informal space (Fig. 5.71).

Modularization—ten modular pods are structurally self-sufficient, interconnected and stabilized by steel tubular conduits. The legs of the pods are telescopic and this allows the entire structure to be elevated. These interconnections allow for variability in deployment, not unlike the elevated jet ways passengers use to embark and disembark airliners.

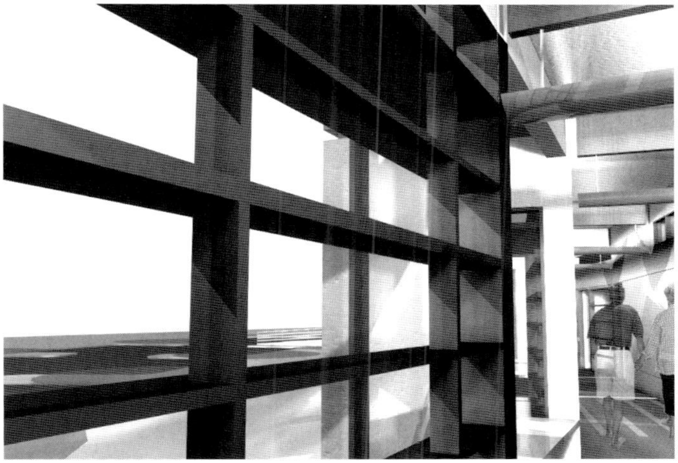

Fig. 5.71

Sustainability—the building minimizes its sole reliance on costly mechanical HVAC systems through the use of passive solar design techniques, including sunscreens, roof overhangs, and a geothermal system. The building maximizes "green" building materials, furnishings, and fixtures throughout (Fig. 5.72).

Human Scale/Decentralized Seating Pods—the building is intensely human in scale. Small pockets of seating throughout reinforce the primacy of the patient; this is especially germane on busy clinic days. Five or six individuals can sit in a single seating alcove. This helps ameliorate the stress often associ-

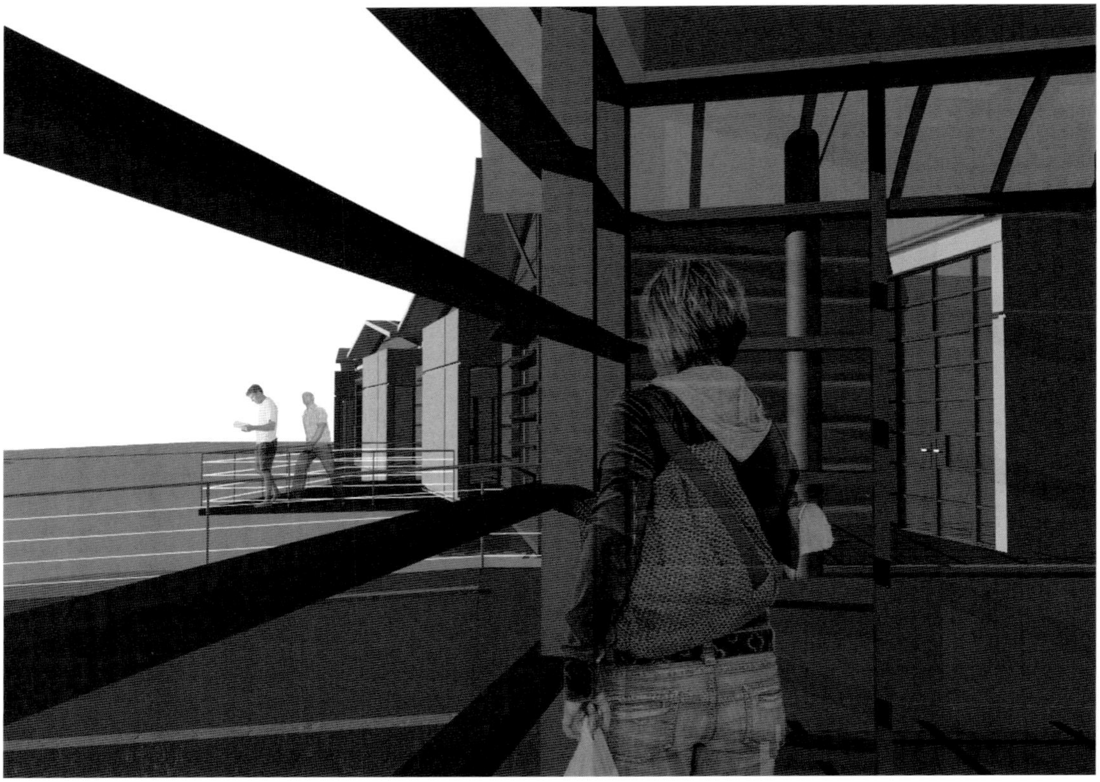

Fig. 5.72

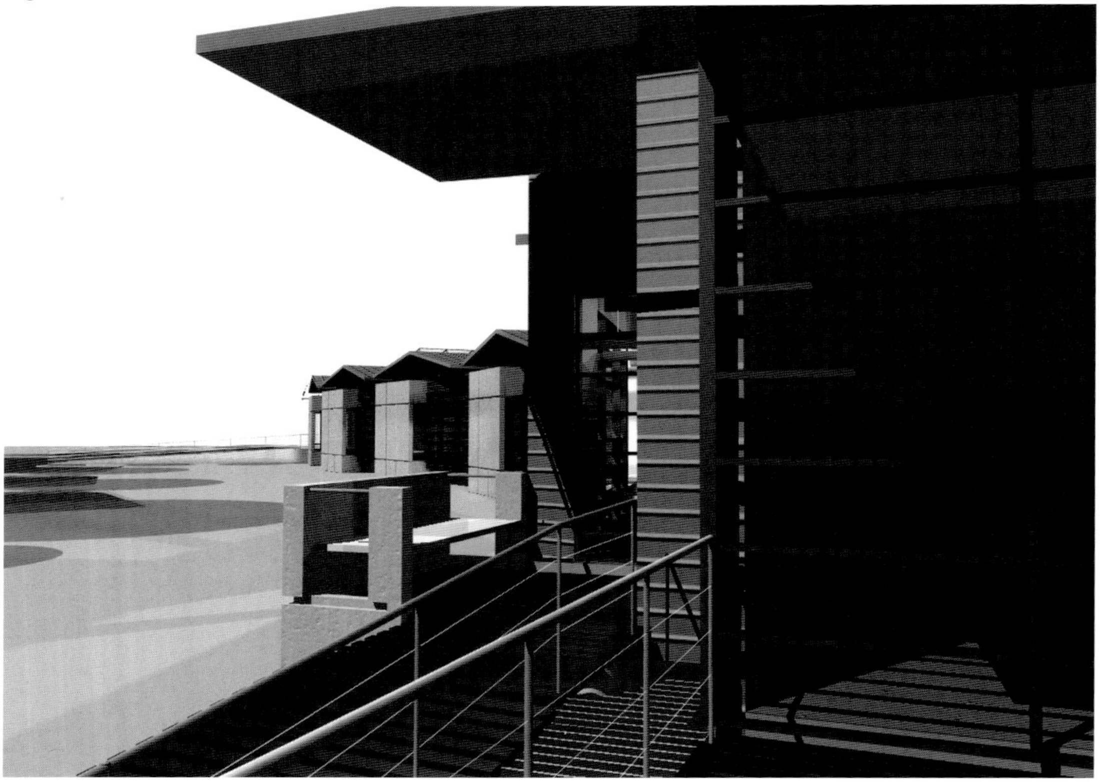

Fig. 5.73

ated with spending time in a large, impersonal waiting room. To achieve this, six window-seating bays are arrayed along the undulating pedestrian spine. A seventh seating pod is positioned on the exterior adjacent to the terrace (Fig. 5.73). These are positioned to allow staff and patients to interact informally, reducing pressure on the traditional reliance on the exam rooms for conversations between patient and caregiver.

Flexivity: Intake—each office provides space for transactions that occur between the patient, and the intake clerk. Walls are demountable and re-deployable, as needs dictate. Examination Rooms, similarly, are adaptable to seminar rooms for up to ten persons, convertible with the aid of mechanically activated, moveable acoustic/visual screens. Each exam room is 15 percent larger than a conventional exam room to allow space for the nurse or physician's administrative work.

Communal Spaces—the WIC kitchen doubles as subwaiting room and staff conference room. A multipurpose community health education room is housed in the environmental health wing. This unbuilt proposal was developed in 2002.

Procedural Steps in the SFI Process

Architectural design, including a building's composition, color palette, ambient qualities, wayfinding amenity, and siting, can be overlooked by a client primarily driven by fiscal cost control.[13] With respect to health disparities among the medically underserved in the U.S., it has been demonstrated repeatedly in the research literature there is a direct correlation between low income patients and low-quality healthcare.[14] However, the fields of architecture and public health have each failed to devote attention to this crisis despite the growing healthcare-gap in the United States.[15] High-quality architecture requires an investment, and the relatively small but growing number of practitioners who advocate and practice evidence-based design for health care facilities argue that a high-quality architectural setting is positively correlated with a higher quality of care and higher level of patient satisfaction.[16] With this said, the SFI protocol is presented below, including a discussion of its key strengths, weaknesses and opportunities for its application. While firmly centered on architec-

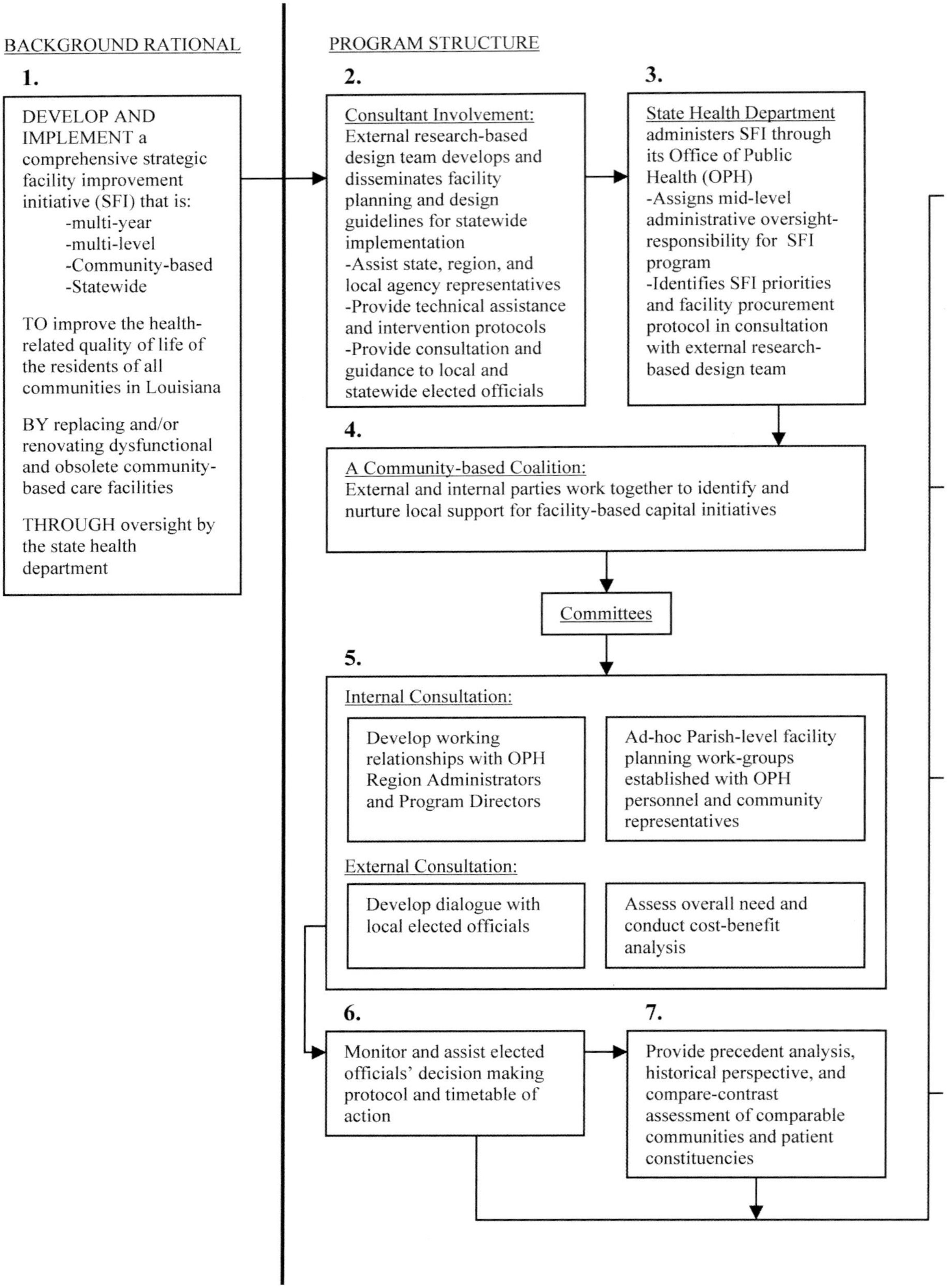

BACKGROUND RATIONAL
1.
DEVELOP AND IMPLEMENT a comprehensive strategic facility improvement initiative (SFI) that is:
-multi-year
-multi-level
-Community-based
-Statewide
TO improve the health-related quality of life of the residents of all communities in Louisiana
BY replacing and/or renovating dysfunctional and obsolete community-based care facilities
THROUGH oversight by the state health department
PROGRAM STRUCTURE
2.
Consultant Involvement:
External research-based design team develops and disseminates facility planning and design guidelines for statewide implementation
-Assist state, region, and local agency representatives
-Provide technical assistance and intervention protocols
-Provide consultation and guidance to local and statewide elected officials
3.
State Health Department administers SFI through its Office of Public Health (OPH)
-Assigns mid-level administrative oversight-responsibility for SFI program
-Identifies SFI priorities and facility procurement protocol in consultation with external research-based design team
4.
A Community-based Coalition:
External and internal parties work together to identify and nurture local support for facility-based capital initiatives
Committees
5.
Internal Consultation:
Develop working relationships with OPH Region Administrators and Program Directors
Ad-hoc Parish-level facility planning work-groups established with OPH personnel and community representatives
External Consultation:
Develop dialogue with local elected officials
Assess overall need and conduct cost-benefit analysis
6.
Monitor and assist elected officials' decision making protocol and timetable of action
7.
Provide precedent analysis, historical perspective, and compare-contrast assessment of comparable communities and patient constituencies

PROGRAM INTERVENTIONS

8.

Policy Interventions:
-Provide elected officials with recommended and alternate capital improvement options
-Define project budget and potential cost savings
-Define project scope
-Develop project brief
-Interface with local architect of record
-Provide architectural design facility-sensitive strategic planning leadership

9.

Site Selection/Planning Interventions:
-Assess multiple locations for highest and best use as healthcare program site
-Assess parking requirements
-Assess public transit linkages
-Due diligence of site attributes, utility easements, and necessary infrastructure
-Meetings with elected officials, local OPH staff, and community representatives

10.

Architectural Interventions:
-Provide decision makers with knowledge of state of the art with respect to community health facility planning, design and management
-Consult with contracted architect of record throughout project
-Provide plan review oversight
-Provide design alternatives
-Conduct periodic post occupancy evaluations of existing facilities, and new or renovated facilities statewide to validate and/or revise and extend existing knowledge base

11.

Program/Service Interventions:
-Directed at minimizing disruptions in service or decrease in quality of care during capital improvement projects
-Communicating with patients on benefits accrued vis-à-vis' an improved community care environment

PROGRAM OUTCOMES

12.

Improvements in Care Setting:
-Efficient staff and patient flow patterns of movement
-Inviting image, appearance and ambiance
-A facility in compliance with local, state, and federal building codes
-A universal design care setting supportive of spectrum of age groups and individuals with physical abilities/disabilities
-A highly visible civic symbol and resource

13.

Improvements in Quality of Care:
-Increase in number of patients served, i.e. a more supportive facility capacity utilization ratio
-An empowered staff, i.e. improved retention, morale, and productivity
-An empowered patient as result of an architecturally supportive care setting

14.

Replication:
-Addition to existing knowledge base for public-policy makers in public and private sectors
-Risks and threats faced in future SFI efforts can be ameliorated
-Case study of successful partnership between community-based, region, and statewide agencies and elected officials
-Transferability of SFI protocol to allied state and local organizations nationally and internationally

ture, this protocol in many respects parallels the procedural protocol employed in a study of diabetes treatment outcomes in an inner urban setting.[17] The SFI consists of fourteen separate steps (Fig. 5.74). These steps are interdependent and generally occur linearly.

Background/Rationale/Structure (Steps 1-7): Seven core components emphasize, first, the program's background rationale and structure. The fundamental aim is to improve health outcomes through the use of evidence-based planning and design knowledge in the renovation and construction of community-based public health facilities (Step 1). Second, it is important to convey to all parties involved the nature of the SFI team's long-term role, from a project's inception to completion, in working with in-house agency staff in a consultative capacity (Step 2). The sustained support and administrative oversight provided by the primary client agency is critical in terms of providing administrative leadership and in establishing capital improvement priorities (Step 3). The solicitation of the involvement of community advocacy groups and interested local citizens in the capital improvement process is equally important to the success of the SFI (Step 4). Effective internal and external communication channels need to be established at the outset with in-house liaison agency committees as well as effective communications with parish-based elected officials (Step 5). The creation of a project review team to assist local elected officials and other concerned parties in the implementation phase can be of great assistance and result in a much more successful architectural outcome, and more timely completion of the construction project, than would otherwise likely be the case (Step 6). It has proven useful to communities to be able to compare and contrast within-state trends, and to assist them in developing their facility improvement strategies locally (Step 7). The ability to compare alternative exam room layouts and equipment options, for example, or the most effective signage system for wayfinding in a clinical setting, can save a great deal of time and effort later on in unnecessary and costly retrofitting of a newly completed building.

Intervention (Steps 8-11): Components 8 through 11 consist of key interventional steps, each focusing on the importance of policy interventions that identify alternative capital improvement options. It is important to conduct cost-benefit analyses of the advantages of new construction versus alternative strategies, such as renovation, and to provide general guidance and architectural counsel to local elected officials and health agency personnel (Step 8). This step also includes the development of functional space program briefs. In defining a project's mission, size, and scope it is essential to identify and select the most suitable site for a replacement facility. The highest and best use of a given site must be assessed, including selecting a site in close proximity to public transportation (Step 9). In many cases, the consulting team is called upon to provide schematic design services as well at this point. It is essential to maintain oversight of the entire SFI process, including scheduling, areas of responsibility, the monitoring of change orders, owner's representative obligations, and frequent review of the construction budget. A post-occupancy evaluation may be necessary at the outset to determine whether to build new or to renovate (Step 10). Regardless, every reasonable measure should be taken to minimize the degree of disruption typically caused by a construction project. Similarly, every reasonable effort should be made to keep things running smoothly in an uninterrupted manner during the period of construction, which may last as long as fifteen months to two years in complex, multi-phased projects (Step 11).

Outcome and Performance Assessment (Steps 12-14): Components 12 through 14 consist of post-construction interventions to ensure the completed project's successful performance over time. These measures consist of the assessment of improvements made following a three to six month "shake out" period during which fine-tuning and various facility management modifications typically occur. Also, the facility must be in full compliance with local, state, and federal building codes on an ongoing basis, and the needs of physically and cognitively challenged patients must be fully supported (Step 12). It is important to assess the extent to which the new or renovated facility yields an increase in the number of patients served daily, weekly, and monthly (Step 13). Similarly, it is important to inculcate in clinical and related program staff, and in officials responsible for site and facility maintenance, a willingness to function as the stewards of their own facility (Step 14).

Performance

A summary of all capital improvement projects completed in Louisiana as of December 2003 is reported below (Fig. 5.75). A total of fifty-five projects were completed during this period (1991-2003). Of these, thirty-eight resulted in com-

Figure 5.75. Statewide facility improvement initiatives (1991-2003).

Region[a]	Completed Projects	Replacement Facility (Y/N)	Renovation (Y/N)	Adaptive[b] Use (Y/N)	Planning[c] Phase (months)	Construction[d] Phase (months)	Square Feet[e] New Construction	Square Feet[e] Other	Expenditure[f]
1(12)	5	Y(1)[g]	Y(3)	Y(1)	8.4	11.3	12,250(12,250)	8,881(44,404)	780,240(3.90M)
2(9)	5	Y(4)	Y(1)	N(--)	14.8	9.6	7,513(30,050)	3,000(3,000)	750,000(3.01M)
3(11)	7	Y(4)	Y(1)	Y(2)	10.9	11.7	9,900(49,500)	4,067(12,200)	610,127(6.71M)
4(17)	6	Y(6)	N(--)	N(--)	12.2	12.8	8,328(49,970)	--- (---)	1,100,177(6.60M)
5(10)	6	Y(4)	Y(1)	Y(1)	20.7	10.4	10,837(54,185)	3,940(3,940)	1,288,571(9.02M)
6(11)	4	Y(2)	Y(1)	Y(1)	9.7	10.2	9,320(37,280)	--- (---)	898,213(4.49M)
7(14)	5	Y(2)	Y(1)	Y(2)	10.3	10.7	7,800(15,600)	10,593(31,780)	587,857(4.12M)
8(12)	9	Y(8)	N(--)	Y(1)	14.1	13.6	10,178(81,425)	3,250(3,250)	875,909(9.63M)
9(11)	8	Y(7)	N(--)	Y(1)	15.9	9.6	6,889(34,445)	7,767(23,300)	1,190,000(5.95M)
Total (107)[h]	55	38	8	9	13.0	11.1	9,224(364,705)	5,928(121,874)	897,899(53.4M)

[a] Project data reported through 12/31/03. Number in parentheses denotes total freestanding program sites in Region (with exception of school-based clinics).
[b] Certain projects involve combination of either new and/or renovated or adaptive reuse strategies.
[c] Mean across projects reported (in months).
[d] Mean across projects reported (in months).
[e] "New Construction" data reported as Building/Gross Square Feet (BGSF). Number in parentheses denotes total BGSF. "Other" category consists of renovation and adaptive reuse projects. These data are reported as Departmental Gross Square Feet (DGSF). Number in parentheses denotes total DGSF.
[f] Mean total project cost, including land acquisition, site improvements, parking areas, access drives, signage, landscaping, furnishing equipment, and building expenses (in millions). Number in parentheses denotes total capital expenditure in Region (in millions).
[g] Y denotes decision to replace community public health facility since 1990-1991 Fiscal Year (FY). Number in parentheses denotes total number of facilities built in Region.
h A total of 25 program sites have been closed or consolidated with existing DHH-OPH facilities since 1990-1991 FY.

pletely new replacement facilities, eight in renovations or expansions to existing facilities, and nine resulted in adaptive re-use of a "new" existing building for use as a community public healthcare clinic. The average project-planning phase, from project inception to groundbreaking, was thirteen months. The average length of time required for actual construction from groundbreaking to opening day was 11.1 months.

With respect to the amount of construction activity across the nine administrative regions, the average size of a new facility was 9,224 square feet. This represented 364,705 total square feet in new construction. Other building projects, consisting of renovations and adaptive re-use of existing buildings, averaged 5,928 square feet per project. This represented 121,874 total square feet in this category. With respect to fiscal expenditure, the average capital improvement project was $897,899 (unadjusted for inflation). Total capital improvement expenditures during the period reported across the nine OPH regions totaled $53.4 million (unadjusted). Despite the considerable volume of construction activity during the twelve-year period reported, it is noteworthy a total of twenty-five program sites were closed outright or consolidated due to administrative restructuring.

The performance of the SFI program is reviewed annually, as is the architectural performance of each facility. A composite facility performance rating is assigned, based on three types of data: first-hand appraisals by its end user occupants (patients and full-time staff), the assessment of the region administrator, and information acquired in the field by the SFI team. Together, this information is translated into a four-point scale to reflect the degree of architectural intervention required. This rating is based on five factors: 1. Site context and neighborhood; 2. Aesthetic appearance; 3. Degree of functionality from the standpoint of internal patterns of use and occupant and materials flow; 4. Patterns of facility maintenance; and 5. Environmental control factors (heating, ventilation, and air conditioning, and electrical systems). The four levels of ranking for priority improvement are: (1) urgent priority, (2) high priority, (3) moderate priority, or (4) no change. A between-region (R1-R9) before/after rating of each clinic and program support site in the network is reported at the twelve-year interval (Fig. 5.76). The before rating, therefore, is the pre-intervention rating (1990) and the post-architectural intervention rating is cumulative

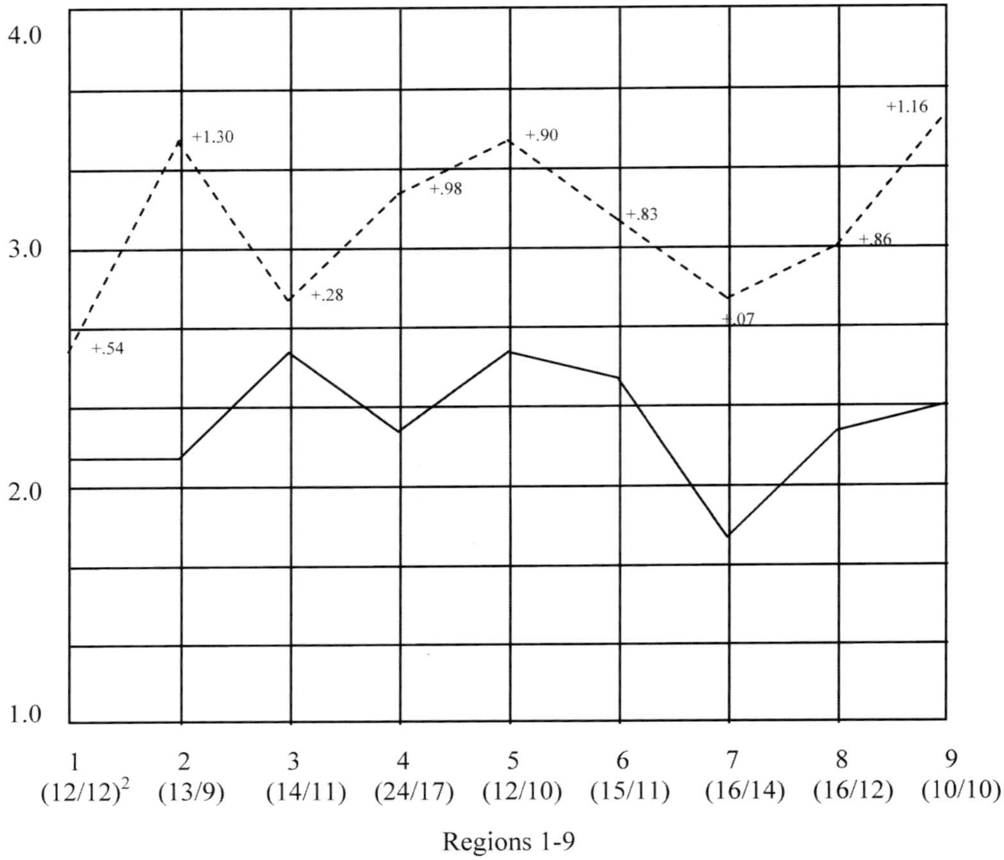

Figure 5.76: Statewide Capital Improvement Priority Rankings[1]

——— 1990-1991 Fiscal Year
- - - - - - 2003-2004 Fiscal Year

1 Four point assessment scale: 1= urgent priority; 2= high priority; 3=moderate priority; 4= no modification required at time of assessment.

2 First number in parentheses denotes number of freestanding program sites in Region in 1990-1991 fiscal year (FY). Second number denotes number of freestanding program sites in 2003-2004 FY (figures reported do not include 16 school-based clinics).

as of December 2003. This method of evidence-based facility review has been consistent with the collective architectural quality of facilities markedly improving during this period, with the most significant improvements achieved in Regions 2, 4, 5, 8 and 9 (Fig. 5.76).

In 2000, a slightly altered statewide survey from 1990-91 was re-administered with one significant modification.[18] The respondent group was greatly enlarged to a total of 1,143 full-time DHH-OPH personnel (see Appendix B). This longitudinal strategy made it possible to discern broad trends, and in many ways reaffirmed the significant progress made during the decade. Also, these data have since been of use in tandem with post-9/11 anti-terrorism programs initiated by the CDC and the Office of Homeland Security. The SFI initiative has improved the architectural environment for the delivery of community healthcare. Nevertheless, a minimum of fifteen clinics in the statewide network remain in urgent need of replacement as of July 2005. To date, no instances have been reported of the SFI protocol having an adverse impact on the quality of or the untimely completion of any capital improvement project. As mentioned, this architecture-based protocol shares certain attributes not significantly dissimilar from CDC-sponsored public health program initiatives.[19] This initiative, in the broadest sense, is therefore not dissimilar from research efforts to reduce the incidence of chronic diseases in communities, as it endeavors to express the needs and aspirations of patients, families, direct care providers, agency administrators, elected officials, and advocates for improved access to health services among disadvantaged populations.[20]

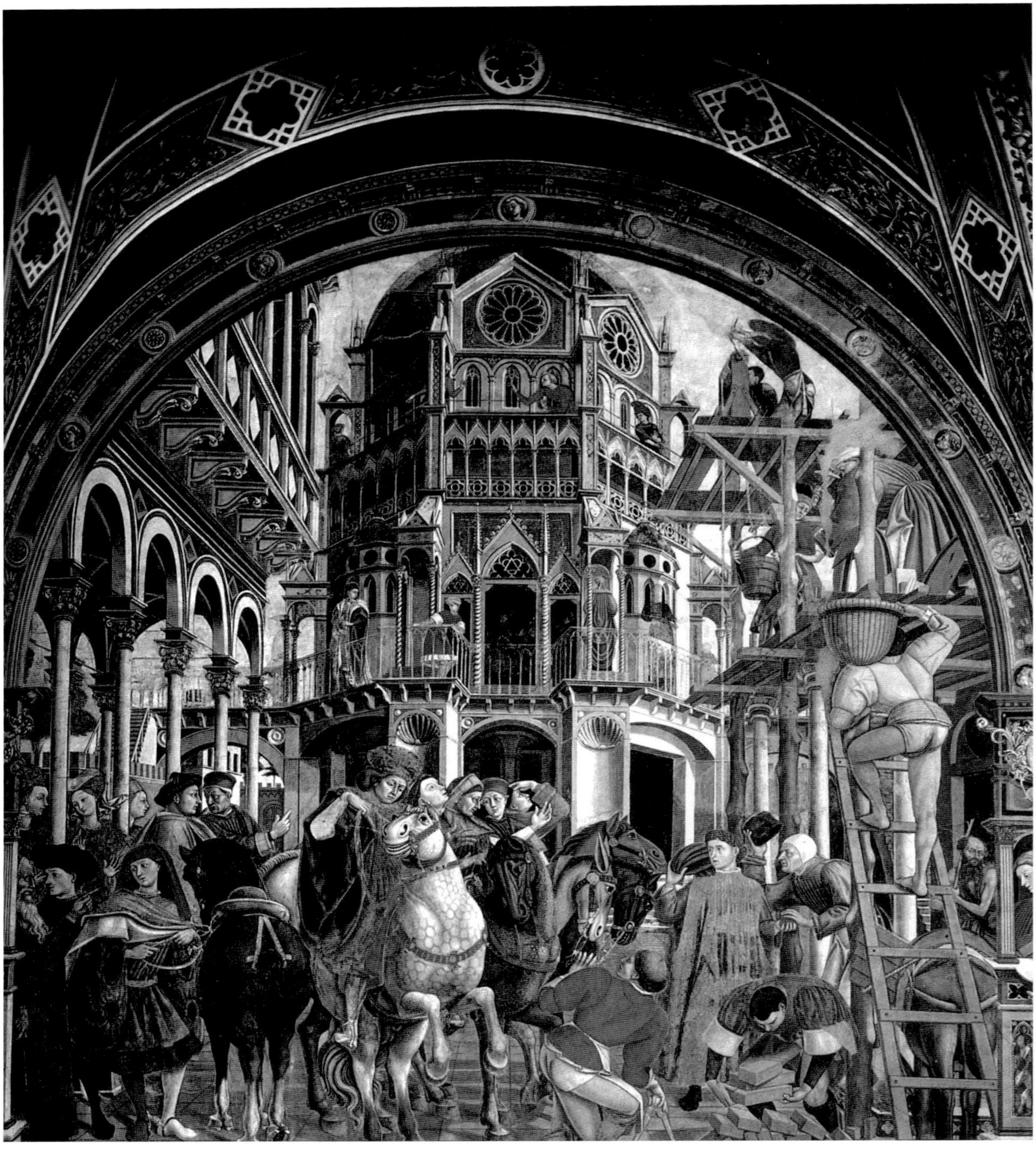

Chapter 6

In Praise of the Occupant

The client pays for a building, although, all too often, meeting the client's wishes on the part of the architect remains an axiomatic proposition. Historically, two precursors to the contemporary outpatient community care clinic, the hospital and the insane asylum, provide insight. The client, usually either a wealthy benefactor or a sponsoring patron "Friends" group, was accorded high status compared to the ignominious status of the lowly occupant—the end user. Then, as now, the paying client seldom, if ever, set foot in the completed building. In a sixteenth century view of the civic preparations for the opening of the new hospital in Sienna, Italy, a painting depicts a collective community effort involving common workers as well as the architect and the institution's sponsoring patrons (Fig. 6.1). This romanticized interpretation of events, while intriguing, is rather misleading. In reality, decision-making was tightly controlled by a select few at the pinnacle of the healthcare power pyramid.

Today, as then, a paying client, that is, an individual, group, or organization that sponsors the services of the architect, often remains disengaged, aloof from the day-to-day realities and peculiarities encountered by the daily occupant—the physician, nurse, assistant, the patient, and the visitor. Paradoxical as it is in many respects, throughout history it has been the rare exception for the paying client, the hospital patient, and the direct caregiver to be the equal focus of the architect. The situation in Louisiana reaffirmed this (Fig. 6.2 and Fig. 6.3). On the questionable status of the user in architecture in the public realm, the British architectural practice collective known as Fat assert:

> The user, like a child, prods the soft underbelly of architectural myth, asks many questions—questions that touch raw nerves, and raise to the surface difficult paradoxes and unpalatable truths. For the user contaminates space and yet is not willing, nor seems able, to partake of the more esoteric debates about what he soils. Lurking within the question of the user is the ugly spectre of elitism and after all, in our . . . age . . . who can afford to be seen as an elitist? A prevailing but useful myth would have it that space is the tool of the architect, that the architect is the manipulator of space . . . this [is based] in numerous conceits . . . that architects manipulate all other determinants outside of ar-

> chitectural space—the spaces of economics, geopolitics, bureaucracy—in other words, precisely those spaces over which architects constantly complain they have no control. In seeking to capture [an] unadulterated architecture via the eradication of its pollutants, the contaminants . . . were also done away with, lest they should leak . . . [in] and thus undermine its purity.[1]

The modernists sought to liberate architecture of the epidemiological impurities of the everyday cultural milieu: the grime, chaos, and vulgarity of the Industrial Age city. In shedding what was then thought to be the restrictive ornamented garb of history, architecture, in the pursuit of a purer formal expression of the Machine Age, sought to purge the user of any contaminating aesthetic influences, unhealthful impurities, and imperfections. The outcome was no less than the cleansing—purification—of the everyday occupant:

> The first of these [problems] assumes that the exclusion of the user from esoteric and therefore, exclusive and specialized debates about architecture, which influence the creation of the environment that the user inhabits on an everyday basis, is a political matter—an issue of power relations between those who create space on their own terms and those who are forced to inhabit it. The second problem is that attempts to address this issue, and which ally themselves to a politics of liberation, tend to locate themselves within a discourse of art, itself a highly specialized and exclusive language. And what of use itself . . . for architecture is peculiar . . . unlike other art forms, it exists not merely as an object of contemplation but is used. . . . [The object] is the basis of the privileged position of aesthetic discourse within architecture and the starting point for the exclusion of the user.[2]

Institutional buildings, and especially large urban hospitals, would increasingly be commissioned by agencies for generic, faceless end-user constituencies. Fiscal or salutary rewards for the architect would be few for paying close attention to the habitual inhabitant compared to the special interests of wealthy patrons, private charities, public councils, and government clients. The day-to-day inhabitant was almost always thought of in the aggregate, with patient and end-user staff representatives on planning committees the rare exception. In the case of hospital architecture, this perverse, medieval-like caste system prevailed throughout the twentieth century.

On the current dismissive connotations of the term user in architecture:

> The word 'user' itself, has moral overtones. It connotes a mercenary practice in human relations and carries undertones suggestive of drug use, and thus intensifies the apparent existence of impurity inferred by the presence of the user. Hence the user is suspiciously perceived as a reprehensible and contemptible character and is treated as such. And, are not the desires and tastes of the user important determinants in the debate which seeks to locate architecture within high culture and which disdains the inclusion of mass or popular culture within its margins? But surely, we architects . . . have the democratic spirit at the heart of our enterprise? . . . [and] as true believers in free speech, can we not bring ourselves to elicit even the slightest whimper. . . . Or would this, in a liberal climate which endorses all kinds of shallow worthiness, contaminate our purest and most heart-felt inclinations?[3]

Architects are notorious for privately castigating their public-sector clients and the end users of their commissioned buildings alike with verbal brickbats, such as "They don't know what they really want, anyway," or "They could not recognize good design if it hit them over the head." Pent-up frustrations become vented in the form of behind the scene inside jokes: "I've shown them ten different designs and they rejected them all," or, "They keep telling me I don't understand their needs, but they are the ones who really need to be educated." Such passive/aggressive behavior is perhaps a topic worthy of psychoanalytic research, and as such is beyond the scope of the present discussion. Nonetheless, here, the psychiatrist would be well advised to begin with questioning the architect's sense of

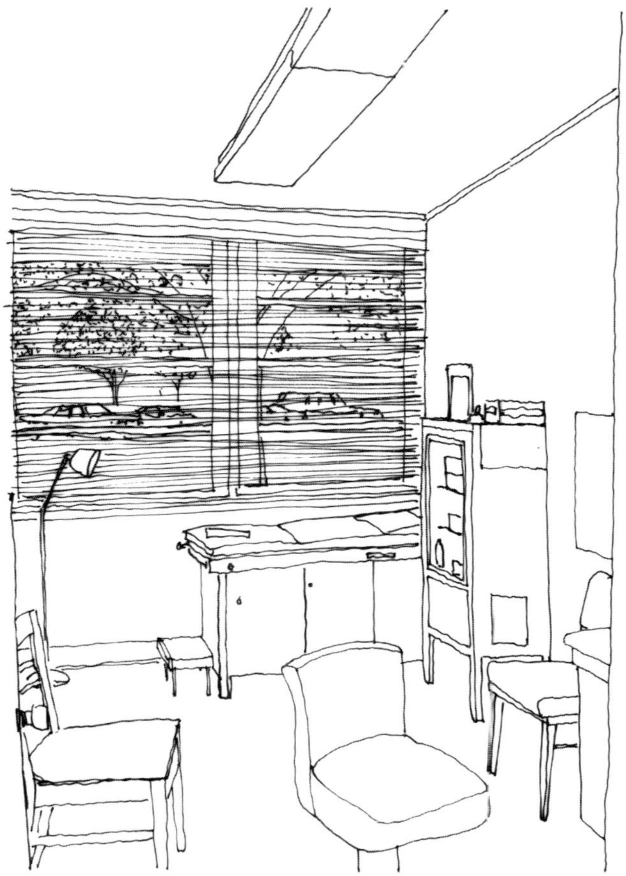

Fig. 6.2

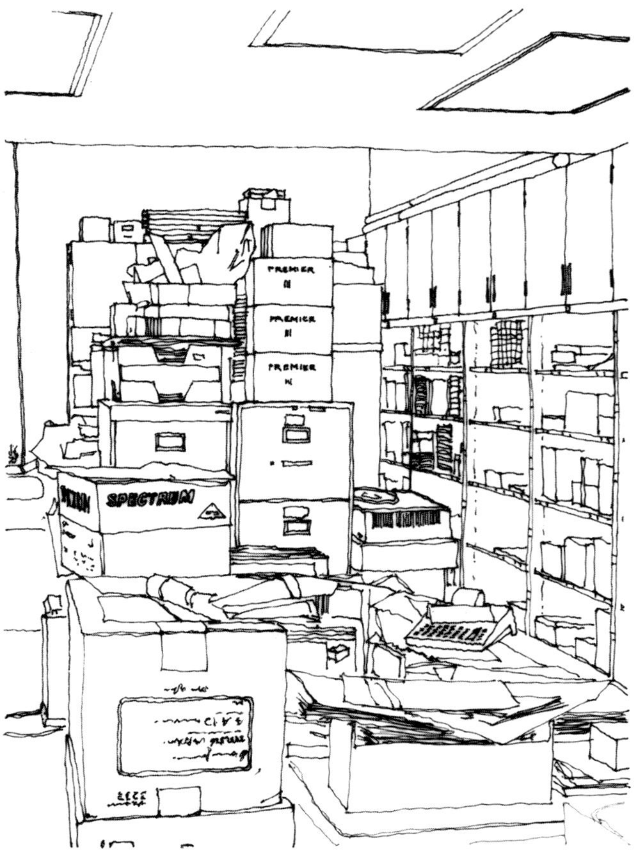

Fig. 6.3

self-worth and how this relates to one's self-sense of proprietorship, control, and influence over one's clients: "Do you think the buildings you create remain *yours or theirs* after they are completed and occupied?," and "For whom are they designed, the person that pays your invoices, or the end users?" The outpatient, especially any recipient of "indigent care," continues to be viewed, unfortunately, as an architectural contaminant of sorts. Therein lies a deeper irony.

Architects deeply engaged in design, in the midst of designing, are experts on distancing themselves from the reality of this so-called user-contaminant. A common method is to simply employ a homunculus—an idealized conception of the end-user-as-inhabitant of the given building when it is completed. This entity exists in the subconscious realm of the designer's mind during the process of design—as iterative, imprecise processes played out in waves of graphic musings sketched on trace paper or as digitally transcribed with a computer. The entity for which one designs is therefore at first abstracted in order to be realized as real persons at a later juncture. Acclaimed, internationally respected architects have openly stated the importance and value of precisely this type of cognitive distancing from the grist of reality, if even momentarily, as essential to their design process and to creativity itself.[4]

In the Machine Age, the end user was reduced to that of functionalist, faceless analog. As passive, purified participant, he or she was subject to the will and whim of the architect and the paying client-sponsor, and the situation in Louisiana reflected this neglectful attitude toward the occupant (Fig. 6.4 and Fig. 6.5). This predilection ran deep: early formulators of modernism, such as Gottfried Semper, argued persuasively for the dominance of the building's formal properties over what (or whom) it was to contain.[5] Later, Le Corbusier argued for the universal acceptance of modernism, cross culturally.[6] Pure functionalism, driven by dictums such as "fitness for purpose equals beauty," however, revealed a deficient comprehension of the full breadth of culture, human behavior, social factors, and vernacular traditions.[7] Hannes Meyer first introduced behavioral science courses to the curriculum at the Bauhaus in Germany in the early 1930s. He taught the topic of housing from a minimalist perspective—as the provision of a basic set of functions: sex, sleeping, eating, dining, personal hygiene, and so on.[8] It would be logical to apply this rationalization to the modern machine hospital. In the megahospitals of the late-twentieth century the habitual inhabitant—be it the patient, nurse, or technician—was thoroughly dehumanized.

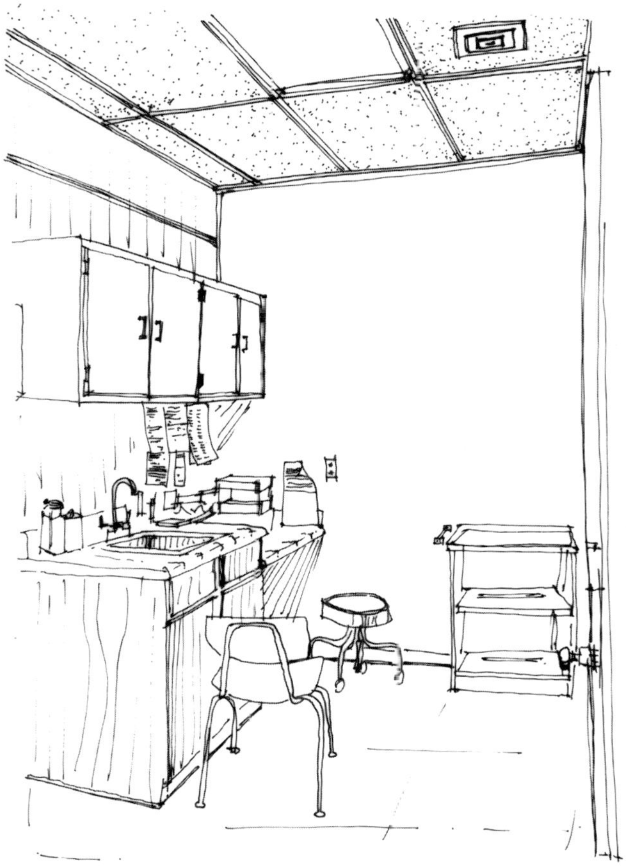

Fig. 6.4

Owen Hardy and Lawrence Lammers, in their influential 1977 book on hospital facility planning, personified this ambivalence toward the value of obtaining grassroots input:

> Internal review of planning documents and design drawings can become an extremely tedious and time-consuming process unless it is handled proper-

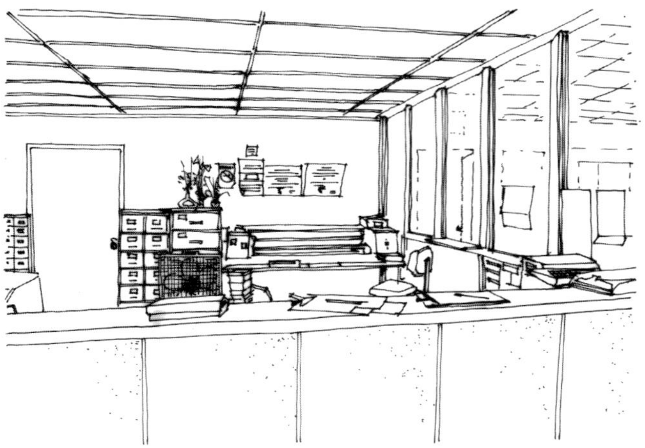

Fig. 6.5

ly. An appropriate review mechanism . . . must be broadened to include certain groups to which no decision-making authority has been delegated. For example, certain user representatives should be asked to review documentation, assess alternatives, and submit recommendations. The decision-making authority relative to those recommendations should be retained elsewhere, with either the director of planning, the building committee, the special user committee, or the governing board . . . it is not necessary to seek out hypotheses regarding needs or functional planning theories from staff members.[9]

Hardy and Lammers further addressed the importance of not questioning too closely the fundamental structure, or rocking the boat, of the top-down political landscape of the megahospital. By inference, it was deemed impractical to consult any patient whatsoever on matters of facility planning or design, as this may somehow contaminate perceptions, cause restlessness among those in the trenches, or set unrealistically high expectations. Anyway, shouldn't the experts already know what the daily occupant wants, what functions best, and what the building is to look like? The situation in public health in Louisiana, at least on the part of parish elected officials and despite the comparatively small role of the buildings, too often personified this attitude of institutionalized indifference (Fig. 6.6 and Fig. 6.7).

In the 1960s, as one urban medical center after another devoured its neighborhood under the dualistic rationalization of medical science expansionism and urban renewal, an alternative paradigm was unfolding in the work of Christopher Alexander.[10] The pattern language he and his students developed opted for people versus users, as in "people like to have gardens" . . . "people need to be able to open their windows to take in fresh air" . . . "buildings with uniform grids of fluorescent overhead light fixtures make people crazy over time" . . . "people need to be able to walk to their nearby neighborhood health center."[11] To him, user denoted a far darker, dehumanized, controlling construct.[12] The New Urbanists, similarly, owe Alexander a debt of gratitude.[13] In architecture, one might conclude that this position would have been long-accepted by now.[14] In reality, evidence-based research and design, as a percentage of the total number of buildings built each year, for health or otherwise, remains outside the mainstream, although in healthcare, this may finally be beginning to change.[15]

The tacit acknowledgement in many influential quarters that modernist megahospitals were failures from a humanist perspective gave rise, in part, to the patient-centered care movement of the 1980s and '90s.[17] More needed to be done to improve buildings planned and built for health.[18] This revisionist attitude and the ongoing spate of large-scale mergers and acquisitions in the for-profit healthcare industry between 1985 and 2000 affected building types of all kinds of scale and complexity, from small outpatient clinics to tertiary teaching hospitals. Because of this, one might expect evidence-based projects to be commissioned on a regular basis by now.[19] In the United States there are now more multi-site outpatient care providers than ever.[20] Evidence-based knowledge of the architectural performance of, for example, a national network of fifty outpatient kidney dialysis centers, or a network of sixty outpatient women's oncology centers located throughout the Southeast Unites States, can undoubtedly provide the client a competitive edge.[21]

Comparative data on the successful facilities provides numerous obvious advantages.[22] If this is the case, why do so few architects support this position in professional practice? Habitual inhabitants are the ultimate benefactors.[23] Urban planners realized their past mistakes in the aftermath of the public housing fiascos in the latter third of the twentieth century.[24] They forged ahead of architects in adopting participatory theories and methods expropriated from the social sciences.[25] Planners also became more actively involved in the consumer rights movement during these years.[26] By contrast, architects, lacking a genuine tradition

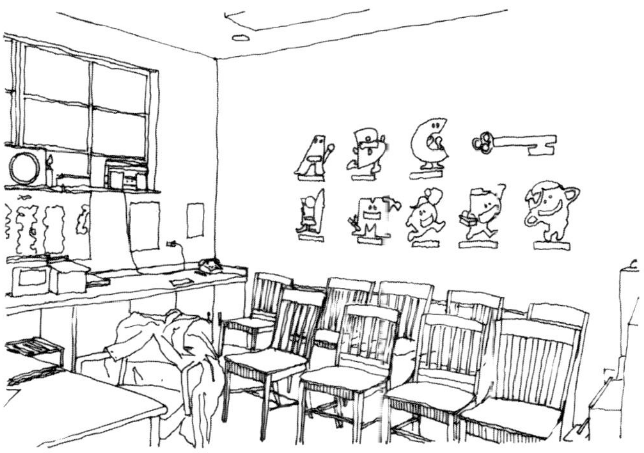

Fig. 6.6

of advocacy or research, for the most part remaineded disinterested in the work of environmental psychologists.[27] The engagement of architects hinges on acknowledging at least these two implicit assumptions:

1. *The primacy of the underserved patient*—Patients, many of whom are medically uninsured, are buoyed by architects' interest in their functional and symbolic requirements in a nation with as many as forty-seven million uninsured persons as of 2005, and with most members of underrepresented minorities. It has been found in nearly every community that patient use/utilization levels increase by approximately 15 percent in new parish health units compared to the old facility. This has occurred even in cases where the new facility was exiled from Main Street to the far edge of town. In some cases, the "halo effect" of the new versus the old has resulted in a 20 percent increase.

2. *The primacy of the care provider*: The evidence-based architect is from the outset more closely attuned to the daily responsibilities of the staff, and their day-to-day requirements. The facility itself is no longer dismissible as a mere commodity on paper within the matrix of organizational management priorities. Moreover, staff, and by inference, patients, are empowered when the architect takes the time to listen to his clients. For staff, the inability to affect change in their workplace/healthplace often results in an environmental docility syndrome.[28]

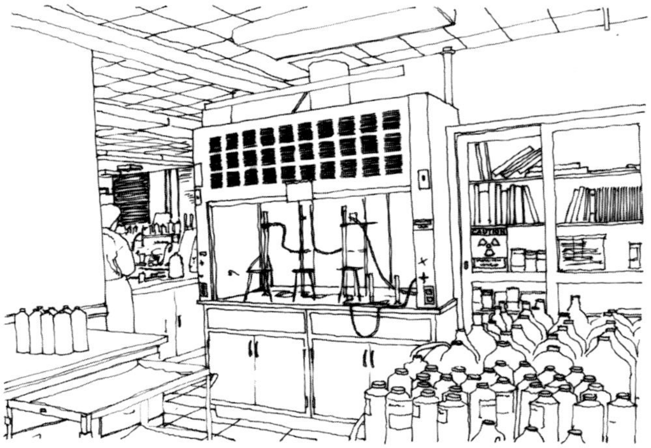

Fig. 6.7

When one believes there is little incentive to improve the way things are done, architecturally or otherwise, or believes that nothing will occur even if they speak up, little changes.[29] Indeed, without incentives for the architect as well as the client and resultant inhabitant, little will change.[30] In an open, competitive marketplace, if it remains acceptable architectural practice to dismiss or sidestep evidence-based research and design, one's competitors will probably thank you in the long run.[31]

When viewed in a broader global context, the theoretical foundation of EBR&D for health remains woefully underdeveloped, even elitist. Market and competitor-driven rationalizations of the value of EBR&D are receiving much attention from the for-profit sector of the U.S. healthcare industry at this time. Unfortunately, the manner in which it has been marketed to healthcare administrators in the for-profit sector tends to skew the focus away from genuine social engagement on issues of cultural diversity. This bias, unfortunately, ignores deeper societal and cultural forces and therefore runs the risk of dismissing more subtle potential interactions between design decisions and their predictive effect upon health outcomes and this is a particularly acute problem in the case of underrepresented monority patient constituencies. In other words, it would be regrettable if EBR&D came to be the sole province of wealthy, privately funded healthcare organizations, such as boutique hospitals. It would be equally unfortunate if it were to consist primarily as the provision of high-end design amenities for wealthier patients. The current dominance of the for-profit sector in the sponsorship of EBR&D threatens to distort the fundamental, initial socio-cultural imperative of EBR&D as it evolved from the fields of environmental psychology and environmental design research in the 1960s. As a result, the real possibility exists that the medically underserved patient will continue to be dismissed. Such narrow market-driven conceptualizations of EBR&D are open to attack on the grounds of being hyper-capitalistic, and in the extreme, culturally hegemonistic. Should the aim be to market this paradigm to healthcare clients as a means for them to increase their profits, as an approach that will, above all, save a hospital millions of dollars? As history has repeatedly illustrated, in the wrong hands, this profit motive can undermine and erode even the best of intentions.

It is naïve to view EBR&D as an autonomous phenomenon, as if disconnected from its historical precursors, or as if cultural specificity or socio-economic equanimity need not be its explicit aims. An example of the latter is the work of Florence Nightingale, who was perhaps the first modern practitioner of EBR&D. Her work with enlisted "commoner" soldiersin the adapted barracks hospital in Scutari, Turkey, in the late 1850s was translated into two seminal texts, *Notes on Nursing* (1858) and *Notes on Hospitals* (1859), and the design concepts presented therein were most certainly based on empirical field-tested evidence. And what of cross cultural interpretations of EBR&D? Virtually no research has been reported on this subject in healthcare settings. Didactic, hegemonisitc models of EBR&D emphasizing an obsessively capitalistic-driven aesthetic run the risk of being branded as elitist, especially as compared to the present situation in less developed nations. The problem lies in blind transference. For example, a carpeted patient room considered to express home-like and residential qualities to an American designer may be dismissed as over-designed to a non-American designer trained in minimalism. As stated, most EBR&D initiatives to date have been commissioned by for-profit healthcare organizations. By contrast, a paucity of EBR&D work has been devoted to the improvement of care settings habituated by the medically underserved. If this is to change, public sector organizations, including government agencies, must enter this arena with both feet, and must provide adequate research funding for systematic EBR&D initiatives. The for-profit sector cannot alone be counted on to advance compassion in healthcare architecture, as this will likely result in the further autonomy of, or worse, trivialization, of EBR&D.

For these reasons, EBR&D is at a crossroads at this time. A theoretical view of an empathic socially-engaged paradigm for EBR&D is presented below as a response to this dilemma (Fig. 6.8). At the base of this diagram are four basic components of an empathic paradigm for the future of EBR&D. The influence of the prevailing political system cannot be ignored. Local, regional, and national political structures provide a framework for the delivery of any healthcare to the members of a society. Neither can the role of technology be overlooked. Medical, architectural, scientific, and product technologies are constantly re-shaping the delivery of healthcare and the settings where it is dispensed. The degree to which a society's citizenry has access to effective care is also a fundamental issue that must not be sidestepped. Cross-cultural determinants are of utmost importance to address and set the global context for the flouirshment of EBR&D in the coming years (Fig. 6.8).

A second tier of concern is the functional imperative, or purpose, for which an EBR&D initiative is created and implemented. This imperative is interwoven with three areas of concern. These consist of a theoretical imperative, a premise which can give rise to a meaningful form-making language. The importance of placemaking, nature, and landscape is essential here, as is the influence of historical precedent. These dimensions vary with a second tier of concerns. This tier consists of the need for the EBR&D initiative to be in full support of sustainable environmental design policies and practices. Related to this concern is the language of materiality in architecture, that is, the palette of materials and objects within a room or building, as these must be of primary concern in identifying the appropriate degree of person-environment fit. Related to this, the acuity adaptability of a given building, department, room, and the elements within a room is endemic to the formulation of an empathic socially-engaged EBR&D initiative. These dimensions of concern relate to the degree of reciprocity between person and setting. As such, these dimensions, taken together with the fist tier foundational concerns, comprise a potentially useful paradigm. Initiatives that are aesthetically enhancing from a design perspective, and life enhancing from the standpoint of human health and well being, represent, in theory, the full realization of EBR&D as such initiatives and outcomes will express compassion, clarity of purpose, and social and medical relevance. In so doing, EBR&D will ethically and responsibly advance architecture and the allied design disciplines for the betterment of society.

Five Points

A building does not just go away when it becomes dysfunctional. It cannot be treated as an old carton of milk or soda can.[32] Neither can an architect's blind adherence to his or her own personalized conception of the homunculus-as-end-user any longer be viewed as acceptable in an increasingly fragmented, pluralistic society.[33] Five points are described below, centered on the primacy of the habitual inhabitant:

1. *Preparation*. Start early. The earlier the architect enters the planning process, the better. Do the necessary due diligence. Do the background homework necessary to ensure the highest quality outcome. Review the literature for new knowledge to be gleaned through case studies. Encourage elected officials, agency administrators, staff and patient care advocates to visit recent comparable facilities.
2. *Participatory Engagement*. Involve all key constituencies from the outset. Do not pay too much attention to any core constituency. Otherwise, resentment, mistrust, and related problems will surface later, possibly with unfortunate ramifications for the project. Embedded in the triumvirate of the end-user patient, end-user staff, and the agency-client is involvement. The specific nature of each constituency's involvement should be clearly defined. For example, a

bleak windowless pre-manufactured steel building cannot be considered acceptable.

3. *Coordination*. In close consultation with key constituencies, select the site, help establish the construction budget, and establish the project scope early on. The architect is then in position to function as the orchestrator, from a concurrent grassroots and organization-wide perspective. Do not allow untrained laypersons, i.e. policy makers or politicians, to ascertain project need or scope. It can be difficult for the architectural team to be brought in after major decisions shaping the building's scope, content, size, budget, site planning determinants, and so on, are a fait accompli.

4. *Commitment*. Attend all key meetings, or send a representative. This insures continuity and reinforces one's engagement and role as a member of the team. Remain cognizant of the shopworn adage, "out of sight, out of mind." Identify advocates at the local community grassroots level who can make your case better than you can, and persevere. In the public sector the layers of bureaucracy and red tape can be voluminous and overwhelming. Take one step at a time, political and otherwise. Monolithic, "fell swoop" all-or-nothing approaches are doomed to failure.

5. *Construction and Performance Assessment*. Each successfully completed project speaks for itself as a symbol of reaffirmation, of a renewed commitment to community health. Build upon successes. Learn from mistakes and missteps. Conduct post-occupancy and facility-management evaluations to assess performance. Establish a track record. In the haste to produce a building the credibility of the architect or facility management specialist will suffer.[34]

Many healthcare organizations and third-party insurers in the United States are recasting the underrepresented patient into the role of a healthcare consumer. As the federal government's Medicaid and Medicare programs, and Social Secutiry, fall under increased scrutiny in order to rein in soaring fiscal expenditures in a rapidly aging America, the term "welfare" has come under attack. Self-anointed elected officials and media pundits speak in vaguely condescending, coded terms of a society of individual stakeholders vested in the virtues of privatization. Meanwhile, as discussed in Chapter 1, the workplace/healthplace, as a humanist construct, is threatened by reductive conceptions of architecture as it relates to facility management:

> The current slippery nature of the term 'user' coincides with its increasing importance. As shifting or multiple and conflicting definitions pervade, and

> as electronic zones exert a greater presence in physical space, the architectural conception of 'user' will be forced to accommodate, negotiating [among] real and virtual identities.[35]

An architect cannot become well versed in the habitual inhabitant's genuine needs and aspirations without meaningfully engaging him or her.[36] Neither can the intermediate users be dismissed, those who pay for the building and who wield control from a policy making, financial, or facility management standpoint.[37] The architect must be equally engaged in environmental advocacy. For example, Leadership through Energy Efficient Environmental Design (LEED) certification through the United States Green Building Council should be a priority.[38] The health administrator must remain cognizant of the time-tested adage "out of sight, out of mind."[39] The time required to plan, design, and construct can be agonizingly slow. Even a fast-track project may take years longer to finish than anticipated. Organizational resolve is prerequisite to surmount political hurdles, staff turnover, and evolving building codes.[40] Evidence-based architectural standards need not be unduly costly, and can yield far more than the mere minimim outcome.[41]

Leaders of state and local public health agencies are well advised to make site visits to recently opened EBR&D-produced buildings before initiating their own capital improvement projects. Agency representatives and local elected officials are equally encouraged to solicit community input.[42] The civic realm and architecture are inseparable.[43] Public health agencies, in this regard, need to become more attuned to architecture.[44] A well-designed facility supports an increasingly informed healthcare consumer.[45] Underserved patients around the globe at the present time receive care in overcrowded, dysfunctional buildings.[46] Despite this, the chronic under-financing of buildings built for public health is only likely to escalate, particularly in communities with chronic health disparities, unless positive programs are undertaken.[47]

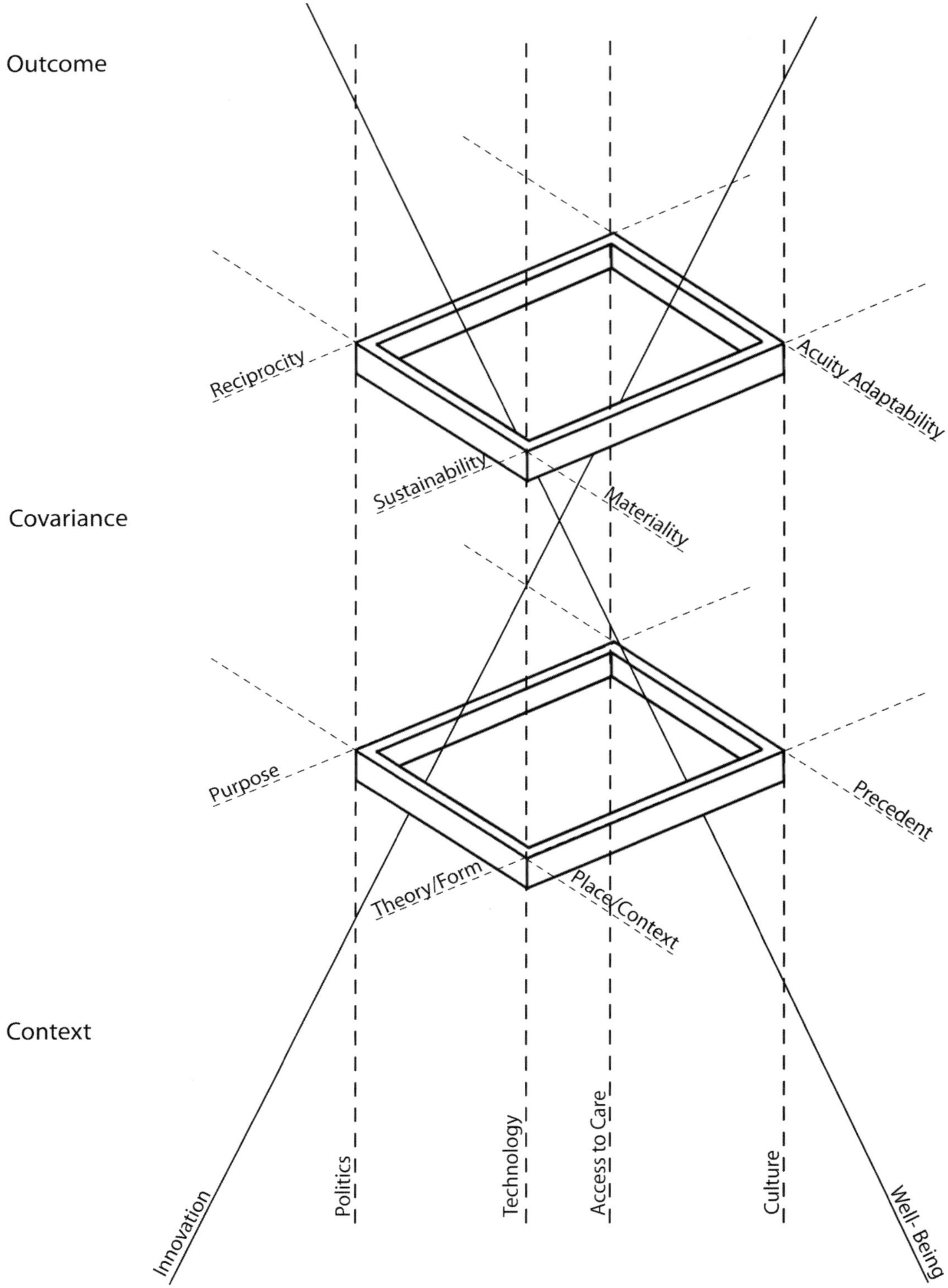
Outcome
Covariance
Context
Reciprocity
Acuity Adaptability
Sustainability
Materiality
Purpose
Precedent
Theory/Form
Place/Context
Innovation
Politics
Technology
Access to Care
Culture
Well-Being

Fig. 6.8

Chapter 7

Compassion as a Professional Concern

> Every day, one, two or three people . . . show up at my bedside to make up the difference between what my insurance company will pay for and the care I truly need. . . . Bone deep, I hunger for life, for love . . . worldwide, faith-wide, race-wide, planet-wide, universe-wide. Love. And peace. And justice. And compassion . . . I am grateful for every manifestation of human compassion. It is a sin to draw lines so that unequal portions are doled out based on dogma or doctrine, gender or politics, ethnicity, or any other artificial division we humans cling to century after century.
>
> *-Delle Chatman, a young mother of a seven-year-old and a victim of cancer, speaking from her hospital bed*[1]

Compassion is fundamental to human existence. The toothless skull of a 1.77 million-year-old homo sapiens recently discovered, deemed that of an elderly male, may attest to our species' oldest known example of human compassion for the elderly and the handicapped.[2] Humans have withstood devastating diseases, epidemics, world wars, totalitarian rule, famine, apartheid, genocide, and catastrophic natural disasters. Brazen, dispassionate rulers, acting with intense hatred and brutality, have left their stain upon the landscape of human history. Despite this, through the centuries, most societies have exhibited the capacity to endure, through acts of compassion expressed through architecture. Architecture is capable of uplifting the human spirit and nurturing the psyche. At its worst, it can exert a deadening effect on human well being, thoroughly denigrating the human condition. Architecture, in the civic sense, has had a somewhat checkered past in America. It has been deployed to perpetuate cultural and social divisiveness, such as the divisiveness that prevailed during the Jim Crow era of institutionalized racism in the American South. Then, public buildings, as discussed in the previous chapters, including all parish health units in Louisiana and throughout the South, were designed with separate entrances, waiting rooms, and restrooms for "coloreds only." Examples abound, but particularly indelible and lasting images include schools, churches, and places of social entertainment.

The relationship between passion and compassion in architecture is complex, timeless, and contradictory. The modernists of the early twentieth century were no less passionate than the persons and institutions who designed and built the great civic edifices of ancient Greece and Rome.

An architect's "signature" style may passionately express compositional elements, colors, materiality, fenestration, the siting of a building, and so on. Passion in architecture can invoke a building's developmental narrative as much as the physical end result. Recent examples are to be found in the self-authored developmental narratives of large-scale civic projects by Norman Foster,[3] such as his Hong Kong and Shanghai Bank (Fig. 7.1) and Frank Gehry, such as his provocatively composed Disney Concert Hall in Los Angeles (Fig. 7.2 and Fig. 7.3).[4] Both architects have become internationally renowned for their use of passionately complex, inventive formal and technical vocabularies facilitated by elaborate computer software algorithms, combined with unorthodox and exotic building materials and construction methods.

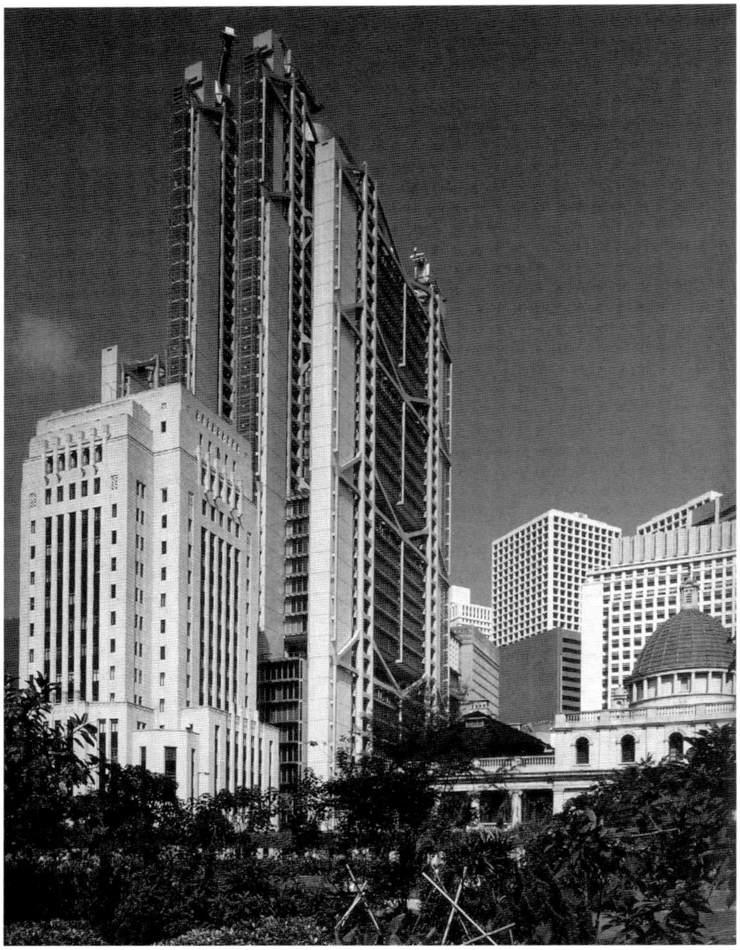

Fig. 7.1

Many a passionately conceived and executed building is upheld for critical praise essentially for its aesthetic or tectonic quotients, not its social engagement quotient. In architectural discourse, compassion is rarely cited as a virtuous attribute per se. Often, by comparison, within

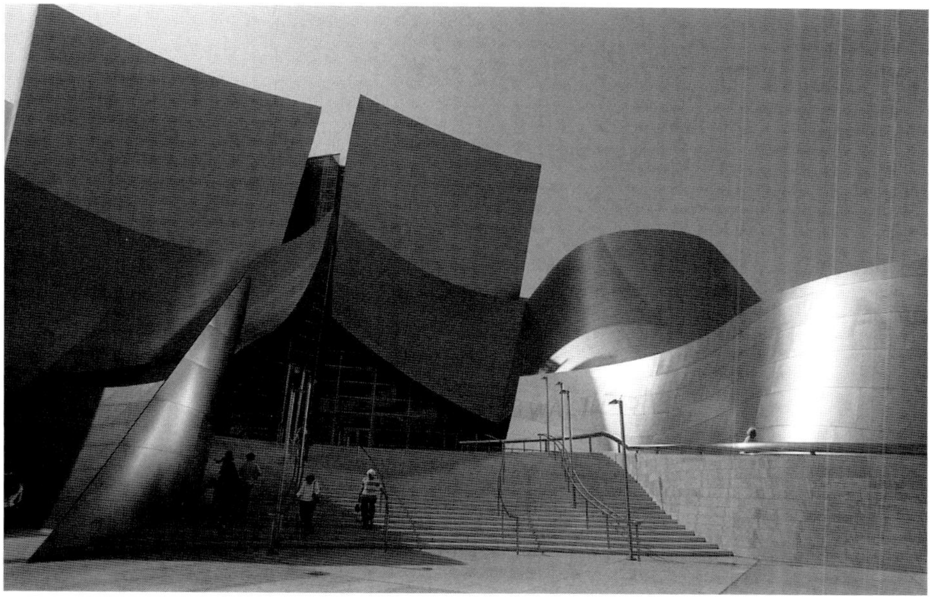

Fig. 7.2

the mainstream architectural press, it seems to matter little if the building explicitly speaks to issues of social empathy regarding groups who are generally disadvantaged or underserved by architecture. The compassion quotient expressed in a building or environment may therefore be glossed over, politely sidestepped, or dismissed outright.[5] *Webster's Dictionary* only obfuscates the nature of passion and how it may or may not relate to compassion in architecture. Webster defines passion as "the state of being subjected to or acted on by what is external or foreign to one's true nature . . . an uncontrollable display of emotion . . . a strong liking or devotion to some activity, object, or concept . . . intense, overwhelming, driving emotion."[6]

By contrast, compassion is defined as far less opaque in nature—"literally, suffering with another; fellowship in feeling sorrow or pity excited by the distress or misfortune of another; commiseration; sympathy . . . deep awareness of the suffering of another coupled with the wish to relieve it."[7] Compassion, by definition, would appear to be subordinate to any salient passionate qualities in a work of architecture. Many of the most enduring civic buildings constructed in history, however, have expressed both sensibilities as a seamless duality in

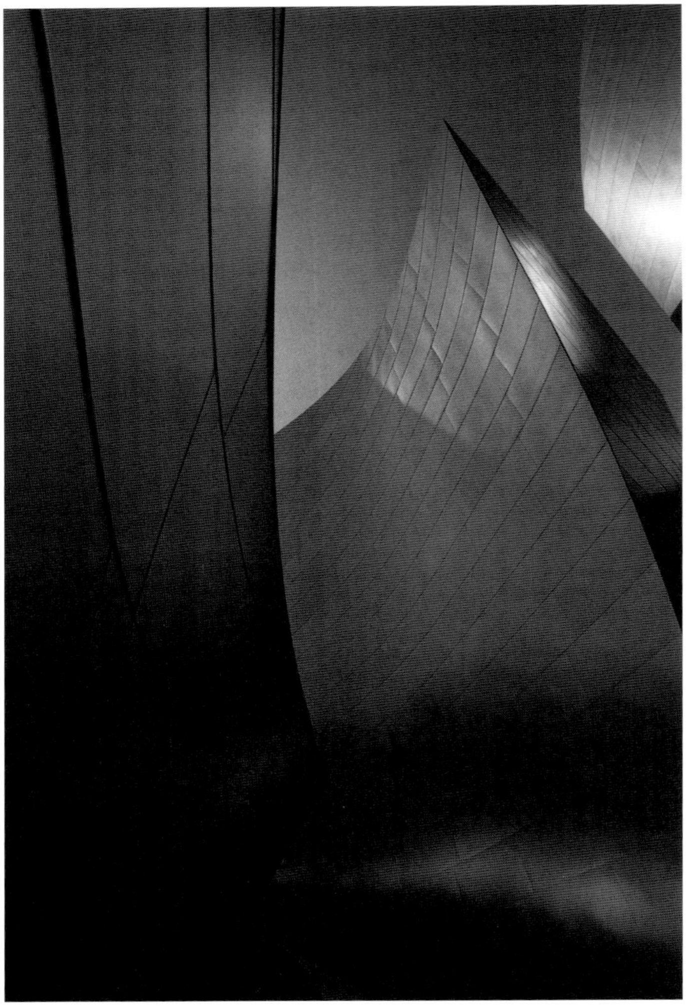

Fig. 7.3

their intent and in formal terms. A building is a cultural investment. But what does recent architecture say about our present cultural condition in relation to compassion? Conspicuous consumption is a predominant trait in American culture and recent surveys indicate Americans are anxious about maintaining their current quality of life. In 2004, unemployment in the United States hit an eight-year high while the savings rate of Americans hovered near zero. States nationwide faced their worst budget deficits in fifty years. In the aftermath of the transformative events of 9/11 an increasing number of employers are outsourcing jobs to overseas markets, and the digital age is radically altering everyday American culture.[8] In architecture, can compassion survive?

Everyday ordinary buildings and places are planned, designed, built, expropriated, celebrated, despoiled, and often eventually discarded. These phenomena have been studied as a function of politics, social class, race, gender, and the "hidden histories" of place and building type, for example, the depravity of Japanese-Americans during World War II in internment camps with scant amenities.[9]

In this sense, architecture expresses the reality of the habitual inhabitant.[11] Empathic architecture, in a social and civic sense, is becoming rare in the ordinary everyday built environment.[12] This is because passion and compassion, in architecture, threaten to become divorced from one another in a dispassionate consumer culture. Most buildings in our everyday lives are banal and lifeless, and this fact cuts to the heart of the problem. Professions generally seek to do good as they define it, often in ways to increase the power, status, and income of their members, through "benevolent professional imperialism."[13] This approach, unfortunately, is not always in the best interest of the client or the end user.[14] Benevolent imperialism is impossible to hide or obscure in architecture. Anything-goes pluralism in popular culture and with respect to what gets constructed in the everyday built environment is a knife that cuts both ways.[15] In the revisionist language of postmodernism, a colorful Lucky Dog hot dog stand in New Orleans' Vieux Carré was ordained as being an equally appropriate subject of critical inquiry as the nearby St. Louis Cathedral.[16]

Milton Rokeach, a sociologist, has described social systems as a series of interrelated hierarchies comprised of personal, institutional, and societal constructs. Personal constructs are unstable and constantly being modified to respond to the ever-changing influences within one's life. Institutional value constructs such as education, religion, and government are more stable in nature and one responds to these societal influences more slowly. The third type, societal value constructs, while being the most stable of the three, are the most deterministic, as they affect both personal and institutional value constructs. In addition, two types of values—terminal and instrumental—exist. Rokeach defines terminal values as being the "end state of existence" such as freedom, equality, self-respect, and security. The value constructs within a society are few, he asserts, perhaps no more than two to three dozen.[17] Instrumental values are defined as the "mode of conduct" we utilize in our quest to attain the terminal values—end states of existence. These values are also relatively small in number, somewhere in the range of three to four dozen. Instrumental values—ambitiousness, broadmindedness, honesty, responsibility, and logic—are more unstable in nature than terminal values and as a consequence are subject to being in a constant state of flux. Rokeach believes these values are determinants of all social behavior, including a group's actions, attitudes, ideologies, moral imperatives, comparisons, and in its attempt to influence.[18] Jay Garrott asserts:

> It is clear that the architect immerses in the societal ambience of value systems in every aspect of his [her] personal and professional existence. He [she] is

> at once a respondent to the value system milieus within which he [she] exists, as well as an influence upon those very same value systems. Consequently, it is in the architect's attitudinal response to this dichotomy . . . that becomes the essential characteristic in determining [the] architect's role . . . two architect role models [exist]—the 'egoist' and the 'pragmatist.' The egoist architect role model is . . . the 'I-give-them-what-I-want' approach to practice, while the pragmatist is attitudinally described as the 'I-give-them-what-they-want' approach.[19]

A third role for the architect, the "I-give-them-what-I-can" modus operandi, is a middle ground, an in-between stance whereby the architect-as-facilitator values both aesthetic autonomy (passion), as well as social engagement, empathy, and equanimity (compassion). The egoist architect characteristically values the former highest and the latter much less.[20] Garrott summarized the egoist's approach as paternalistic, whereby the pragmatist, on the other hand, is essentially entrepreneurial. By contrast, the midpoint perspective (this book's thesis) is that of interpreter, aiming for a nuanced balance between extremes, including the reconciliation of one's own world view with these extremist positions.[21] The accumulated political power and cultural hegemony of the modernist architect (hospital architects included) led to an attitude of dispassion, and, in the extreme, even contempt, toward the public-at-large and especially toward the politically disconnected building occupant.[22]

The Private Sector Bias in Architecture for Health

Specialists in architecture for health have both fueled and perpetuated this dilemma more often than not. Three trends were clearly discernable prior to 9/11. The first might be best described as a loss of social conviction among healthcare architects. Architects have always been quick to proclaim their work is compassionate and caring although in reality such claims soon diminish to clichéd marketing brochure sales pitches. Such overworked clichés, particularly among architects and firms specializing in the area of healthcare, included "high tech/high touch," "user friendly environment," a "caring setting," and so on. More recently, the terms "therapeutic design" and "restorative environments" have been in vogue. Such claims, if unsubstantiated with reliable facts, in the long run actually do a disservice to the profession unless they can be backed up by credible evidence.

A second discernable trend was the hyper-corporitization of healthcare architects, and to some extent, even architectural researchers in this specialized sector of the architectural profession. Many large healthcare clients in the private sector were bought out or merged, and this had a major impact on the way in which architects adapted and competed with one another for plum commissions. In some cases, these firms funded third-party research, although this research often reflected the agenda of its sponsor. On the other hand, clients compared various architectural firms' responses to their RFPs (requests for proposals) and with the firms' track records, with an unusually keen eye on the bottom line. The process widely known as "value engineering" can send shivers down the spines of any healthcare design architect. Every aspect of one's design, from the flooring materials, the shape of the ceiling, the color palette, the fenestration, and virtually every quantifiable design attribute was now subject to the microscopic scrutiny of item by item "value-added" analysis (as opposed to its aesthetic or social engagement quotient) disconnected from either its inherently passionate *or* compassionate virtues within an overpopulated architectural profession, as services were viewed more than ever before as an instrumental commodity to be purchased, procured, not unlike a new washing machine for the hospital's central laundry. The cost of the building "package" was now being equated by clients, at least in theory, with the housekeeping costs incurred in the cleaning of its sheets and pillowcases. Compounding matters, downward pressures on architects' fees in the 1990s, combined with the increasing need to convince the client of the need for more "caring" and "therapeutic" buildings, eventually would have a whipsaw effect of pitting marketing slogans directly against tangibly therapeutic environmental outcomes .

A third unfortunate discernable trend in the waning years of the century was an alarming lack of conviction among healthcare clients and related decision-makers on the value of building high quality architecture for health as a civic investment in the public realm. More and more, decision-makers, and the organizations they represented, appeared to have become complacent, disinterested in the civic quotient of architecture for health in its broader sense. For example, why are so few hospitals LEED certified in the United States? In short, the healthcare industry in the United States was, prior to 9/11, by and large, preoccupied with its own health. Did architects practicing in this specialized sector aid and abet, willingly or otherwise, this trend? In the United States, health care lobbyists on both sides of the managed care debate, for example, reported $230 million in lobbying expenses in 1997 and 1998 alone while as of 2005, an estimated 47 million Americans lacked health insurance.[23]

For the architect practicing in the realm of architecture for health, too little time and creative energy is directed to the actual everyday occupant, the habitual inhabitant. Why? For one thing, too many "healthcare firms" chase only those clients with the deepest pockets, sometimes, neglecting "poorer" clients and fiscally or socially marginalized client constituencies. Second, relatively few architects practicing in this area of specialization proactively engage in shaping public governmental policy to influence the quality of the built environment for health in the civic realm.[24] As a result, a disproportionate share of design investment, including evidence-based design investment, is commissioned by for-profit healthcare clients as discussed in the previous chapter. Case in point: architects working for healthcare clients over the ten-year period from 1990 to 2000 were increasingly obsessed with private-sector corporate clients, evidenced by the projects they submitted to peer-reviewed recognition programs.

In a study conducted by this author of *Modern Healthcare* magazine's annual design awards program, 2,047 submissions were examined over this ten-year period.[25] Of the 149 projects receiving an award or a citation, the fewest awards (only fifteen) were given to public sector governmental client-sponsored projects. The largest number of awards (forty-eight) was bestowed upon private-sector corporate projects. Across the decade a clear upward trend occurred in the number of corporate-built winners, with a corresponding downward trend in the number of not-for-profit public governmental sector sponsored award-winning buildings. Not surprisingly, only eight awards (5.4 percent) were bestowed on publicly financed community outpatient clinics during the entire decade even though the number of such buildings built was rapidly escalating annually nationwide, such as outpatient women's oncology centers and kidney dialysis centers. As discussed in the previous chapter, the challenge for EBR&D for health at this time is to not dissolve into an elitist self-referential area of research and practice. The first and foremost challenge is to expand the scope of concern and expand the range of critical inquiry from the standpoint of attaining excellence in design on multiple levels of use and interpretation.

The Crisis of Disengagement

What is the future of architecture for health in the political realm? In other words, what is the future, in a larger sense, of architecture in the civic realm? A nation benefits from having an extensive and active civil society, and the evidence is mounting in support of the position that citizen participation in our democratic system is on the wane.[26] Americans vote, serve on juries, pay taxes, consume, and work, but beyond these activities, involvement is in precipitous decline.[27] These and other ingrained civic activities generate valuable byproducts, including social trust, political competence, and community spirit. The sociologist Robert Putnam has argued for the re-centering of our collective definition of community in American public life, because the performance of our social institutions are directly influenced by the quality and depth of our involvement as expressed in the norms and networks of our civic engagement in the public realm.[28] This thesis of societal disengagement was captured in his research on the collective and individual loss of "social capital" in contemporary America.

This diagnosis of civic decline, as a cautionary note, speaks to the future risks of a depleted stock of social capital. Americans who came of age during the Depression and World War II were far more deeply engaged in the civic life of their communities compared to the generations that followed. And the empirical database from which he drew his analyses, including studies dating from the 1950s on our use of leisure time, consumer behavior, memberships in organizations, and involvement in local government, point, to a large extent, to a collective loss of confidence in the meaning and authority of civic institutions as enforcers of social and civic norms. This thesis was echoed in the final report of the National Commission on Civic Renewal (1999), which stated, in part:

> On the eve of the twenty-first century, America is prosperous, secure, and free. With lower levels of unemployment, opportunity is expanding. In recent decades, important social movements have helped protect individual rights and have brought long-suppressed voices into our public dialogue. While racial, ethnic, and class divisions persist, we are a more inclusive and tolerant

nation than we were a generation ago . . . but when we assess our country's civic and moral condition, we are deeply troubled . . . political participation is at depressed levels last seen in the 1920s. Public trust in our leaders and institutions has plunged. Never have we had so many opportunities for participation, yet rarely have we felt so powerless.[29]

Critics charge that one very prominent and unpleasant feature of contemporary middle-class morality is a "perverse pleasure in powerlessness."[30] Is the architectural profession part of the problem? In a time that cries out for architects' involvement in the civic realm, we are in danger of, in the words of the National Commission report, becoming a nation of spectators:

> We complain about the influence of popular culture on our young people, but as parents we do try very hard to monitor the programs our children watch and the music they hear. We desert neighborhood organizations and then lament the fraying of community. We elect, and then re-elect, leaders for whom we profess mistrust. We say we do not have time for civic life. But in fact we enjoy more leisure than ever before. . . . And too many of us spend too much of it watching television. . . . Yes, leadership matters.[31]

This view can be directly extended to the architectural profession, as having become a profession of spectators. The unexpected best-selling book *Reinventing Government* (1992), by David Osborne and Ted Gaebler, presented an incisive thesis on the changing role and function of government in society. They critiqued the by-then worn out mentality of 1930s New Deal politics, a mentality so badly outdated that an entirely new paradigm was called for—one in which government borrowed heavily from entrepreneurial ideas and practices in business and industry. They argued that elected officials with the freshest ideas and the ability to transform their ideas into reality were often new to public service. Many were young; many had previous careers as journalists or business leaders, or as social activists. This gave them a freshness and vitality previously woefully lacking in the vast majority of career politicians.

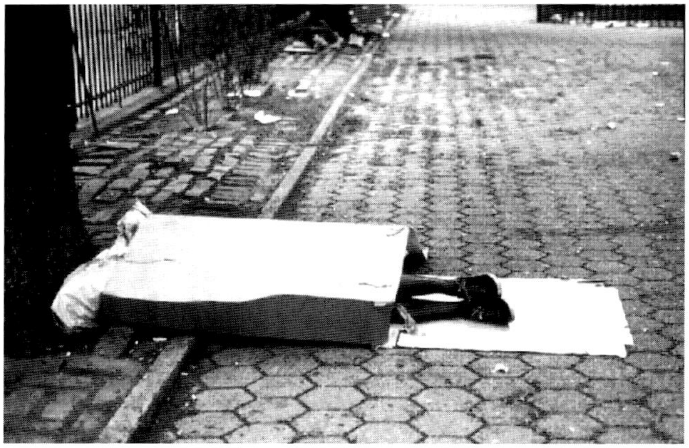

Fig. 7.4

Their book contained many examples of this thesis, drawn from all levels of government, local, state, and federal.[32]

As a nation too much emphasis is placed on presidential politics and the politics of national government, with too little attention given to local government. Elected political leaders now act like their corporate counterparts, having become the public sector equivalent of private sector entrepreneurs.[33] Leadership became a buzzword in the 1990s. Leadership, however, is quite different from managerial acumen: Leadership engages followers in the joint pursuit of mutually agreed upon goals. These goals represent significant, rather than merely incremental change. By contrast, managerial acumen centers on the ability to get the trains to run on time.[34] Result: The image of the ideal political leader has converged with that of the ideal business leader.[35] Meanwhile, in Louisiana, a legacy of unbridled political corruption continued.[36] A brain drain ensued, as 140,000 residents left the state between 1990 and 2000, and politicians surreptitiously profited from the healthcare system in Louisiana.[37] By 2000, the state had the largest percentage of children living in poverty of any state in the United States, and the second highest percentage of persons uninsured.[38] Nationally, the public health system was being challenged in the face of epidemiological, population and management crises.[39] This requires rapid, ethical, empathic responses.[40]

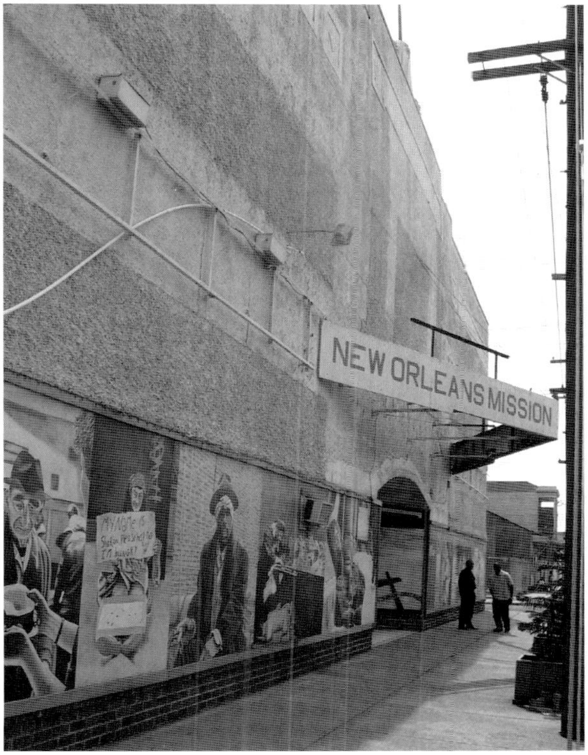

Fig. 7.5

Architecture and Civic Well Being

It is well-documented that the construction of public housing ghettos in American cities in the latter half of the twentieth century was a failed experiment in social engineering. Although initially conceived as utopian, even compassionate, by the 1960s these places had dissolved into dystopian, crime-infested slums. Highly unsafe housing projects epitomized the failure of dispassionate public policy.[41] Since, social programs for the poor and the homeless have struggled for decades with the question, "Where should the poor live?" Many social theorists have viewed the poor as deviant, arguing that they elect to pay little or nothing for housing. Further, they blame poor persons' imprudence, lack of judgment, and outright ignorance for their inability to afford adequate housing. The belief that the poor do not value housing in the same way as the middle class ignores the fact that the poor have much less income and therefore vastly fewer options to choose from. With less income, a poor person is not able to make the same choices as is a middle-class person.[42] The growth of an underclass which is systematically denied access to the political and economic mainstream continues to rise. This rise in poverty is due in large part to the growing discrepancy between rental rates and incomes.[43] As the present political structure disproportionately favors individuals and families with higher incomes, significant income improvement among the poorest classes is the only way to actually end the present housing crisis in America, although this prospect remains remote at best.[44]

The rebalancing of compassion and passion in architecture is urgently needed in a manner that strives to eradicate the sense of fear and uncertainty in the built environment. The New Orleans Mission provides job training for hundreds of persons each year (Fig. 7.4). Homelessness is the result of a convergence of many factors (Fig. 7.5).[45] The homeless elderly are one segment of the underserved population who are particularly inattentive to matters of self-health and sickness prevention, counseling, and related social support services. They tend to be particularly susceptible to unresolved psychological problems that lead to anger, guilt, pain, regret, isolation, and low self-esteem. In many cities, hostels and shelters accommodate homeless persons of all ages, but it has been learned in the United Kingdom and in America that many older people, and women, will not use the facilities for fear of violence and intimidation from younger, male residents. A few service providers in Europe and elsewhere have therefore developed hostels specifically for older homeless people. These have included the Zambesi Project, in Birmingham (United Kingdom) which provides housing for persons aged forty-five and older in several interconnected houses with a twenty-four-hour support staff. Since 1986, the Dwelling Place in

Washington, D.C. has provided well-designed accommodation for those aged sixty or older in single rooms.[46]

The Committee to End Elder Homelessness (CEEH) was established in Boston in 1991 by a group of professional women who were committed to eliminating homelessness among older persons in the city. Housing and social assistance is provided at four sites throughout the city to persons over age sixty who are homeless or at risk of being homeless. The objective, both socially and architecturally, is to promote independence and a sense of community among residents, many of whom were considered "unhousable."[47] A not-for-profit company in Melbourne, Australia, provided a high-quality architectural environment for elderly homeless men in aesthetically sophisticated residential care facilities. In setting a new standard of housing for the homeless aged in Australia, this initiative has received international acclaim, in part for its expression of traditional Australian vernacular architecture, which older people relate to postitively. This residential campus has six houses, each providing a home for five to seven men. [48]

In New York City, a record 37,000 homeless persons slept in city-sponsored shelters as of October 2002—this number had risen from 21,000 in 1998. The city's commissioner of services for the homeless at the time proposed that retired luxury cruise ships be purchased by the city for use as homeless shelters. Homeless advocates immediately attacked the plan as outlandish and unnecessary, demanding the city instead provide affordable permanent housing.[49] Other countries are working on promising housing solutions in a more compassionate manner. In Senegal, West Africa, architect Nader Khalili's vision of a city for the homeless built with sandbags and wire could become a reality. The government of Senegal wants to build a town of roughly 20,000 houses using his innovative design for bee-hive-shaped adobe dwellings.[50] Meanwhile, the the United States in 1999, students of a UCLA urban planning course constructed a small city sleeper structure, using only found materials. The professor who directed the project said the goal was to "get them to know how it feels walking in someone else's shoes." One student found a sturdy, wooden museum shipping crate and wrapped it in plastic.[51] These exercises, however, tend to be more patronizing than compassionate in their intent and subsequently have had very little impact.

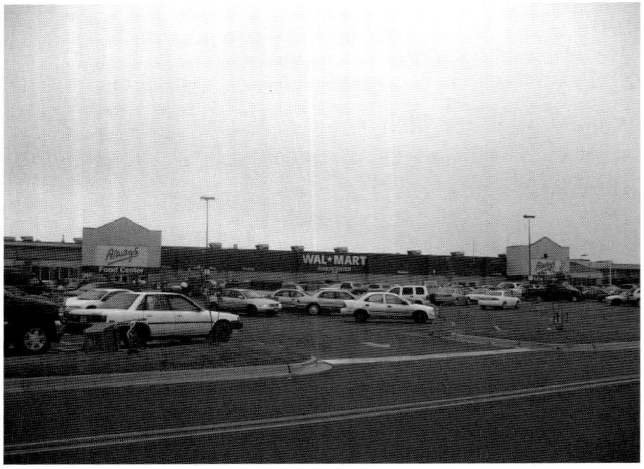

Fig. 7.6

In Japan, Shigeru Ban's "Community Dome Project" provided a meeting place for victims in the aftermath of the severe dislocation caused by the Kobe earthquake in 1995. Architectural interventions in the wake of natural disasters have become a high profile issue, especially in light of the 2004 Indonesian tsunami. Regretably, architects around the globe, however, have been slow to adopt a leadership position in this area of concern. Conferences have produced useful publications on the topic of transportable architecture.[52] These efforts focus attention on the emergency shelter needs of victims of earthquakes, floods, hurricanes, tornadoes, avalanches, severe drought, and more recently, terrorist attacks.[53] The International Red Cross and the Pan American Health Organization have published reports on disaster mitigation shelter needs.[54] Are practicing architects listening? Are the community-based architeectural schools listening? A prototype design for an HIV/AIDS mobile health clinic has been developed by the Architecture for Humanity organization.[55] Government-sponsored programs to build flood-responsive housing in Bangladesh have been only somewhat successful to date.[56] Critics charge that too little planning and architectural research work on this topic is being funded at present.[57]

A newfound balance between compassion and passion is equally needed with respect to the function and architecture relative to management of the earth's finite and non-renewable resources. For decades now, the chronic dispassionate treatment of the earth has been well documented as having deleterious environmental consequences, including the depletion of fresh water supplies, deforestation, and potentially, long-term climatic change. Suburban sprawl, meanwhile, remains largely unchecked. Each year, the equivalent of many moderately sized cities are constructed on previously open, undeveloped land, but the parts represented by these new communities do not add up to anything of lasting meaning. These developments remain little more than loose aggregations of uncoordinated parts. Zoning laws, many obsolete, virtually guarantee an outcome characterized by a gangling array of meandering, overburdened roadways and diffuse relationships between buildings. This condition is avoidable if the basic ingredients—the houses, commercial establishments, office centers, civic institutions, and roads—are assembled in an architecturally more intelligent manner.[58] Alternatively, compassionately planned and built communities share certain timeless attributes. These include a clearly defined center, short walks via pathways from one's work or residence to the center, a pedestrian scaled street network, narrow versatile streets which promote human interaction, mixed land and building uses, and the setting aside of "landmark" sites for civic buildings, including places for health.[59]

Unlike the traditional neighborhood model, which evolved organically, sprawl is a dispassionate artificial system, itself unsustainable. Unlike the traditional neighborhood, sprawl is not healthy growth: it is essentially self-destructive. It consumes land at an alarming rate, while producing insurmountable traffic problems and exacerbating social inequity and isolation.[60] In Japan, architectural sprawl is practically nonexistent because 90 percent of the population is able to live on only about 10 percent of the nation's land area. Unfortunately, unsustainable public policies in the United States are the rule rather than the exception.[61] Recently, suburban politicians have begun to build careers by attacking the sources of sprawl and advocating intelligent, smart growth policies.[62] Conservative majorities at present populate many so-called commuter communities.[63] It is paradoxical, however, to vote to build more roads while espousing anti-growth sentiments.

Megastore discount chains, led by architecturally and environmentally dispassionate Wal-Mart, have only exacerbated the architectural sprawl syndrome. Wal-Mart's influence on the United States economy has reached levels not seen by a single company since the nineteenth century rise of Standard Oil.[64] Its massive, unsightly stores sprawl across open

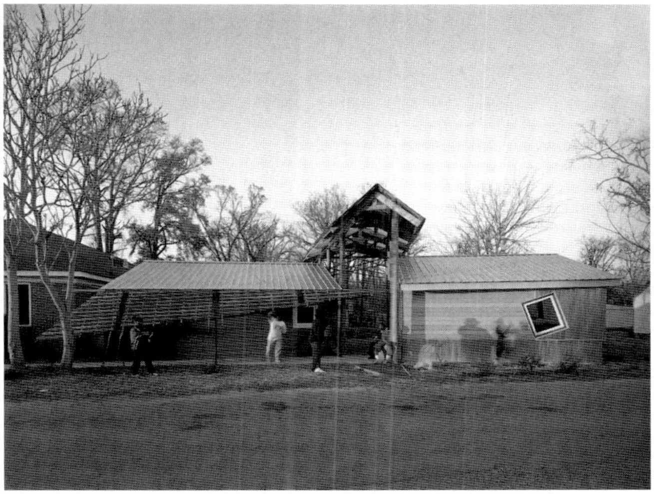

Fig. 7.7

farmland at an alarming rate. At the same time, the giant's fierce competition and relentless price wars are decimating architecturally historic town centers. In terms of facilities, the expansionism of the company's stores from first generation Wal-Marts into metamorphosed Super-Wal-Marts is having deleterious consequences both environmentally and socially, with many unanticipated consequences on the quality of life. In town after town, the opening of the local Wal-Mart on the town's fringe signals the end of its Main Street (Fig. 7.6). Will the local Wal-Mart become the new civic hub, or the new civic attraction, to the detriment of formerly prominent places such as the town's movie theater? Long before Wal-Mart began to dismantle rural American downtowns, the American movie palace was little different from the parish health unit of the 1940s and '50s, also on Main Street. Each served an important civic function. Architecturally, both contributed to the civic and architectural fabric of the town.[65] In Louisiana and elsewhere in America these places are being reclaimed, with the help of architects, as performing arts centers.[66] In New Orleans, the former Carver Theater is now a community care clinic.

Historic preservation programs in Louisiana and elsewhere can take a leadership role in compassionately documenting meaningful historic buildings for the Historic American Buildings (HABS) survey. HABS drawings document endangered buildings across the everyday cultural landscape.[67] This is nothing new, however. Edicts to protect old buildings date as far back as Emperor Majorian, in 458 CE Rome, and ever since have been in harsh contrast with the unrelenting forces of commerce, war, and dispassionate development.[68] Preservation versus demolition decisions must be based on common sense, integrity, and the compassionate balancing of practical needs with the preservation of heritage as "social capital."[69] American building contractors, not known for acting particularly compassionately towards the environment,[70] are also starting to rethink their role with respect to their compassion towards the environment.[71]

Architectural Education and Civic Life

The Design/Build Studio, as a pedagogical model, has emerged in the past five years as a popular tool for fostering social and civic engagement in the architect. It converges passion and compassion in architecture. The Rural Studio, founded by the late architect and educator Samuel Mockbee, is perhaps the most well known. Mockbee worked and taught architecture in one of America's poorest rural settings. His leadership of the Rural Studio at Auburn University, and the students' projects, centered in Hale County, Alabama, resulted in the design and construction of nearly thirty projects. Completed work consists of houses, civic centers, a chapel, a children's center, parks, play fields, a farmer's market, a community theater, and a boys and girls' club.[72] Andrea Oppenheimer writes:

> When Mockbee founded the Rural Studio in the early 1990s, American architecture had retreated from social and civic engagement to a preoccupation with matters of style. The architectural stars, swept up in the new global economy and entranced by new technologies, were designing increasingly ambitious buildings for affluent clients worldwide. Mockbee instead was digging in at home in the Deep South, focusing on the design and construction of modest, innovative houses for poor people. . . . Naïve as it may sound, Mockbee, a MacArthur 'genius grant' recipient in 2000, is battling for convictions. One is that the architectural profession has an ethical responsibility to help improve living conditions for the poor. Another is that the profession should 'challenge the status quo into making responsible environmental and social changes . . . (and) to sowing a moral sense of service to the community.[73]

Gradually, the Rural Studio inscribed its mark on the ordinary everyday landscape of Hale County. The studio designed and built inexpensive, striking structures made from inexpensive salvaged or donated materials. Mockbee presented architecture as a discipline rooted in civicness. In his words, he told his students "as architects their goodness was more important than their greatness, their compassion more eventful than their passion."[74] The Hero Children's Center, completed in 1999, is operated by the Hale County Department of Human Resources (Fig. 7.7). The department's family resource center, district court and district attorney office, police department, and the county sheriff's department for examining use it and evaluating children suspected of abuse. A playground is adjacent.[75]

The Rapid Response Design Studio pedagogical model presents a second kindred option for re-engagement with the needs of communities. It is premised on studios devoted to pressing needs in the community where the school is situated. In the aftermath of 9/11, the design studio continues to occupy a position of centrality and prominence in the nation's architecture schools. Rapid response implies a proactive, anticipatory stance and a willingness to address a pressing external issue. The digital age is characterized by relatively long periods of dramatic change punctuated by brief periods of constancy. This cultural state is defined as punctuated chaos—constant upheaval marked by brief respites. In light of this, too many architecture schools appear to be afraid too break out of static, time-tested, normative (conservative), studio teaching formats.[76] Perhaps a pro bono fieldwork residency should be required of every architecture student.

On the fractured relationship between clients and architects, Sarah Goldhagen writes:

> Even when clients have the basic knowledge to choose quality architecture and inspired urbanism, they are often reluctant to do so . . . architects and urban designers have earned the public image, not always unfairly, of being impractical, ego-driven money spenders . . . [those] who maintain credibility with corporate and public clients have often done so by acceding to their conservatism, thereby sacrificing social responsibility, aesthetic innovation, and sometimes just plain good judgment to expedience, the familiar, and the bottom line. Thus, they have created a blander, poorer architectural and urban landscape, setting low aesthetic standards that further reinforce the disinclination of governmental and corporate clients to create good, let alone great, architecture.[77]

Goldhagen asserts that postmodernism's influence, as reappraised in the aftermath of 9/11, has had both positive and negative consequences for the learning and the practice of architecture. This is because certain core assumptions have rendered it problematic to envision what values the civic realm should ideally express. And, as discussed in Chapter 2, Foucault's observations have influenced many influential intellectuals who subscribe to postmodernism's pluralism, a position its critics maintain as inherently nebulous, in assuming that all institutions, even when administrated by well meaning individuals, or, in Goldhagen's words, "agents," are "structured to dominate in insidious ways." She asserts that this condition makes it very difficult for architects to take a positive/positivist (compassionate) stance, toward government, civicness, and commercial bastions of power. It is these institutions, nonetheless, which remain perceived as the embodiment of the harbingers of selfish, self-sustaining, unbridled financial gain at any social cost, and the accumulation of raw power, whether resulting in fiduciary corporate gain, bureaucratic gain, or both.[78] The truth remains that it is difficult to design compassionately when one believes the institution one is designing for is harmful to society.[79]

THE FUTURE

A growing chorus of critics claim that American culture is experiencing a decline similar to the one that afflicted and finally extinguished Rome. Frequently cited indicators of this malaise include low literacy rates, political apathy, cynicism, spiritual alienation, eroded civility, rampant consumerism, and the rise of global corporate hegemony on the part of American corporations. These forces are viewed as exerting a suffocating effect on our intellectual aspirations and abilities, hypnotizing Americans with kitsch, gadgetry and placid mass entertainment. This corporate hydra, exported internationally, has been dubbed McWorld.[80] Morris Berman takes this view further, as tantamount to the coming of a new Dark Age. In this even, new monastic individuals will be entrusted to preserve our learning and critical thinking, our humanistic habits of mind, our refined and beautiful ideas, our arts and sciences, ethics, and virtues, before they are completely eclipsed or extinguished.[81] Contemporary America is the most affluent, wasteful society in history. In point of fact between the year 2000 and 2020 Americans between ages thirty-five and fifty-three will inherit $12 trillion from their parents. In what way will the benefactors opt to reinvest this accumulated capital? Will self-interest rule? Nothing of this financial magnitude has ever occurred—in this society or any other.[82]

But what good is it to extend the quantity of life if its quality will be significantly diminished? Harry S. Dent, Jr. writes of quality of life changes in the cultural landscape of the twenty-first century:

> The prosperity of the coming decade and new communication technologies are going to make new lifestyles possible well before and into your retirement . . . our life expectancies have made tremendous gains over the last century, more than at any other time in history . . . people who live longer learn more, earn more, spend more, and contribute more. The average life expectancy is expected to have been around 22 to 25 for most of biblical times forward. It started rising in the 1700s, moving toward 35 by 1800 and then to around 47

> by 1900. Then in just one century it advanced 30 years! . . . the coming wave of genetic technologies is likely to cause another wave of faster expansion . . . this would occur from around the 2010s into the 2060s and our life expectancies could advance toward 110 to 120.[83]

We aren't just living longer, but the quality of our life and health into older age ranges has been improving and yet questions arise as to whether this can continue.[84] The question remains, for whom? Will everyone share equally in a "higher" quality of life in the face of this upwardly spiraling age trend? Will society be able to afford a healthcare system where everyone equally reaps the benefits of new forms of medical care? Will everyone have access to routine full body CT scans?[85] Of course not. Health disparities will persist as long as global access to healthcare resources remains disproportional, geared towards the "haves." Most indicators point to the stark reality that health disparities between the haves and the have-nots portend to only increase, magnifying, worsening the quality of life gap between the classes. The risk is that the under classes will become further marginalized, only now across a longer lifespan than ever before.

Medical costs are once again rising rapidly, and the U.S. healthcare system is on the verge of a crisis. Yet other advanced countries manage to spend much less than the United States while getting better results. In 2002, the latest year for which comparable data are available, the United States spent $5,267 on healthcare for each individual patient. Of this, $2,364, or 45 percent, was government spending, mainly through Medicaid and Medicare. Canada, alternatively, spent $2,931 per person, of which $2,048 came from the government. France spent $2,736 per person, and the government financed $2,080. Despite this, Americans have a substantially lower life expectancy and higher infant mortality rate than most advanced nations. The United States scores high on expensive high-tech equipment, such as MRIs and CT scanners, but on more fundamental measures—physician visits and in-hospital stays—America is average or below average. There is also growing evidence that the same diagnostic or surgical procedure costs far more in the United States than in many other countries.[86]

Architects are not alone in the need to soul search. The medical profession has been engaged in its own brand of soul searching. Medical schools and the health sciences professions have come under fire recently for physicians' insensitivities in their interactions with their patients and with patients' families. One such recent study sought to identify personality traits common to physicians considered to be compassionate and empathic in their practice. It was found that although these attributes are desirable they are not essential in order for one to rise within the professional hierarchy.[87] The function of compassion in community-based family practice physicians has also been studied. It was concluded that many more public-private partnerships will be needed in the coming years in order to overcome persistent inadequacies in the provision of quality healthcare to the indigent and the uninsured.[88] The practice of discrimination remains prevalent against Chinese-American patients in outpatient clinics. This was concluded to be the result of the lack of compassion on the part of the "majority culture" care providers who staff these clinics.[89] Medical schools now realize that inculcating the ethics of compassion in future physicians requires coursework on the history of the ethics of caring in past societies.[90] Should architecture schools do the same? In the field of community psychiatry, the budget cutbacks of the 1990s led to a documented shift in the public's attitude, one of increasing indifference, toward mental healthcare.[91] A parallel occurred in architecture with the closure of community design centers that were operated by architecture schools in the 1960s and early '70s. This led to sharp decline in architecture schools' pro bono community work, as the schools became seduced by postmodernist theory.[92] In both cases, these empathic interventions died for lack of funding.[93] Against this backdrop, two questions come to mind:

1. Is the discipline of architecture up to meeting the challenge in the new millennium to exhibit compassion for the less fortunate?
2. Is the discipline or architecture capable of overcoming self-defeating, internal turf wars, ideological and otherwise, to aid a society sorely in need of its knowledge and expertise?

Stanford Anderson, writing on the preponderance of theoretical discourse at the expense of learning about the making of buildings, concluded:

> Architecture has turned in on itself—or worse, on a limited vision of itself. It is time to 'reground' architecture. There may be many ways to give substance to this notion of regrounding, but we may start with a few recognitions: Ar-

> chitectural production is political. The position of architecture within the remarkable world of political events of today demands attention, even as it must also be seen within the current inane political condition of America. We must reinvigorate the knowledge of making. Attention to architecture as politics, as physical and cultural environment, and as materiality are three of no doubt many ways to move out of the seductive but finally arid autonomy of architecture. . . . In that awareness [resides] . . . a non-elitist and socially engaged discipline.[94]

Compassionism is a both/and, not either/or condition. It must be simultaneously grounded in design innovation as much as in the well being of the community. It must be both utopian and pragmatic. It is about doing good, including through pro bono work, for its intrinsic as much as its fiduciary rewards.[95] Of course, entities such as the judicial system and the labor market control our daily lives, and these systems are mediated for us, three-dimensionally, by architecture. Breaking the code of dispassion in architecture, as mediated and presently controlled by these systems, is tantamount to decoding the underlying structure of an empathic society.[96]

A 2005 editorial essay by Robert Ivy, "It's in the Air" in *Architectural Record,* noted that a new movement in community-based design is emerging, or, in his words, "blossoming" once again. It is a trend not seen since the 1960s, and newfound interest among architecture students in community engagement is putting designers in direct contact with real clients and real contexts, often away from the isolation of the college campus. A number of organizations are now devoted to the mission of bringing architecture, via students' active social engagement, to people and places heretofore dismissed by most architects.[97]

Compassionism is as much about concern for human well being as concern for the well being of the planet. In America, a new civic zeitgeist is needed in architecture, transcending formal aestheticism as a Ground Zero condition in the societal dislocations caused by 9/11. Similarly, dislocations caused by environmental degradation demand no less. The challenge for architects is to make legible, coherent, and rationally transparent the fundamental meaning of the institutions, politics, and social values at the heart of civic life without the individual falling prey to Foucault's thesis of cynical antiauthoritarian detachment. In point of fact, since the mid-eighteenth century, politically driven power relationships have spawned virtually every new institutional building type, healthcare notwithstanding. This typology eventually was transposed into corresponding modernist dogma.[98] The same threatens to occur with regard to postmodernist dogma. Architecture is a stage for highlighting that which is wrong as much as that which can be righted. Individuals and groups who experience quality of life and health disparities in America deserve attention. Do something.

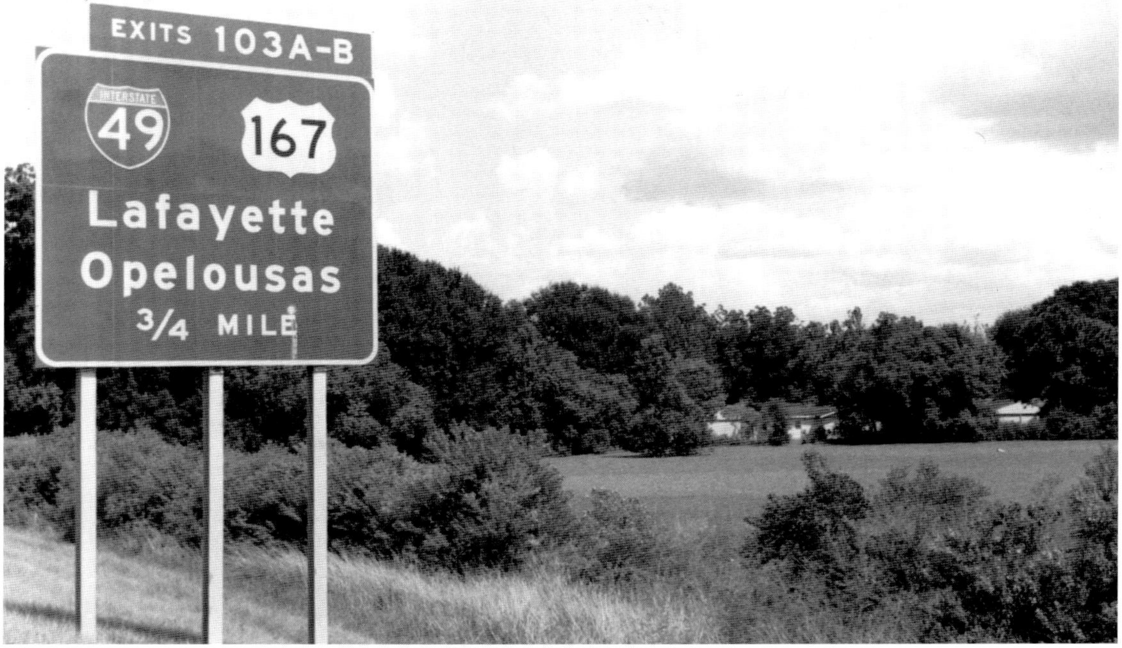
EXITS 103A-B
INTERSTATE
49
167
Lafayette
Opelousas
3/4 MILE

APPENDIX A

ORIGINS OF THE BUILDING TYPE, 1800-1945

New Orleans' port was the main source of the many diseases that plagued the region from its earliest days as a European outpost. New Orleans was the region's first urban center. Doctors soon discovered that many outbreaks followed the arrival of ships from Havana and Central American ports, where yellow fever, in particular, was rampant. In 1804, Gov. William C. C. Claiborne lost his wife and a daughter in an epidemic. His second wife died when the disease hit again in 1809. The situation in New Orleans and the surrounding region was one of near panic from a public health standpoint:

> As the population of New Orleans grew, the toll became higher. A popular, and in a way logical, explanation for the recurrence was the utter filth of the city. Visitors called it the most unsanitary urban area in the country. Few streets were paved, and drainage was far from adequate in a town that lay largely below sea level and had an annual rainfall of nearly sixty inches. An adequate sewerage system would be a development of the twentieth century. Nightsoil was collected from outhouses and simply dumped into the river. The current also would have flushed away the accumulated filth from a densely populated city, but careless residents either dumped garbage into gutters or deposited it on the batture, the area between the levee and the water's edge. They would not walk the extra few steps needed to throw the matter into the water, where it would be washed away.
>
> The yellow fever epidemic of 1853 in New Orleans stands as one of the worst medical catastrophes ever to befall an American city. About half of the population of 150,000 rushed away when the enormity of the outbreak became evident, but as many as 9,000 of the stay-behinds—who were mainly the poor, of course—had fatal attacks . . . the outbreak turned New Orleans into a ghost town, the streets almost deserted and most businesses closed. Whole families, along with their servants, were wiped out. In the cemeteries the scenes were hellish. Bodies were delivered by the hundreds, some in caskets, others only wrapped in sheets. Overwhelmed gravediggers did their best to get the dead into the ground with a thin covering of soil. But they fell far behind and putrefying bodies piled up, their stench adding to the horror. The shallow graves

> quickly filled with water, causing coffins to float . . . at night, by the light of crude torches half-drunk laborers stood in water up to their waists as they tried to provide burial places. Estimates of the number of New Orleanians who were stricken run as high as 40,000. The survivors, of course, became immune, with the result that in 1854 and 1855 the death toll was only about 2,500 persons in each year, since the fever had fewer potential victims. By 1858, however, the number of non-immune residents had risen . . . [and] 4,856 died.[1]

The situation was no better in other parts of the region:

> Carried in large part by refugees fleeing New Orleans, the 1853 epidemic spread over the state from corner to corner, attacking some areas that previously had been spared. In Thibodaux, for instance, 224 persons, about 15 percent of the population, died. Tiny Washington recorded 100 deaths, causing panic in nearby Opelousas, from which as many as three-fourths of the residents fled. The tragedy of yellow fever could be felt in a village as well as in a big city. . . .
>
> In 1873 the fever struck north Louisiana with unaccustomed ferocity. At Shreveport, about half of the town's estimated 9,000 residents evacuated. Of those who stayed on, some 3,000 contracted the illness and at least 759 died. Travelers in the northern parishes reported going for fifty miles and seeing hardly a white person—all had fled to the pine hills, only the blacks remaining. (It had long been observed that blacks were far less susceptible to yellow fever than were whites. The reason, unknown until well into the twentieth century, was that the disease originated in Africa, where many generations of exposure had given blacks a measure of resistance to it. In especially virulent epidemics, however, blacks too died in large numbers.) The disaster was economic as well as physical. Surrounding communities quarantined Shreveport . . . rail service ceased. . . .
>
> [In 1873] smaller towns such as Donaldsonville, Morgan City, Plaquemine, and Thibodaux were also hard hit. The epidemic that year ravaged the entire Lower Mississippi Valley. . . .
>
> The economic costs of the fever had long influenced the handling of an outbreak. At the first report of a case in New Orleans, cities in Mississippi, Texas, Alabama, and elsewhere, as well as other towns in Louisiana, clamped an embargo on shipments from the port, with costly results to business interests. If fever did exist, the pressure was on the medical community to conceal it. Interests outside of Louisiana did not trust health authorities of the state to give honest reports. Once it became known that Yellow Jack was back in New

> Orleans, trains leaving the city were met at stations along the line by armed citizens who threatened to shoot anybody leaving the cars.[2]

In subsequent years the epidemics were recurrent but generally were of somewhat less devastating impact. The fear of a recurrence of the public health crises of prior years had had a direct bearing on the establishment of community-based public health clinics. On the origins of the parish health unit in Louisiana as a building type, Barbara Cole writes:

> By directive of Article 296 of the 1898 Louisiana Constitution, each parish and municipality in Louisiana was to establish a board of health. Act Number 192, titled the 'Batchelor Board of Health Bill,' gave instructions for implementation of Article 296. These instructions included reorganization of the State Board of Health and the specifics for establishing local boards of health in each town, city and parish. The city council of each town and city was to appoint the members of the city boards of health and the respective police juries were to appoint the members of the parish boards of health. The chairman, to be called Parish Health Officer or City Health Officer, of each board of health, was to be a physician. By 1910, sixty of the sixty-four Louisiana parishes had complied, leaving Allen, Beauregard, Evangeline and Jefferson parishes non-compliant. By 1915, these four parishes had complied . . . the board and its President, Dr. Oscar Dowling, felt the best way to deliver health services was through full-time parish health units rather than local boards of health, and they begun efforts to establish full-time parish health units. Due to the costs involved, the police juries met their efforts with resistance. In 1915, with funds provided by the police jury and school board, Calcasieu Parish hired a full-time district health officer. In 1917, Rapides Parish began a full-time public health program. In 1921, the police juries of six parishes, Natchitoches, DeSoto, Caddo, Beauregard, Ouachita and Washington, appropriated funds for full-time public health programs.[3]

On the role of sanitation programs in the earliest parish health units:

> The Louisiana State Board of Health delegated to one of their bureaus, the Bureau of Rural Sanitation, the supervision of these first health units and the management of the funds. The International Health Board of the Rockefeller Foundation lent a staff member, Dr. P.W. Covington, to Louisiana to assist in the establishment of these health units. Dr. Covington was the Director of the

> Bureau of Rural Sanitation. To help the people understand the work the parish health units would be doing, and the benefits of the work to the citizens, Dr. Covington conducted lectures in communities in the parishes. At the end of each lecture, forms, called 'agreement blanks,' were given to some of the prominent citizens attending the lectures, for distribution and signing by the citizens. These 'agreement blanks' stated the work the parish health unit would be performing, the benefits to be derived by the citizens, what was necessary from the citizens for success, and that the first three parish health units to be opened would be determined by the three parishes having the largest percentage of signed 'agreement blanks.' The project began with the establishment of five full-time parish health units in 1921. Carpenters were hired to work part-time to build sanitary privies . . . the director, nurse, and sanitary inspector in each health unit were required to furnish their own transportation and pay the associated costs. They were reimbursed a flat $50.00 per month.[4]

In 1922 the name of the Bureau of Rural Sanitation was changed to the Bureau of Parish Health Administration. By 1926 there were fourteen full-time parish health units in Louisiana.[5] In 1927 nearly the entire lower Mississippi delta experienced a catastrophic flood caused by the raging floodwaters of the Mississippi River. The floodwaters covered approximately 200,000 square miles and 1.5 million people were displaced. The states that experienced the worst devastation were Louisiana, Arkansas, Mississippi, Missouri, Tennessee, and Illinois. This event would have a profound impact on the rise of the parish health unit as a building type in Louisiana and elsewhere. On the aftermath of the flood:

> Fourteen Public Health Service officers were working in the field within ten days of the beginning of the flood, assisting the state health officials. The floodwaters reached Louisiana about the middle of April 1927. Beginning May 1, 1927, numerous breaks in the levee of the Mississippi River occurred. According to conservative estimates, over five million acres in Louisiana flooded in twenty-six parishes, with approximately 325,000 people experiencing severe losses . . . the American Red Cross began emergency procedures and coordinated their efforts with the U.S. Public Health Service, the Army, and Navy medical services, state medical societies, the American Medical Association, and the state health departments of the seven most severely affected states. Fifteen other state health departments, in states not affected by the flood, sent staff to assist. The first objective was to move the people whose homes were

> flooded to safety, and provide shelter and food for them. The American Red Cross established thirty-three camps in Louisiana to provide shelter . . . twenty of these camps were staffed with physicians, nurses and sanitary personnel . . . sanitary management for eleven of the camps was delegated to full-time Health Unit Directors.[6]

Personal hygiene and proper sanitary procedures were soon established in the camps. The administrative records of the camps contained the following account of the types of care:

> Amazingly, there were no severe outbreaks of communicable disease in the camps. This was largely attributed to the strict enforcement of sanitary conditions, along with medical care, feeding and clothing of the people [living] in the camps. Thousands of vaccinations were given. Listed are some of the functions provided by the teams in the affected states: 500,000 typhoid fever immunizations; 140,000 smallpox vaccinations; 149 refugee camps established; 6,449 sanitary pit privies dug; 40,000 pounds of unslaked lime distributed as disinfectant; 40,000 pounds of chloride lime distributed as disinfectant; 230,000 gallons of crude oil used to dispose of dead animals; 225,000 gallons of spraying oil and 191 spraying cans. Some of the activities performed in Louisiana were: 98,000 typhoid fever inoculations; 72,000 smallpox vaccinations; 31,500 quinine capsules distributed; 11,000 water wells chlorinated; 20,000 privies restored, constructed or repaired; 612 houses completely screened; 1,997 screen doors installed.[7]

As the floodwaters receded and people gradually returned to their homes, health workers directed the cleanup operations. A major problem was the progressive impact of the floodwaters: as the floodwaters in the northern part of the state receded, the middle part of the state flooded, later, the southernmost part flooded; as the high water raged ever southward. Not until the end of July 1927 did the floodwaters recede. The flood had inadvertently resulted in a boom in the creation of new parish health units.[8]

Cole continues:

> A national committee comprising representatives from the Red Cross, the U.S. Public Health Service, the Rockefeller Foundation and state health officers from the states affected from the flood, met on June 5, 1927 and developed a

> plan to finance and establish parish-county health units in Louisiana, Arkansas, Mississippi, Missouri, Kentucky, Tennessee and Illinois over an eighteen month period. The estimated cost for the first year was almost one million dollars . . . [in Louisiana] the U.S. Public Health Service and the Rockefeller Foundation provided more than 40 percent of the funding, with the State Board of Health and participating parishes providing the additional funds. . . . The process of hiring employees for new health units revealed that few people had previous public health experience. The Rockefeller Foundation established a Field Training Station at Indianola, Mississippi, and offered their services in training physicians, nurses, and sanitary inspectors. Louisiana employed and sent [the newly hired personnel] to Indianola, for four to six weeks [of] training.[9]

In 1927 alone, thirteen parishes established and opened parish health units, and by the end of the year there were twenty-three full-time parish health units in Louisiana.[10] It was understood that each year funds from within the state would be increased gradually so that eventually the state would be the sole supporter of its burgeoning network of parish health units. From the outset, however, the parish police jury in each parish was responsible for half of all operating costs, with 25 percent coming from the state, and 25 percent in funds split between the Rockefeller Foundation and the U.S. Public Health Service. By the end of 1929 out of the total of thirty-one full-time parish health units five of these had ceased to be dependent upon funds from these last two agencies. The personnel in these thirty-one facilities numbered 114.[11] The public's interest was high in the services provided at their new parish health unit, and this translated into a high level of compassion for and support of its services.

On the problem of funding during the depressed 1930s, Cole writes:

> The amount of funds available determined the types and numbers of services provided by each parish health unit. In 1928, the Governor and the legislature ceased the practice of the State Board of Health providing state funds to the parish health units. Instead, the money was to be appropriated by the legislature each year. This money was sent to the Bureau of Parish Health Administration for distribution . . . federal funds for this purpose were [similarly routed] . . . appropriations for the following years vary. The depression years were very difficult for the parish health units. Some parishes were unable to provide their share of funds, so the International Board of Health of the Rockefeller Foundation continued to provide some support. Effective July 31, 1932,

> all employees in the health units had a salary reduction of 15 percent . . . millions of people were out of work. In an effort to provide employment, the federal government created the Works Progress Administration [WPA] in 1933 . . . one of the Louisiana projects . . . was the construction of privies. During [a] four-month period [they] built 26,099 privies in Louisiana. But even in these financially troubled years twelve new full-time health units were opened.[12]

These clinics were specifically charged with monitoring potential causes of sickness and disease in the community. In the late 1920s, it was envisioned that every parish would soon operate a full-time health unit. But this would not become reality for three more decades. The earliest such centers were located in the basements of the parish courthouses. The clinic and the attached office for the parish sanitarian were cramped and severely lacking in amenities. The staff made the best of their very modest working conditions.

The Bureau of Parish Health Administration ceased to exist in 1940. The State Board of Health from that point received funding from a combination of federal and state sources and local parish government. About half of its entire budget was for the health units. In 1940 and 1941 eight new parish health units opened.[13] World War II was a busy period for the parish health units. They were severely understaffed due to the loss of staff to the military services, but the population was increasing, due in no small measure to the presence of new military bases in the state. The parish health units performed blood tests for persons reporting for duty in the military, and in a few parishes, the health unit physician director performed physical exams for military personnel stationed locally. As a result, larger and more modernized facilities were needed. Through an application Louisiana filed with the Federal Works Agency, under the Lanham Bill, the federal government provided construction funds for nineteen new parish health units.[14] Five new facilities opened in 1942 alone and the staffs were immediately welcomed into their communities.[15] No health units were opened during the rest of World War II with the exception of St. John the Baptist Parish.

Appendix B

Post-Occupancy Assessment

A longitudinal profile is provided below of the network of OPH facilities described in the preceding chapters. Data obtained in 1990-91 were compared and contrasted with parallel data obtained in 1999-2000. This represented an interval of ten years. A ten-page survey was distributed to each program site in November 1990. At the time of Survey 1, 1990 (T1) 138 facilities were open. This number had declined to 106 by Survey 2, 2000 (T2). Similarly, the number of full-time employees had dropped from 1,600 to slightly over 1,200. The survey assessed:

1. Physical size, condition, and aesthetic appearance
2. Availability and proximity of parking and security measures
3. Monthly building operating cost and maintenance issues
4. Occupant and user attitudes towards the building's location
5. Occupants' daily patterns of use within the facility
6. The condition of environmental control systems
7. Facility performance in relation to agency policy

The T1 survey was eleven pages in length. The T2 survey's length was reduced somewhat (9 pages). Some questions were deleted, others were condensed or restructured. In both 1990 and 200, a pretest was conducted in the field at pre-selected program sites. The input of staff at this stage proved critical in order to fine-tune question-phrasing and content. The questions in the T2 survey therefore were a combination of the modifications suggested at the completion of the T1 survey, and also reflected new facility-related issues, which had arisen during the preceding decade. The reporting of these data illustrated a shift in strategy between the 1990 and 2000 surveys away from a less voluminous but equality representative strategy—a one respondent-per-facility strategy—to one where as many as a dozen staff persons assessed a given facility separately and confidentially. In all, 1,147 DHH-OPH employees completed the T2 survey. If was found that occupants were much more satisfied with their facility in 2000. The completion of many SFI projects contributed to this finding.

Patient Utilization and Annual Operating Expenses

It was found that a new facility or a renovated existing facility resulted in an increase of as much as 20 percent in monthly. Between 63 and 70 percent of respondents reported that the new or improved facility did result in greater usage levels as reflected in average total monthly visits. As for operating costs, the largest buildings, not surprisingly, whether new or old, were identified as the most costly to maintain. This included HVAC costs, monthly lease payments by the state, to a parish, or to a private sector leaser, and operating expenses, including landscaping maintenance expenses. As for the differences between T1 and T2 surveys, annual operating expenses increased the most (adjusting for inflation) in the operation of the main health unit facilities (Table B.1).

Parking Provisions

Respondents deemed the new facilities' parking lots satisfactory. This is likely attributable to the fact that replacement clinics were built in the 1990s on considerably more acreage. The sites vacated were generally dysfunctional in this respect: overcrowded with few parking spaces, and lacking designated spaces for the handicapped (Table B.2).

Occupant Satisfaction with Facility

At this point in the survey, the focus shifted to occupant satisfaction with the interior spaces of the health unit clinics. Arrival areas, staff clerical areas, clinic, and staff support spaces were evaluated. The quantity of each room type was identified, as was the average size of a given room type. This was followed by data on whether or not a given room type served multiple functions, such as a staff lounge pressed into double duty as a nutritional education demonstration kitchen (Tables B.3-B.5). In the oldest, most dysfunctional facilities certain room types were prone to being used for three or more different functions in a given day. These data were followed by an inventory of those rooms deemed most securable, i.e. able to be locked in order to protect patient confidentiality in the case of patient medical records. Respondents rated the rooms individually within each facility on a four-point preference scale, with 1.0 the lowest (least preferred) rating and 4.0 the highest (most preferred) rating. T1 and T2 data were statistically compared. For main health units, it was found that for every room type, the facilities had been greatly improved by 2000. This was further affirmed insofar as ten statistically significant differences were identified.

Satellite and branch health units yielded four statistically significant differences between T1 and T2 surveys. Higher T2 ratings indicated that in all cases, with the exception of storerooms, the facilities were much improved in 2000. The evaluation of occupant satisfaction yielded improvement in the quality and size of entry reception areas. Also, medical records storage rooms, patient specimen restrooms as a means to increase patient privacy, and the creation in many cases for the first time of fully equipped, separate, nutritional education demonstration kitchens.

Facility Performance in Relation to Public Health Policy

This question, added to the T2 survey, was phrased as "Have any of the following events occurred in the past ten years in your facility and/or community?" Each respondent provided a *Yes*, *No*, or *Don't Know* response. These same items then provided the basis for inquiry into the influence on the community's use of a given facility: "If you answer *Yes* to any of the above questions, please rate the impact of such events to the increased utilization of public health services provided by your parish health unit/OPH facility." The following six survey items were each rated on a seven-point scale, with a rating of 1 denoting minimum impact, and a 7 denoting maximum impact on outcome (Table B.6).

> *Decrease/Increase in Staffing in Facility:*
>
> Past Policy Decisions—In the case of health units and specialty clinics, respondents were unanimous on this point. Among respondents this pattern held constant when asked if staffing had been increased during the past decade. In no case, statewide for a particular building type, had staffing levels been increased, when all facilities of a given facility type were viewed collectively.
>
> Impact on Community Use—Respondents indicated that staffing reductions had had a significant negative impact on their work performance many cases.

Availability of Public Transportation to the Clinic:

Past Policy Decisions—Staff in the main public health unit facilities indicated an improvement in public transportation access in the 1990-2000 period (53.2 percent responded yes). Specialty clinic staff indicated an even larger improvement, with 88.2 percent indicating yes. By contrast, satellite health unit staff indicated a decrease in public transportation service.

Impact on Community Use—The most striking finding was that neither improvement nor curtailment of public transportation access has a strong impact on clinic facility use one way or the other. People in need will find a way to get there. As for wheelchair patients, these families often own their own lift-equipped vehicle.

Accessibility of the Clinic or OPH Support Facility via Parish Roads:

Past Policy Decisions—Statewide, respondents indicated there was no improvement in access to their facility via new road construction or due to any upgrading of existing roads to the facility over the ten-year period. Specialty clinic respondents were split on this issue due to the relocation of two clinics to new sites adjacent to major access roads. In numerous instances the status quo prevailed, and in some cases, access roads to the facility had deteriorated.

Impact on Community Use—For the patients of the specialty clinics, particularly the Children's Special Health Services clinics (CSHS) respondents indicated the poor quality of access roads as having a moderate to maximum negative impact on access to care. Respondents in other facility types indicated this factor to have had a moderate impact on patients' access to care at their facility.

Emergence of New or Expanded Health Programs:

Past Policy Decisions—Respondents reported significant growth in the range of community care, wellness, and sickness prevention programs offered during the ten-year period.

Impact on Community Use—The CSHS staff in these specialty clinics reported program expansion and the emergence of new programs to have had a dramatic impact on increased numbers of patients and patient visits to their facilities.

Designation as Health Professional Shortage Area or Medically Underserved Area:

Past Policy Decisions—The majority of staff respondents in main public health unit and specialty clinics reported their "catchment area," as designated as a medically underserved community. Data reported by respondents elsewhere statewide were either split equally on this point, or indicated that no such designation had been made in their local community.

Impact on Community Use—Such designations had had a moderate to significant impact on utilization for the three types of public health unit clinics. This pattern was most pronounced for the main public health unit facilities. This is most likely due to their being the only parish health unit in many parishes, particularly in rural parishes so predominant in the northern part of the state. Also, not surprisingly, this was the region with the largest percentage of parishes designated as medically underserved, and with only one public community healthcare site in the parish. The infusion of funds and in a few cases new staff, such as the home health visitation program, and increased "marketing" of the federally funded WIC program for nutritional education had an impact on bringing more patients into the clinics for care during the ten-year period.

Increase in Local Community Funding for Health and Sickness Prevention Programs:

Past Policy Decisions—In no instance did survey respondents report an increase in local community funding for the delivery of services. This survey item pertained to direct services only, not to funding for the facilities themselves nor for staff salaries. This pattern was pervasive during the decade experienced increasing operational expenses.

Impact on Community Use—The one exception to this pattern was in the case of the twenty-five respondents in seventeen main public health unit facilities where the local police jury or parish council had provided increased funds during the decade. Respondents at these locations reported that this had a positive impact on their ability to deliver community health programs. In these clinics the staff had therefore evolved into a mixture of core staff paid by the state working side by side with healthcare professionals employed by the parish. Anecdotal evidence obtained in the field often indicated this to be a productive, mutually beneficial arrangement.

Appendix B

Tables

Table B-1: Monthly Patient Utilization of Facility

Type/Attribute	Region[1] X(SE)[2] 1990	2000	X(SW) 1990	2000	X(N-C) 1990	2000	State X(N) 1990	X(N) 2000	S.D.
1. Main PHU									
a. Patient Visits[3]	1,153	1,397	1,435	1,524	1,184	1,225	1,258	1,382(61)	.72(.80)*
b. Increase (% Yes)[4]	57.9(2)	66.3(11)	84.6(6)	83.5(11)	51.7(8)	59.8(15)	64.7(16)	69.9(37)	.95(.77)*
c. No Change (%)[4]	42.1(2)	33.7(8)	15.4(2)	16.5(2)	48.3(1)	40.2(14)	35.3(5)	30.1(24)	.80(.86)
2. Branch PHU									
a. Patient Visits	968	1104	610	726	845	866	808	898	.81(.77)*
b. Increase (% Yes)	50.0(3)	59.3(4)	66.7(5)	72.6(4)	100.0(3)	---	70.0(11)	65.9(8)	.92(.84)*
c. No Change (%)	50.0(5)	40.7(4)	33.3(3)	27.4(2)	---	---	30.0(8)	34.1(6)	.79(.89)
3. Satellite PHU									
a. Patient Visits	187	196	224	233	105	141	172	190	.96(.92)
b. Increase (% Yes)	25.0(4)	60.0(1)	64.3(2)	66.0(9)	60.0(3)	---	56.5(9)	63.0(10)	.92(.89)
c. No Change (%)	75.0(2)	40.0(3)	35.7(1)	34.0(5)	40.0(2)	---	43.5(5)	37.0(8)	.83(.72)
4. Specialty Clinic									
a. Patient Visits	534	529	150	166	295	332	326	342	.93(.77)
b. Increase (% Yes)	42.9(2)	67.5(0)	---	---	25.0(1)	---	30.8(3)	67.5(1)	.76(.85)
c. No Change (%)	57.1(1)	32.5(1)	100.0(0)	100.0(0)	75.0(0)	100.0(0)	69.2(1)	77.5(1)	.89(.78)

[1] Southeast Region (SE); Southwest Region (SW); North-Central Region (N-C).
[2] 2000 data in parentheses
[3] Patient visits per month reported. Region Office and Region laboratory data not reported, as patients do not directly utilize these facilities. In T2 survey, sixty-one Main PHU facilities reporting, nineteen Branch PHU facilities reporting, ten Satellite PHU facilities reporting, twelve Specialty Clinics reporting.
[4] This question was phrased in T2 survey as "If this facility has been replaced since 1990, has this led, in your opinion, to an increase in its use by the residents of this community?" (Yes/No response only). In T1 survey the period assessed was 1980-89. Only facilities that were renovated in previous decade were assessed in both T1 and T2 surveys
* Significant 2-way ANOVA (Region x Time) difference, $p<.05$.

Table B-2: Parking

Type/Attribute	Region[1] 1990(2000)[2] X (SE)	1990(2000) X (SW)	1990(2000) X (N-C)	State 1990(2000) X	1990(2000) S.D.
1. Main PHU	N=19(19)	N=13(13)	N=30(30)	N=62(62)	--- ---
a. Staff[3]	14.3(16.1)	20.7(21.7)	18.0(21.2)	17.4(19.7)	1.01(.66)*
b. Public[3]	20.5(38.7)	23.4(43.4)	25.4(33.4)	23.1(38.5)	.86(.82)*
c. Handicapped[3]	1.1(3.1)	1.5(2.8)	1.3(3.0)	1.3(2.97)	.82(.79)**
d. On-Street	7.8(5.7)	10.0(10.0)	9.4(9.4)	9.0(9.0)	.91(.62)
2. Branch PHU	N=9(8)	N=6(6)	N=6(5)	N=21(19)	--- ---
a. Staff	9.2(8.8)	9.3(9.3)	10.0(9.5)	9.5(9.2)	.69(.79)
b. Public	18.4(17.8)	15.1(15.1)	9.8(9.2)	15.0(14.6)	.78(.84)
c. Handicapped	1.9(1.8)	1.0(1.0)	0.8(1.0)	1.3(2.0)	.96(.92)
d. On-Street	27.1(28.3)	11.3(11.3)	2.3(2.1)	15.5(16.7)	.94(---)
3. Satellite PHU	N=4(1)	N=14(7)	N=6(2)	N=24(10)	--- ---
a. Staff	5.5(5.2)	2.8(2.4)	2.7(2.9)	3.2(4.0)	.82(.74)
b. Public	21.7(20.7)	16.5(14.1)	9.3(10.0)	15.6(14.2)	.93(.80)
c. Handicapped	1.0(1.0)	1.3(1.0)	1.5(1.5)	1.3(2.0)	1.02(.98)
d. On-Street	4.5(6.5)	2.5(2.5)	0.6(1.4)	2.3(4.4)	.99(.79)
4. Specialty Clinic	N=10(6)	N=2(2)	N=5(4)	N=17(12)	--- ---
a. Staff	6.8(7.7)	2.0(2.0)	14.0(15.5)	8.3(9.2)	.92(.94)*
b. Public	9.5(8.5)	12.5(12.5)	24.0(25.3)	14.1(15.4)	1.04(.97)
c. Handicapped	0.8(1.2)	---(---)	1.6(2.0)	0.9(3.0)	.82(.77)
d. On-Street	9.3(12.3)	---(---)	4.4(5.5)	6.8(7.0)	.79(.66)

[1] Southeast Region (SE); Southwest Region (SW); North-Central Region (N-C).
[2] 2000 Data reported in parentheses.
[3] Average number of off street parking spaces for facilities within region.
*Significant 2-way ANOVA (Region x Time) difference, $p< .05$.
** Significant 2-way ANOVA (Region x Time) difference, $p< .01$.

Table B-3: Functional Space/Use Analysis: Main Parish Health Units[1]

	Room Type	Average Quantity	Size[2]	Multiple Functions		Lockable (%)		Evaluation[3]				
								1990		2000		
				Y	N	Y	N	X	S.D.	X	S.D.	t-test
a.	Entry/Reception	1.3	1,045	30.4	69.6	33.3	66.7	2.76(48)	.72	2.91	.77	3.33***
b.	Waiting Room	1.5	768	35.7	64.3	29.1	70.9	2.86(50)	1.08	2.93	.62	2.27
c.	Staff Offices	8.2	1,942	35.6	64.4	66.7	33.3	2.43(56)	1.07	2.96	.54	-3.27***
d.	Medical Records	1.2**	411	31.0	69.0	75.6	24.4	2.13(51)	.82	3.10	.49	-3.41***
e.	Conference Room	1.8**	450	70.5	29.5	60.5	39.5	---	---	2.63	.61	---
f.	Staff Break Room	1.1	245	34.3	65.7	35.3	64.7	2.52(29)	.77	2.79	.79	3.47***
g.	Health Ed. Classroom	1.0	376	85.0	15.0	65.0	35.0	2.27(38)	.92	2.63	.84	-3.79***
h.	Staff Washroom	2.2	135	12.1	87.9	82.8	17.2	2.40(50)	.80	2.47	.54	1.21
i.	Patient Washroom	1.5	74	27.6	72.4	82.8	17.2	2.79(29)	.86	2.83	.49	2.23
j.	Public Washroom	2.3*	149	7.7	92.3	67.9	32.1	2.84(54)	.84	2.89	.62	3.11
k.	Storage	3.8	486	17.5	82.5	79.3	20.7	2.51(48)	.90	2.93	.73	4.22***
l.	Biohazardous Storage	1.0	157	50.0	50.0	75.0	25.0	2.32(3)	.96	2.81	.75	2.41***
m.	Exam Rooms	5.1*	571	54.4	45.6	71.4	29.6	2.64(59)	.79	2.87	.69	-3.26***
n.	Laboratory	1.2	157	46.9	53.1	68.2	40.4	2.37(30)	.78	2.66	.82	4.11***
o.	Kitchen/WIC Education	1.2	291	56.3	43.8	60.9	29.1	2.73(44)	.95	2.82	.66	-3.11***
p.	Immunology Room	1.2	189	50.0	50.0	66.7	33.3	2.67(29)	.98	2.71	.79	2.96

[1] 1990 : N=62; 2000 : N=62

[2] Reported as average total square feet in facility for this room type.

[3] Assessment of occupant satisfaction with the architectural environment. These data are a summary mean computed across survey items contained in Part III, Question 2: size of room, lighting quality, noise level in clinic, quality of furnishings, color scheme, security system quality, location of room within overall facility, views to the outside (if any)from the room, and temperature level.

*Significant regional difference, p. < .05 (1990 only).

** Significant regional difference, p. < .001 (1990 only).

*** Significant 1990-2000 difference statewide, p. < .05.

Table B-4: Functional Space/Use Analysis: Branch and Satellite Parish Health Units[1]

Room Type	Average Quantity	Average Size[2]	Multiple Functions		Lockable (%)		Evaluation[3]				
							1990		2000		
			Y	N	Y	N	X	S.D.	X	S.D.	t-test
a. Entry/Reception	1.0	133	33.3	66.7	33.1	66.7	2.45	.82	2.66	.71	-2.66***
b. Waiting Room	1.0	433	47.4	52.6	33.3	66.4	2.23	.77	2.51	.81	4.02
c. Staff Offices	5.4	1,069	47.6	52.1	73.7	26.3	2.71	.92	2.83	.59	1.31
d. Medical Records	1.3	188	63.6	36.4	60.0	40.0	2.26	.90	2.39	.79	3.22***
e. Conference Room	1.0	352	71.4	29.6	66.7	33.3	---	---	----	---	---
f. Staff Break Room	1.4	435	73.6	26.4	73.6	26.4	2.48	.72	2.63	.58	2.11
g. Health Ed. Classroom	1.0	178	100.0	---	75.0	25.0	2.20	.58	2.29	.66	2.41
h. Staff Washroom	1.7	80	6.3	93.8	76.5	23.5	2.30	.92	2.49	.52	3.11
i. Patient Specimen Washroom	1.4	50	27.3	72.7	90.9	9.1	2.75	.94	3.01	.77	-4.01***
j. Public Washroom	1.9*	124	23.5	76.5	76.5	23.5	2.46	.80	2.59	.88	3.11
k. Storage	2.7	253	27.8	72.2	83.3	16.7	3.06	.77	2.39	.66	2.14
l. Biohazardous Storage	---	---	---	---	---	---	---	---	2.61	.70	---
m. Exam Rooms	3.6*	385	36.8	63.2	68.4	31.6	2.55	.72	2.76	.79	2.93
n. Laboratory	1.0	122	38.5	61.5	69.2	30.8	2.16	.82	2.42	.82	2.41
o. Kitchen/WIC Education	1.0	140	75.0	25.0	60.0	40.0	2.46	.79	2.71	.69	-2.69***
p. Immunology Room	1.0	142	66.7	33.3	83.3	16.7	2.82	.86	2.89	.56	2.22

[1] 1990 : N=62; 2000 : N=62
[2] Reported as average total square feet in facility for this room type.
[3] Assessment of occupant satisfaction with the architectural environment. These data are a summary mean computed across survey items contained in Part III, Question 2: size of room, lighting quality, noise level in clinic, quality of furnishings, color scheme, security system quality, location of room within overall facility, views to the outside (if any)from the room, and temperature level.
*Significant regional difference, p. < .05 (1990 only).
** Significant regional difference, p. < .001 (1990 only).
*** Significant 1990-2000 difference, p. < .05 statewide.

Table B-5: Assessment of Site Context, Exterior Appearance, and Staffing Patterns in Relation to Facility

Characteristic	Main PHU				Branch PHU				Satellite PHU			
	1990		2000		1990		2000		1990		2000	
	X	S.D.	X	S.D.	X	S.D.	X	S.D.	X	S.D.	X	S.D.
1. Location/Access:												
a. Location within the Parish	3.43	.67	3.26*	.77	3.40	.71	3.29	.88	3.39	.89	3.26	.70
b. Sense of safety on the grounds	2.71	.55	2.57	.93	2.85	.79	2.63	.85	2.91	.88	2.80	.81
c. Amount of parking available on the site	2.08	.81	2.20	.82	2.20	.59	2.43*	.79	2.52	.66	2.85*	.49
d. Distance to entrance from parking lot	3.40	.73	2.96*	.69	3.40	.92	3.35	.80	3.30	.71	3.10	.55
e. Availability of public transportation	2.38	.74	2.60	.75	2.43	.70	2.25	.71	1.71	.52	1.55	.92
2. Aesthetic Appearance:												
a. Image of facility in the eyes of community	2.94	.77	2.99	.71	2.75	.66	3.21**	.72	3.04	.64	2.90	.90
b. Appearance and upkeep of the grounds	2.30	.84	2.45	.81	2.27	.77	2.39	.90	2.60	.88	2.75	.91
c. Appearance and upkeep of the building	2.44	.81	2.56	.93	2.15	.84	2.36*	.81	2.78	1.03	2.55*	.85
d. Placement of exterior signage	2.66	.73	2.69	.89	2.80	.89	2.60	.59	3.09	.92	2.90	.81
e. Placement of interior signage	2.43	.69	2.68*	.86	2.30	.98	2.50	.66	2.55	.87	2.40	.94
f. Appearance of neighborhood	2.47	.57	2.55	.87	2.58	.93	2.44	.77	2.95	.87	2.63*	.95
3. Staffing Issues in Relation to Facility:												
a. Reputation of the facility at this time	3.16	.49	3.12	.61	3.10	.69	3.30*	.72	3.26	.93	3.44	.99
b. Ability to recruit staff to this facility	2.69	.77	2.53*	.79	3.00	1.01	2.51*	.88	2.48	.61	2.40	1.02
c. Ability to retain staff at this facility	2.55	.82	2.77*	.59	2.80	.92	2.26*	.79	2.91	.68	2.25*	.73
d. Freedom to modify the physical setting	2.10	.71	2.24	.83	2.27	.79	2.16	.91	2.33	.82	2.41	.89
e. Co-workers' attitudes toward this facility	2.15	.69	2.30	.81	2.25	.81	2.39	.80	2.27	.90	2.31	.95
f. Degree of support this facility provides for the work one does	2.20	.83	2.29	.80	2.29	.77	2.15	.79	2.23	.88	2.35	.94

* $p < .05$ (2 sample students' t-test).
** $p < .01$ (2 sample students' t-test).

Table B-6: Degree of Functional Support Provided by Facility in Relation to Health Agency Policies (2000)[1]

Type/Assessment	Decrease in Staffing	Increase in Staffing	Public Trans.	Access Roads	New/Expanded Programs	Medically Underserved Designation	Increased Funding for Programs
1. Main PHU (%, N)							
Yes	90.0(56)	115.5(7)	53.2(33)	37.1(23)	72.5(45)	72.3(45)	27.4(17)
No	10.0(6)	88.5(54)	43.6(27)	61.3(38)	25.8(16)	24.5(15)	66.2(41)
No Opinion	---	---	3.2(2)	1.6(1)	1.7(1)	3.2(2)	6.4(4)
Rating (X, S.D.)[2]	N=41(2.61, .41)	---	N=43(2.71, .72)	N=40(2.79, .77)	N=36(2.99, .59)	N=31(3.66,.67)	N=25(3.52,.72)
2. Branch PHU (%, N)							
Yes	100.0(1)	11.8(2)	100.0(1)	100.1(1)	100.0(1)	---	100.0(1)
No	---	88.2(15)	---	---	---	---	---
No Opinion	---	---	---	---	---	100.0(1)	---
Rating (X, S.D.)	N=12(2.77, .57)	---	N=14(2.56, .67)	N=14(2.44,.56)	N=14(2.66,.79)	N=14(3.22,.58)	N=1(5.0,---)
3. Satellite PHU (%, N)							
Yes	82.3(14)	---	23.5(4)	35.3(6)	53.3(8)	39.4(5)	17.7(3)
No	17.7(3)	100.0(1)	70.6(12)	64.7(11)	26.7(4)	29.4(5)	64.7(11)
No Opinion	---	---	5.9(1)	---	20.0(3)	41.2(7)	17.6(3)
Rating (X, S.D.)	N=9(2.93, .63)	---	N=13(2.99, .78)	N=12(2.72,.77)	N=12(2.71,.64)	N=12(3.11,.82)	N=3(5.50,---)
4. Specialty Clinic (%, N)							
Yes	100.00(17)	23.5(4)	88.2(15)	50.0(7)	76.9(10)	60.0(3)	8.3(1)
No	---	76.5(13)	11.8(2)	50.0(7)	23.1(3)	40.0(2)	75.0(9)
No Opinion	---	---	---	---	---	---	16.7(2)
Rating (X, S.D.)	N=5(2.77, .80)	---	N=5(2.10, .44)	N=5(3.61,.71)	N=5(3.78,.72)	N=5(2.29,.59)	N=4(3.08,---)

[1] Data reported by facility. Percentage reported, followed by number of reporting facilities (in parentheses).
[2] Each outcome response item rated on a 7-point response scale from "minimum impact" (1.0) to "maximum impact (7.0). "Increase in Staffing" question not reported due to its equivalency to "Decrease in Staffing" survey item.

APPENDIX C

ARCHITECTURAL AND SITE PLANNING CONCEPTS

Community health care should be non-institutional in image and project a spirit of warmth, caring, and human scale. This appendix consists of a compendium of 143 guidelines grouped into eight content areas. The content areas emerged as a result of a series of meetings, discussions, and focus groups. They have repeatedly been "tested" for validity in the field during subsequent years in the context of the SFI process. The guidelines incorporate recent findings from the research literature and recently completed buildings. The insights and appraisals of more than eleven hundred respondents who completed the facility evaluation surveys are also incorporated.

The guidelines and supporting data are meant to assist architects, engineers, interior designers, public health specialists, physicians, nurses, nutritionists, educators, elected officials, and others. They are not intended to be narrowly interpreted or viewed as mere recipes: each one represents the nucleus of an idea which is adaptable in many ways to a set of intentions and logistical realities. Nor are they meant to be exhaustively inclusive, is merely an attempt to see and organize issues the evidenced-based-design team believe warrant attention. The eight content areas are:

1. Community Context (1.1-1.7)
2. Strategically Planned Facilities (2.1-2.10)
3. Site Environs (3.1-3.10)
4. Clinical Realm/Environmental Health/Outreach (4.1-4.55)
5. Regional Support (5.1-5.10)
6. Total Environment (6.1-6.37)
7. Cost Containment (7.1-7.7)
8. Phased Implementation (8.1-8.7)

Within each category, guidelines are generally arranged in a sequence from the community scale (macro), to the architectural scale, to the scale of a room (micro). Each guideline has an introductory statement in boldface type. This statement is followed by a brief background statement of support explaining why it is important for consideration. An illustration accompanies each guideline in an attempt to further illuminate the text, stimulate thinking, and to suggest rather than dictate design solutions. In some instances, the title of the guideline is accompanied by an asterisk. This indicates that the information may only be pertinent to one or two OPH building types, or that the recommendation may not be of equal priority in all situations (ten guidelines were identified in this manner). These guidelines can be used as background information and to compliment and extend one's present knowledge and experience.

1. COMMUNITY CONTEXT

CONTEXT—IMAGE

1.1 PROVIDE A DIGNIFIED HEALTH CARE ENVIRONMENT SUPPORTIVE OF THE NEEDS OF THE COMMUNITY

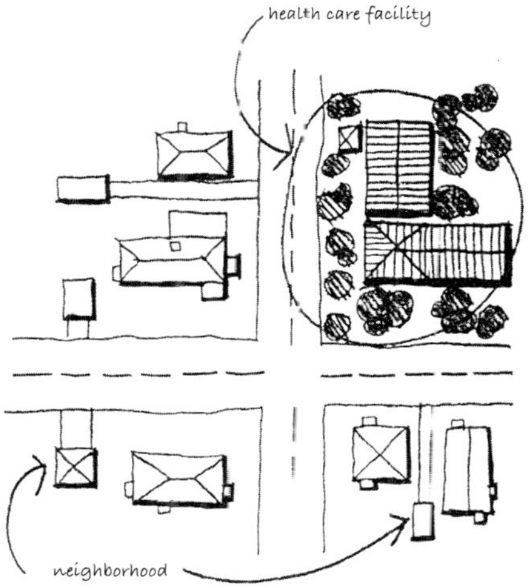

Community health requires sustaining a meaningful relationship between a community and its health care providers. Success in the long term requires a sustained partnership between the public and the private sectors, and between the federal government and state-level government. It is naïve and unrealistic to assume a community will blindly hold in high regard an outpatient health center whose architectural environment brazenly symbolizes a chronic lack of respect for the community. Therefore, steps must be taken to define and address the importance of this transactional bond—the glue—prerequisite to the articulation of a common philosophical language which values a dignified up-to-date facility.

CONTEXT—ADVOCACY

1.2 DEVELOP INCREMENTAL PUBLIC–PRIVATE SECTOR PARTNERSHIPS AS A MEANS OF CREATING SUPPORT IN THE COMMUNITY

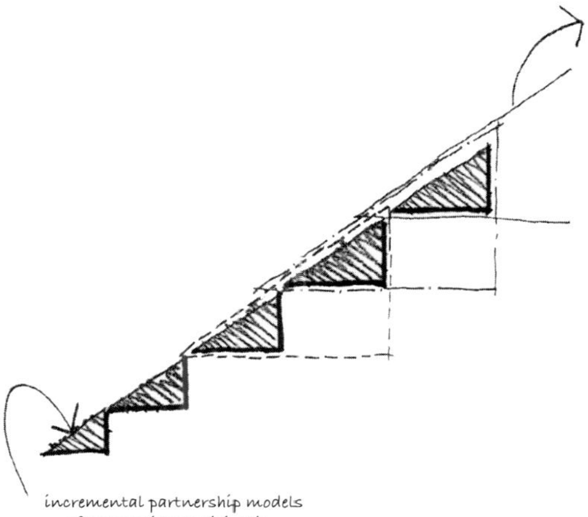

An effective means of achieving shared goals with respect to the community local health center is to identify specific projects or programs that can be successfully up and running in a matter of months, rather than years. This set of goals can serve a valuable aim, especially early on in public-private and interagency partnership process, as positive symbols of effective collaboration and constituency building. A strategy of incrementalization is sometimes much less daunting than defining complex and far-reaching goals from the start. An incremental strategy can still function within a larger strategy for change. Early successes will function as cornerstones for more ambitious projects. Architecturally, this strategy would perhaps translate into the procurement of a new roof for the health unit, a new heating, ventilation, air conditioning (HVAC) system, establishment of a reference library on-site, a new sign on the exterior of the building, and so on. It will not take long for the word to get out in the community that the health center is lifting itself up to be a more valuable resource in the community.

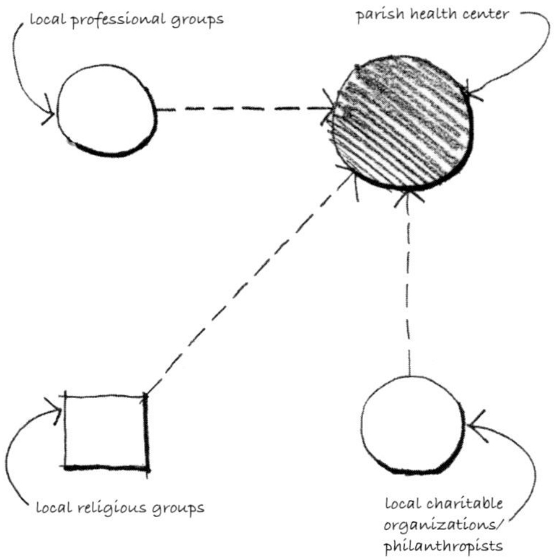

CONTEXT—ADVOCACY

1.3 ESTABLISH A 'FRIENDS OF THE HEALTH CENTER' COMMUNITY ADVOCACY AND SUPPORT GROUP

Increasingly, private sector support of the health center's mission has emerged as an important adjunctive vehicle in promoting the advancement of community public health care. Public taxpayer funds alone will be insufficient in the coming years to meet the needs of an aging patient population. State employed staff will have increasing difficulty in meeting this challenge without the active support of the local community. Therefore, work to establish a community advocacy group to help improve and further enhance the quality of care and its accessibility to the community. Volunteerism is an effective means to foster such involvement. A 'Friends of the Health Center' advocacy group, from a facility support standpoint, can help make the case for needed facility improvements or a complete replacement facility. Volunteers can also assist in community health education seminars, transporting patients without cars to appointments, and the staffing of the indoor and outdoor children's play spaces. Their sheer presence on a sustained basis can therefore greatly help to justify the cost of constructing needed spaces within a health center.

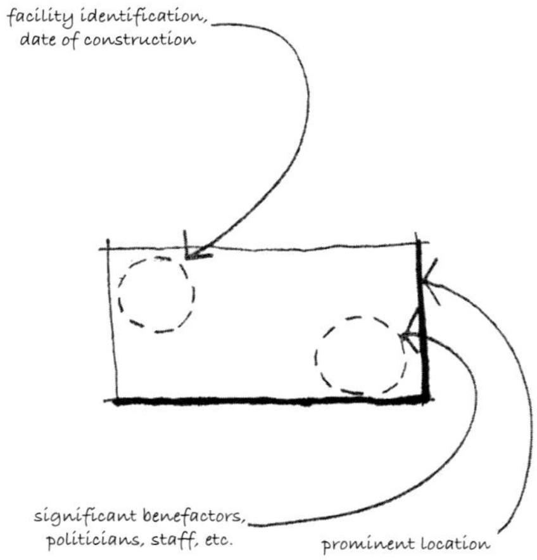

CONTEXT—RECOGNITION

1.4 INCLUDE A BRONZE PLAQUE AT THE MAIN ENTRANCE TO ACKNOWLEDGE THOSE WHO MERIT RECOGNITION FOR THEIR EFFORTS

The construction of a building funded by the taxpayers requires the participation and cooperation of many individuals and constituencies and often takes several years. Throughout history, public buildings have been inscribed with the names of their various benefactors. This information is typically inscribed in a location clearly visible to all who enter. Publicly elected officials, the builders, clients, the staff of the health center at the time of construction, private benefactors, and even luminaries of Western civilization are variously honored in these tributes. It is entirely appropriate to honor those who helped achieve the construction of the health center vis-a-vis the inscription of their names in a commemorative wall plaque. This should be located in a visible location near the main entrance. This plaque should be no larger than 15′ x 24′ or 18′ x 30′. At the top should be the name of the facility, its location, and the date of construction.

CONTEXT—CHILD ADVOCACY

1.5 IN LARGER HEALTH UNITS A SPECIAL PLAY ROOM FOR CHILDREN CAN BE STAFFED BY VOLUNTEERS FROM THE COMMUNITY

In heath units of sufficient size, create a room for children apart from, yet adjacent to, the main waiting room. This space should be separated acoustically, as mentioned in guidelines (see below) on the children's play zone, yet visually connected to the waiting room vis-a-vis a transparent or a semi-transparent wall so parents can view their children from the adult seating area of the main waiting room. Equip this room with carpeting, acoustic tiles on the walls (and perhaps the ceiling), videotapes for children, blocks, puppets, books, toys, a few playpens for infants, child-size chairs and tables, and a storage closet for supplies. This space should be flexible. It is important to equip and staff this room with volunteers drawn from the local community through the Friends of the Health Center advocacy group. This group can take an activity like this on as a special project. It is anticipated that this space would be staffed during all child health, WIC, and family planning clinics. Policies are needed, however, to avoid some mothers from abusing this service by turning it into a private daycare program for their own children. The use policy must be firm insofar as this amenity is available only during one's visit to the clinic.

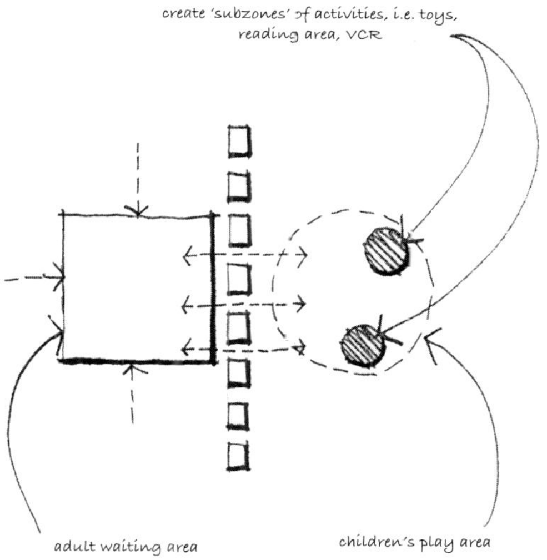

CONTEXT—ACCESS

1.6 ACCESS TO LOCAL RESOURCES IS ESSENTIAL TO SUCCESS IN REPLACEMENT AND RENOVATION INITIATIVES

A health care institution operating in the public sector is increasingly dependent on the support of its community context. This includes the network of local churches, schools, volunteer groups, civic booster groups, social service agencies, physicians, and other health care institutions. If located near a teaching hospital or university medical center, strong ties should be established. Internships and residencies could be developed, and joint research activities may develop in time with respect to, for example, laboratory research projects with a field component based in the regional labs, and similarly, community public health research that is based to some extent in selected health centers. Architectural implications of these activities include the provision of office and lab spaces, reciprocity in library and computer resources, and a multipurpose room for lectures, films, and workshops, which is dividable into more than one room. These spaces will function collectively as the stage upon which community health improvements can be nurtured.

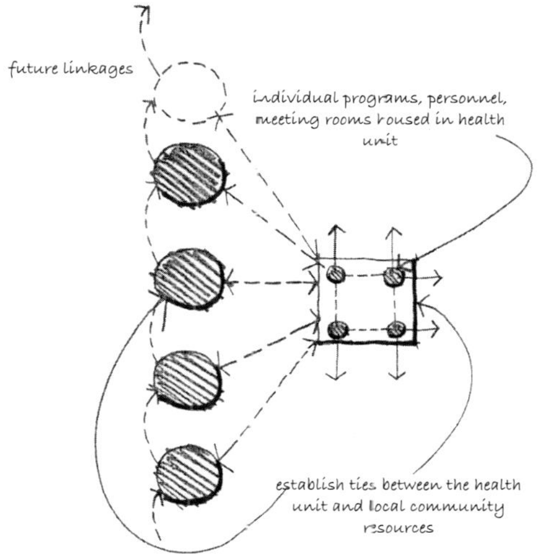

CONTEXT—ACCESS

1.7 REAFFIRM THE HEALTH CENTER'S MISSION BY ENCOURAGING ITS USE BY THE LOCAL COMMUNITY

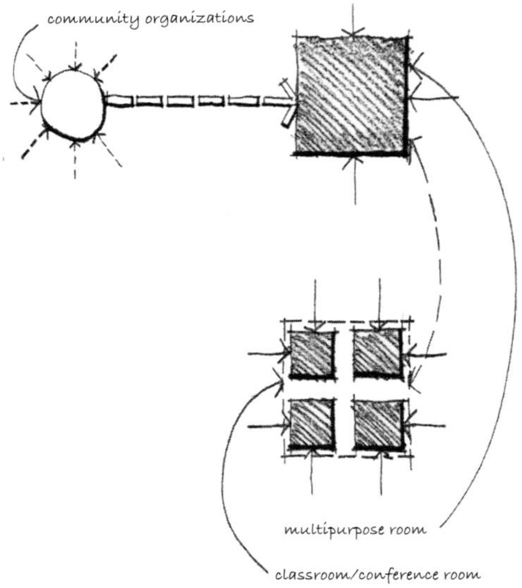

It is very difficult to weave the educational mission and treatment programs of a community health center into the life of its community if the facility lacks adequate physical space. Multipurpose rooms are needed to host a wide range of health education activities sponsored by local organizations such as Alcoholics Anonymous, Alzheimer's disease support groups, in-service seminars for health professionals, support groups for persons attempting to quit smoking, and for films and lectures. Many of these events take place in the evenings. In this manner, the health center's mission is reaffirmed as the key source of new information–a clearinghouse of sorts, for preventative health care. These outreach activities can foster more favorable perceptions in the local community than if it is only perceived as a place to receive treatment after one is already sick, i.e. a place to receive STD or TB treatment. Therefore, provide at least one multipurpose room for health education and related wellness programs. This will reaffirm local support for the promotion of community health.

2. STRATEGICALLY PLANNED FACILITIES

PLANNING—PARAMETERS

2.1 CLEARLY DEFINE THE ROLE OF ALL KEY DECISION MAKERS

Effective organizational leadership is the most important prerequisite in successful facility development. The agencies and governing bodies associated with capital improvement initiatives should clearly identify the key decision-making persons and groups. The representatives who are granted decision-making authority need to develop and sustain a dialogue from start to finish. Their roles should be defined in an organizational chart and distributed to all parties. This facility committee must identify ways to promote oversight of the project. This committee is charged with collectively defining the role and mission of every clinical, epidemiological, educational, and environmental service to be housed in the new or renovated facility. This group should also develop a database of the patient utilization of services on a program-by-program basis. The committee must retain oversight from pre-feasibility analysis to completion. Building maintenance, upkeep, and life cycle operating costs must be addressed. Build in strategic optional courses of action so one gap or unexpected change does not jeopardize the entire project. Create a sense of mutual trust and shared goals, and, if a project's scope requires redefinition midstream due to cost constraints, do not shy away from the task.

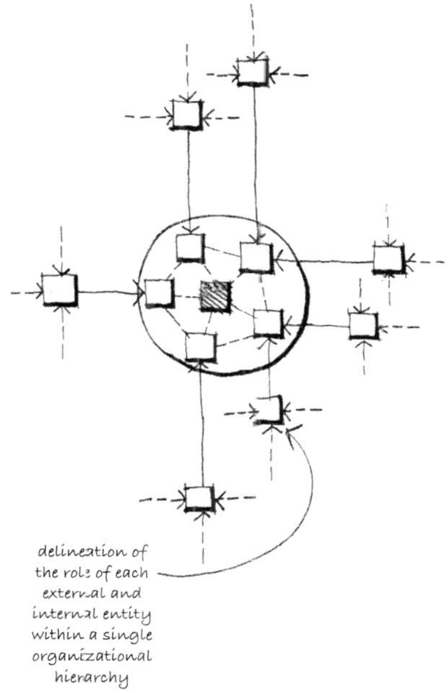

PLANNING—COMMUNICATION

2.2 CREATE AN ENVIRONMENT OF MUTUAL TRUST AND SHARED GOALS THROUGHOUT THE SFI PROCESS

If poor communication exists between agency officials, local elected officials, and community advocacy groups, little can be accomplished. The ultimate loser is the patient who must contend with, at best, the status quo by having to put up with a treatment environment that continues to deteriorate. Therefore, define and nurture an effective communication channel with key decision makers who have a direct influence at the local level including health advocacy groups, the health center's staff, and even with the local media. Respect is a two-way street, and consensus is most satisfying when it leads to positive outcomes. Shared goals, expectations, and a mutually appreciated definition of success should be the by-words, rather than an atmosphere of acrimony, resentment, disrespect, and mistrust. It is critically important that local public government leadership is familiar with and realizes the importance of seeking ways to improve the health status of the community and how the health center can achieve this goal.

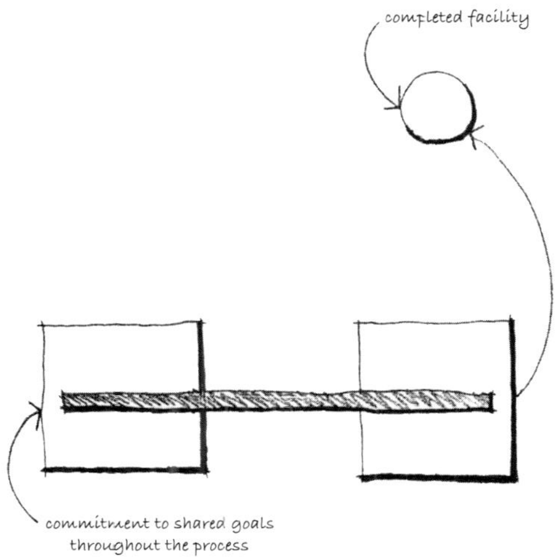

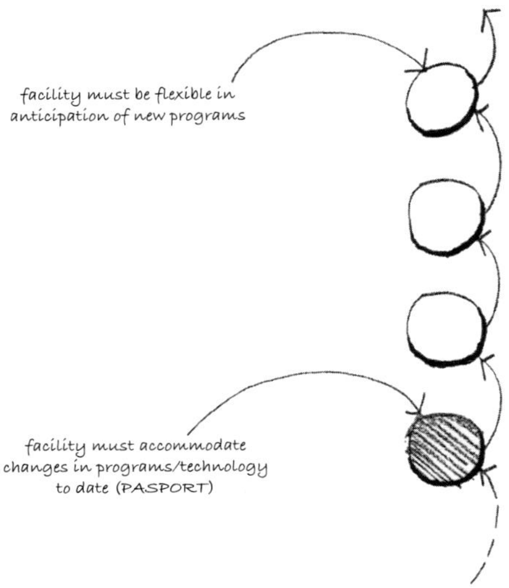

NEW PROGRAMS

2.3 PROVIDE FLEXIBLE SPACES IN ANTICIPATION OF NEW COMMUNITY HEALTH PROGRAM INITIATIVES

In the information age, health centers continually struggle to implement new programs and to improve existing programs, particularly those centered on the implementation of digital technology. Budget cutbacks imposed during the 1990s took their toll on both the ability to attract and retain quality staff and also on many efforts to upgrade public health facilities, of which the latter is a challenging, lengthy undertaking even in the best of fiscal times. In such conditions, it is necessary to take stock of the degree of catching up needed, and what changes in the size, layout, and amenity of facilities is required to accommodate the physical space and equipment needs of new and revised health care programs and treatment procedures. Staffing levels rise and fall depending on budget resources. The facilities themselves remain relatively stable as they are fixed assets, and yet flexible spaces are required to support changing uses in light of the range of new programs added in recent years. These have included HIV/AIDS early intervention clinics, wellness education seminars, case management programs, and home health care programs.

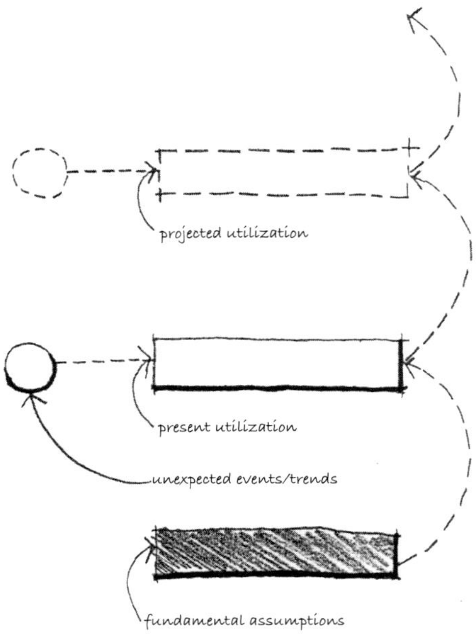

PLANNING—USE

2.4 IN THE PRE-DESIGN PHASE, IDENTIFY UTILIZATION LEVELS AS THE BASIS FOR DETERMINING SPACE NEEDS

Perhaps the most direct, tangible indicator of how much a community care environment is used by the public is its level of utilization. Data on how many patients are seen on a daily, weekly, monthly, and yearly basis can be a powerful tool in making the case for an improved or new community health center. It is prudent to examine discernible trends in the utilization of the facility by going back in the records five years or more to identify salient patterns of use or non-use. This abbreviated history can be merged with population forecasts for the community and the projected utilization of new programs, such as those centered on the treatment of obesity, smoking cessation, lead abatement, and HIV/AIDS. Concurrently assess the tapering off or decline of patient participation in any existing program. Base this facility utilization analysis on the types of services offered at the present time together with projected trends in use by the public. Two ways to report the findings to the community are through workshops and town hall meetings.

PLANNING—FEASIBILITY

2.5 CONDUCT DUE DILIGENCE PRIOR TO SELECTING A TOTAL REPLACEMENT VERSUS RENOVATION STRATEGY

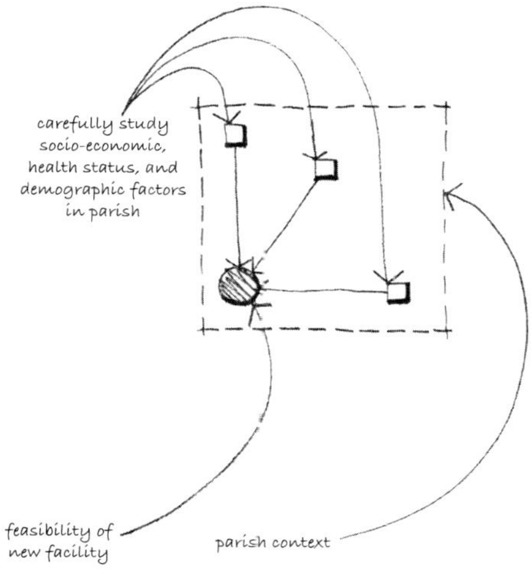

A bad building can be difficult to overcome for even the most dedicated health care professionals. Similarly, for the patient without any other source of care, a run-down, inconveniently located, poorly laid-out setting, lacking in such essentials as patient confidentiality, is a source of stress. This results in the "why bother" syndrome. The staff must self-advocate on behalf of their plight. This background "homework" can be accomplished with the help of community health advocates in terms of increasing public awareness of the need for change. Statistics should be compiled on current utilization and projected growth. Take photographs of existing conditions. Compile statistics on the number of births, utilization by zip code, numbers of Medicaid eligible persons, immunization records, the sewerage permits and health inspection reports filed, median family income, Title XIX recipients, and current local transportation amenities. Build a case on statistical data rather than on innuendo or sweeping generalizations. Decision makers in the local community will respect the effort.

PLANNING—FEASIBILITY

2.6 AVOID MULTI-LEVEL CLINICS BECAUSE THEY ARE AN UNNECESSARY INCONVENIENCE TO STAFF AND PATIENTS

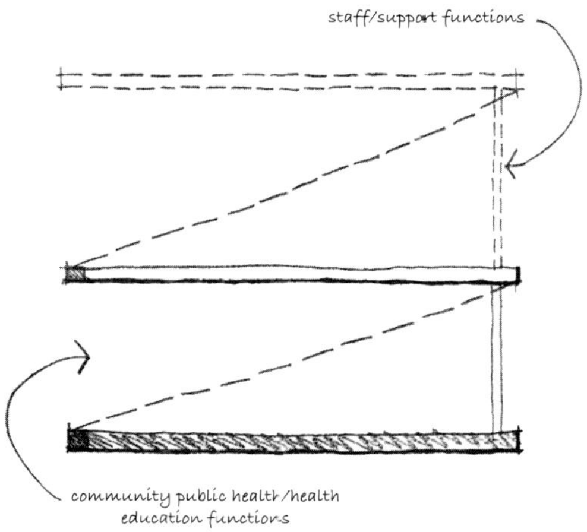

Clinics housed on two levels were documented and analyzed among the case studies conducted during the first phase of field research. In one particularly unfortunate situation the entire clinic was located on the second level, raised up on columns, with parking beneath on the ground level. This configuration may not cause significant stress for staff persons who spend long unbroken periods of time in the clinic, and come and go without children. However, for the parent who must negotiate the level change, often with a child in a wheelchair equipped with cumbersome extension devices, this can pose a significant cognitive, as well as physical barrier. If absolutely necessary due to site constraints, the second level should be designed in a way that maintains a strong connection with the ground level; this can be achieved through the use of more graduated access ramps, an atrium, double height ceilings, an elevator, open stairs, and other means for transporting natural daylight into the heart of the building. It is best to locate the clinic on the first level, with non-patient areas housed above. Minimize unnecessary travel distances, whether in a single or multi-level configuration.

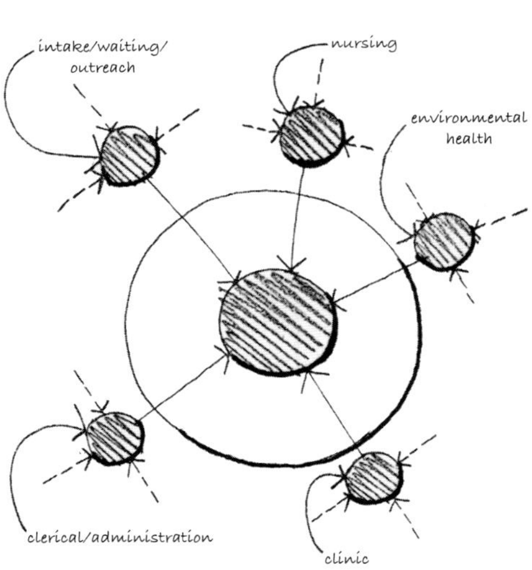

PLANNING—HIERARCHIES

2.7 RECOGNIZE THE UNIQUENESS OF EACH MILIEU WITHIN A COMMUNITY HEALTH CENTER

A typical community public health center consists of five basic interdependent components. These are the arrival, reception and waiting realm, the clerical administration realm, the clinic realm, environmental health services realm, and the health education realm. Architecturally coordinate the specialized spatial and equipment requirements of each realm within a single building envelope, and layer and collage various functions which overlap. Numerous opportunities exist to reinforce the differences between the components of a health unit without creating five autonomous "islands." This does not foster communication among the staff, and in the extreme, each group may want its own break room and its own entrance to the building. This is unnecessary. Therefore, endeavor to spatially weave together these constituent parts into a single, cohesive whole. In so doing, there is no need to assign all functions to one large box. A differentiated yet interconnected massing of elements (wings, creating courtyards) is worth examining in consultation with the staff, local officials, and agency representatives.

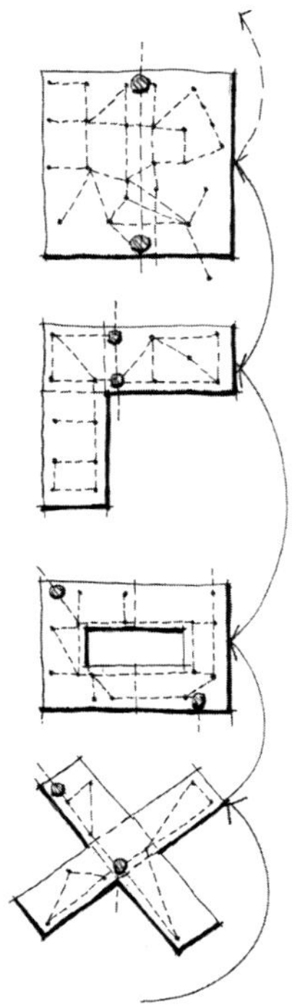

PATIENT-STAFF FLOW

2.8 IDENTIFY AND ASSESS EFFECTIVE PATIENT-STAFF FLOW DIAGRAM OPTIONS EARLY

From the start, the local staff needs to work closely with the architect to work out the most effective staff-patient flow diagram for the proposed facility. This is equally important for units that are undergoing renovation as in total replacement projects. The three major concepts in defining and evaluating staff-patient flow patterns are: 1) minimization of unnecessary trips and travel distances; 2) functional separation where deemed appropriate between staff and patients; and 3) achieving a high degree of fit—compatibility—in spaces shared by staff and patient, such as the examination room. No one "perfect" flow diagram exists, and two or three different types of diagrams may be equally effective depending on the overall shape, or footprint, of the building and site. Architecturally, a given flow diagram may result in a centralized plan versus three or four wings radiating from an administrative core. Multi-level diagrams are not recommended where clinic staff is housed on a different level apart from patient areas. Respect the confidentiality needs of the patient, and reduce the number of decision points, such as at "dead" hallway intersections. This will minimize confusion, which leads to stress.

ADAPTABILITY

2.9 CREATE TRANSFORMATIONAL SPACES IN ANTICIPATION OF NEW PROGRAMS AND TREATMENTS

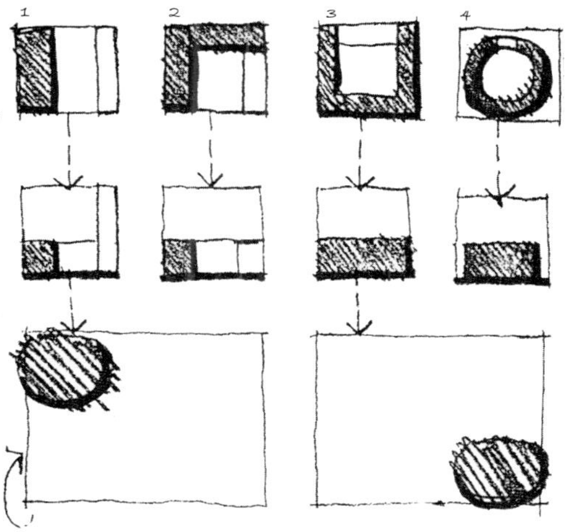

In the past, clinics, hospitals, and other health care buildings were designed as fixed, static entities. Walls, counters, cabinetry, doors, etc. were fixed attributes. When relocation or removal was necessary, renovation costs were considerable. In the Hill-Burton post-war box clinics, interior walls were constructed of glazed tile on bulky masonry walls. This type of construction almost always guaranteed rapid facility obsolescence. This rendered it next to impossible to relocate circulation paths. Therefore, explore methods to create spaces that can be transformed for minimal cost from, for example, a series of small offices to a large conference room, or one exam room being opened up to a space three times its size by means of expansion-contraction strategies within a fixed total envelope. Incorporate new flex plumbing systems in exam rooms, labs, and restrooms. Reception and intake areas should also be designed for flexibility. Fluidity and adaptability is paramount. This strategy may result in somewhat higher (5-10 percent) initial total construction costs, but will yield significant cost savings later in the life of the "flex" building.

COORDINATION—FACILITY MANAGEMENT

2.10 ESTABLISH OVERSIGHT OF THE DAY-TO-DAY OPERATIONS OF THE HEALTH CENTER

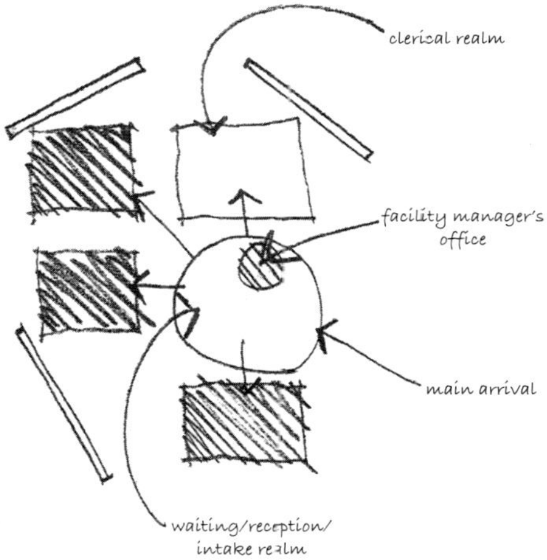

The health centers in the statewide network traditionally had been managed by a triumvirate of three specialists. This group consisted of the parish sanitarian, the clerical supervisor, and the nursing supervisor, with each maintaining oversight for their individual program. This arrangement, ad hoc in nature, led to certain distortions in the actual management of the total care environment. This included situations where personalities clashed, or where one of the three emerged as the dominant spokesperson for the group. In the extreme, one of the three would make sure his/her domain was well taken care of, sometimes barely making an effort to consult the others in terms of their space needs and equipment requirements. Additionally, in capital improvement projects, no one contact person was solely responsible. As a result, the facility manager's duties should consist of overseeing one or more program sites, on a day-to-day basis. This includes scheduling, personnel, building maintenance, grounds maintenance, and the coordination of capital improvements. The facility manager's office should be located near the main entrance, and not in the clinical realm. Provide space for a small conference table and chairs.

3. SITE ENVIRONS

IMAGERY—SITE

3.1 HEALTH CARE ENVIRONMENTS SHOULD BE COMPATIBLE WITH THEIR IMMEDIATE SITE ENVIRONS

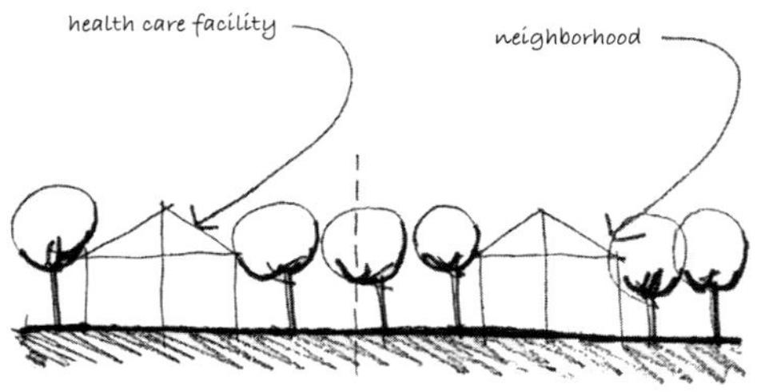

create a virtually seamless connection between the community public health care facility and its neighborhood context

Of the case studies conducted during the early fieldwork phase of the research, no two were alike. A typology was developed, i.e. new versus adapted facility, center of town versus fringe site, old and obsolete versus recent and sophisticated, too small versus over programmed, inaccessible versus accessible, therapeutic versus counter therapeutic, and compatible versus incompatible with respect to its site environs. Site environs denote the immediate neighborhood, streetscape, and the type and condition of the nearest buildings. The presence or absence of trees and landscaping was also recorded. Each case study was assessed in terms of its degree of fit, or compatibility according to these criteria. Therefore, do not locate the community health center in a site context where it will be an awkward fit, or out of synch with the adjacent land uses, imagery, or character of the neighborhood. Work to achieve a seamless connection between building and environs. Provide adequate outdoor lighting for evening activities so people can safely walk or drive to events held in the evening.

SITE—HEALTH CAMPUS

3.2 CREATE A COMMUNITY HEALTH CENTER CAMPUS ON A SINGLE SITE WHEN FEASIBLE

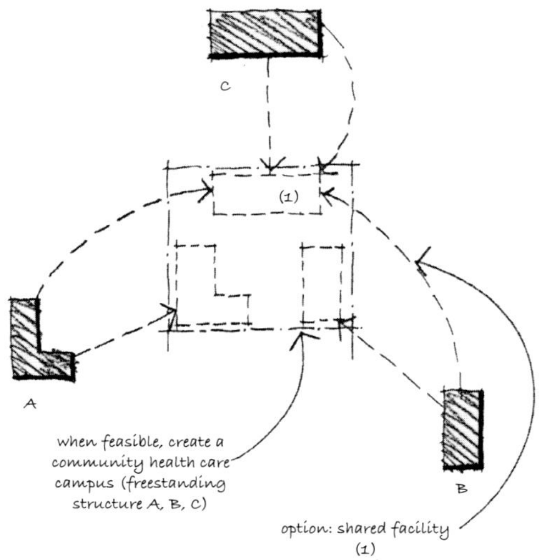

Since the events of 9/11, public health as a field has been under increased pressure to have anti-bioterrorism and related rapid response programs in place. As the need to increase access to services intensifies, and the manifold programs expand, so does the need to centralize services near to one another. Clustering health care services and rapid response programs in the event of terrorist attacks or the aftermath of natural disasters on a single site results in greater convenience to the public. This, in turn, translates into increased utilization and, presumably, improved health. Centralization of allied services cannot occur without planning and coordination among state and local officials representing various agencies. Whether housed in the same building or in separate buildings, work towards creating a unified campus. Construction and operating costs can be reduced by eliminating duplicative spaces, i.e. one multipurpose lecture room rather than two or three, shared support spaces such as restrooms and waiting areas, a common outdoor play space for children, shared HVAC equipment rooms, and the creation of a cohesive aesthetic language.

SITE—IMAGE

3.3 ESTABLISH DIGNIFIED IMAGERY THROUGH THE INCORPORATION OF EMPATHIC WAYFINDING SYSTEMS

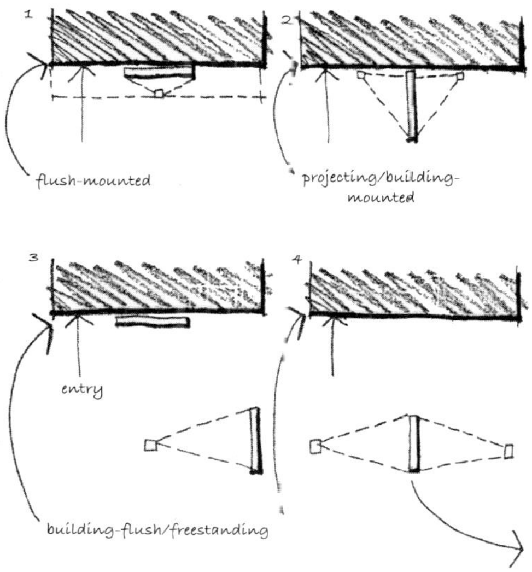

In conducting the case studies, it became apparent that signage is treated ad hoc without any accepted standards or guidelines, beyond the assumption that the facility has to have some sort of a sign someplace. Many were found to be in disrepair. Others had become dysfunctional due to illegible graphics, weathering, or poor initial placement on the building or site. Moreover, directional signs were often lacking indications of parking and entrances. Therefore, design exterior signage to convey a positive first impression and aesthetic image. Staff and patients will tend to respect the building more if it shows it respects them vis-a-vis signage that is legible and dignified. Freestanding signs should be made of durable materials such as concrete, aluminum, and steel. Avoid the use of wood. Letters should be highly contrasted against the background field, i.e. black letters/white background to be legible from a distance. Lighting at night can be internal or provided by external spotlights. Signs should be low to the ground without becoming obscured by bushes, fences, oncoming traffic, and the like.

SITE—SECURITY

3.4 A SUPPORTIVE HEALTH CARE SETTING IS SAFE AND SECURE

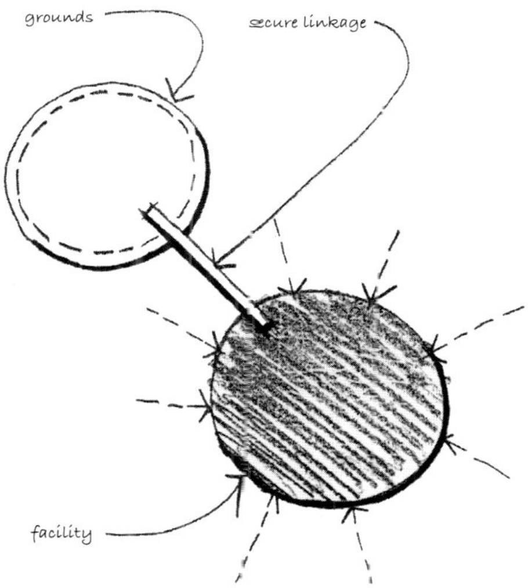

Most of the more than 1,000 respondents to the 2000 SFI survey rated personal safety and security as a very high priority in their facility. In interviews, a number of people had a personal story to relate regarding their own negative experiences. Therefore, create an environment that allows for a freedom of personal choice during the day and at night, both indoors and on the grounds. An environment, indoors or out, where events are unpredictable can be a source of real as well as perceived danger. Incorporate defensible space interventions as a means to provide all visitors and staff a sense of personal safety and protection while on the grounds, and install an appropriate and effective site and building security system to monitor activity. This is of necessity in particularly high-crime areas.

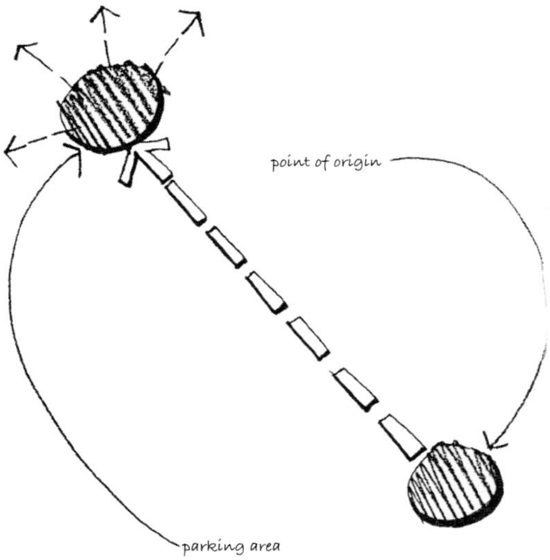

SITE—SECURITY

3.5 PROVIDE SAFE AND DIRECT ACCESS TO PARKING AND LANDSCAPED OUTDOOR AREAS

Parking areas should be decentralized, in order to break down the inhumane scale of large expanses of asphalt. It is also undesirable for parking areas to directly abut the building. The sounds of people coming and going should be visually and acoustically buffered from interior offices and patient care areas. These pockets of cars should be designed to provide safe, direct access from one's point of arrival to one's point of destination. By the same measure, people should be able to easily walk along landscaped outdoor pathways to these parking areas. Minimize unnecessary conflicts between footpaths, paved sidewalks, and highly trafficked vehicular thoroughfares. Minimize the impact of all vehicles on the site. Establish sight lines, which make it possible to see where one must walk between car and main entrance, as this can be a harrowing experience. Ideally, the journey from one's car to the entrance should not require one to cross a driveway. Provide speed reducers to slow down vehicles. Provide a separate entrance to the site for the delivery of supplies. This, combined with having to cross busy driveways, is particularly threatening and stressful to mothers arriving with infants and small children.

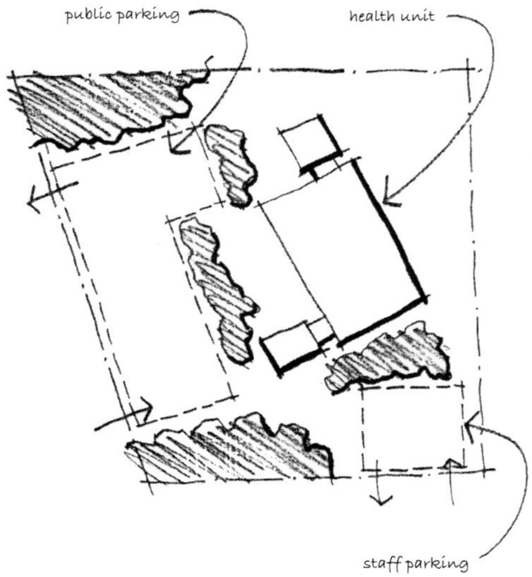

SITE—CIRCULATION

3.6 PROVIDE SEPARATE PARKING FOR STAFF AND PATIENTS IN CLOSE PROXIMITY TO THE BUILDING

People do not like to walk long distances from their car to their destination within the building. Convenience is important, but at what point does the desire to park as close to the building as possible become obsessive? At what point does the minimization of walking distance become unhealthful? In some of the case study sites, the parking areas and sidewalks were found to be awkwardly located and much too close to the building. The buildings were crowded by the cars on the site. This creates a visual sense of over-compression. It is therefore prudent to create a separate parking area for staff apart from the parking area designated for patients. In addition, make every effort to incorporate shade trees and attractive ground landscaping. Such amenities create a significantly less stressful, more attractive environment. Locate these decentralized parking zones and paths near to but not "on top of" the building.

SITE—CIRCULATION

3.7 AUTOMOBILE AND TRUCK TRAFFIC SHOULD HAVE MINIMAL IMPACT ON THE SITE

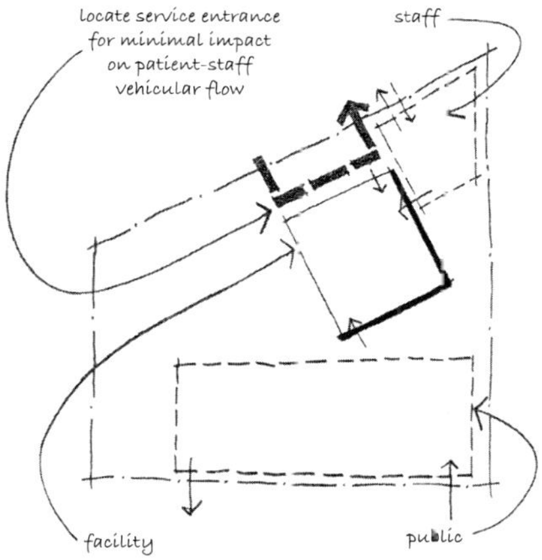

Car and truck traffic on the site of a health care facility have a negative impact from the standpoint of visual distraction, aesthetics, the unwanted noises generated, and the safety and security of patients, visitors, and staff. Vehicular accessibility for emergency and service vehicles is required by local safety codes. However, access is also required for the public and for staff personnel. Regardless, the presence and unwanted consequences of excessive vehicular traffic should be minimized. Therefore, locate service and public access drives at the perimeter of the site, and especially away from the patient arrival areas.

SITE—NATURE

3.8 INCORPORATE LANDSCAPING INTO BUILDING AND SITE DESIGN

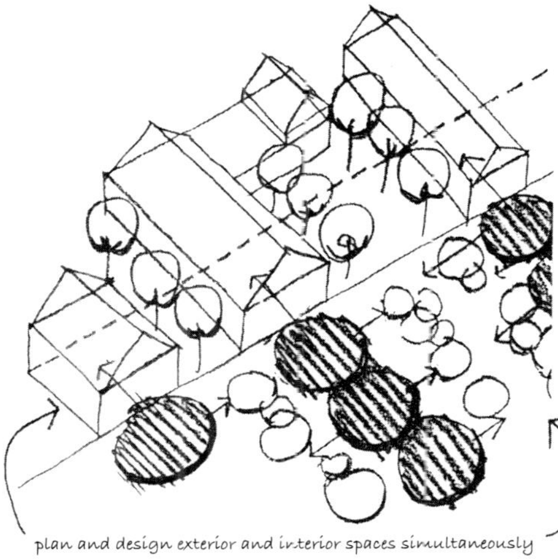

Research in environmental psychology has shown that patients in hospitals prefer visual contact with nature, be it a tree, garden, lawn, fountain, bushes, or flowers, opposed to a view of a blank wall, a totally windowless room, or a room high above the street level. To a large extent, building configuration is determined by basic site planning decisions: a large box, a narrow building with wings, low rise, urban site, rural site, how much parking on the site, and related factors. The footprint of the building is the prime determinant of the configuration of adjacent outdoor spaces. Outdoor spaces should function as rooms in their own right, extensions of the interior realm, as positive contributors to the overall architectural environment. Shaded patios, courtyards, walkways, and screened entries—all are creative landscape interventions and can effectively function as adjunctive architectural design elements. Landscaping should never be treated as an expendable amenity. When the budget becomes tight, retain landscape design interventions, as these provide solace and respite for the building's occupants and enhance its exterior aesthetic appearance.

HISTORIC PRESERVATION

3.9 EXPLORE THE ADAPTIVE USE OF HISTORIC BUILDINGS IN URBAN AND TOWN CENTERS

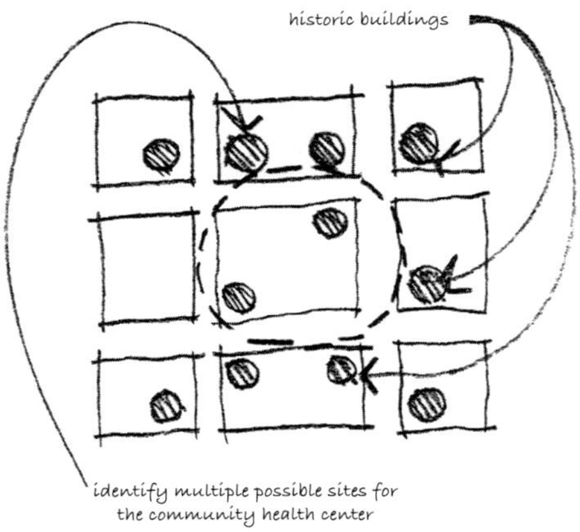

The health centers were founded in the basements of the parish courthouses in Louisiana. As these spaces became obsolete, operations were relocated to the wave of Hill-Burton International style clinics built with federal funds. These buildings were usually built near to the center of the parish seat, on the main street, typically next door to or down the block from the parish courthouse. During these years (1940s through the early 1960s) Main Street was the locus of civic and commercial activity and was the undeniable center of life in their communities. As years passed, Main Street entered a period of precipitous decline and many vacant historic buildings were left to deteriorate. Make every effort to rescue these historic buildings and adapt them to new use as community health centers. Examples include post offices, vacant stores, libraries, banks, and religious structures. These buildings also tend to be within walking distance of the neighborhoods where the vast majority of patients reside—the homes of the working poor who lack health insurance. This strategy of adaptive use of buildings at the urban and town core can help to combat this nation's chronic obesity and chronic disease epidemic.

SUSTAINABILITY—LEED CERTIFICATION

3.10 CREATE SUSTAINABLE, ENVIRONMENTALLY RESPONSIVE HEALTH CARE ENVIRONMENTS

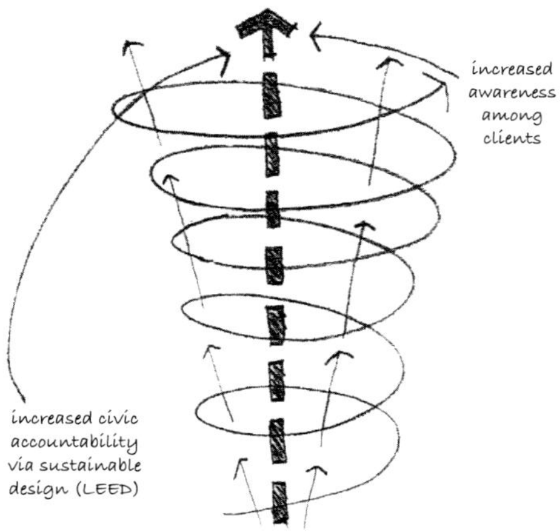

Health care clients need to become better educated with respect to the need to create "green" health care architecture in their communities. Hospitals and related health centers tend to be among the worst polluters. The movement to demand that health care institutions become model citizens of environmental accountability has been slow in developing. The public needs to hold them up to a higher level of scrutiny. There will be no choice but to do so in the face of skyrocketing costs of non-renewable resources such as wood, steel, and other ubiquitous building materials. Therefore, incorporate sustainable planning and design strategies, and obtain Leadership in Energy Efficient Design (LEED) certification. The community health center should become a paragon of environmental sustainability. The rapidly growing LEED certification movement needs to become an integral part of the thinking of health care providers and their architects, in the United States and globally. LEED is sponsored by the U.S. Green Buildings Council, based in Washington, D.C. Refer to their web site, www.usgbc.org/LEED, for additional details, and employ this philosophy from the earliest stages of project development.

4. CLINICAL REALM/ENVIRONMENTAL HEALTH/OUTREACH

ENTRY—TRANSITIONS

4.1 DEVELOP ZONES OF TRANSITION BETWEEN MAJOR DESTINATION POINTS

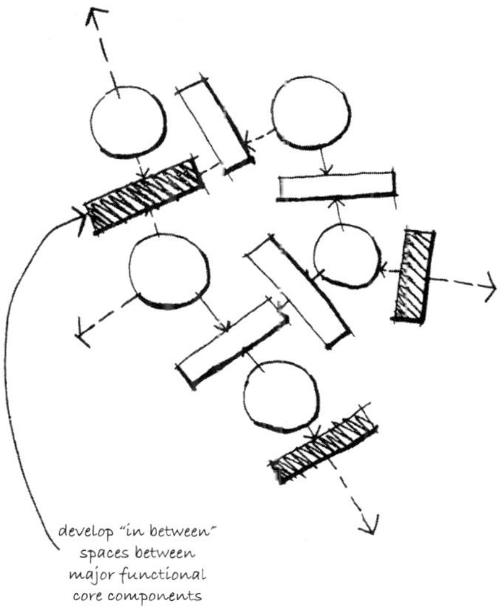

The core is comprised of the clinic's functions: exam rooms, laboratory, consultation rooms, nurses' offices, waiting area(s), charting, and medications storage. Each is integral to the whole. A hierarchy exists with respect to optimal adjacencies among these various spaces and their sizes. However, while these function as anchors, the spaces between provide an equal amount of amenity beyond the matter of mere character and ambiance. Therefore, create hallways, lounges, entry sequences, recessed doorways, and window seats as "in between spaces." These give added hierarchy and contribute to the overall success of anchor functions and provide opportunities for informal interaction among staff, and between patient and staff member. More important, these spaces combat the sense of institutionalism and blandness which exists in too many health care facilities constructed during the past thirty years. Develop strategies to incorporate "in between" spaces without adding significantly to total building costs by creating flexibility, able to be adapted as needs change, i.e. hourly, weekly, or over a longer period of time as needs evolve.

ENTRY—TRANSITIONS

4.2 SATELLITE WAITING ROOMS IMPROVE THE QUALITY OF CARE AND REDUCE STRESS

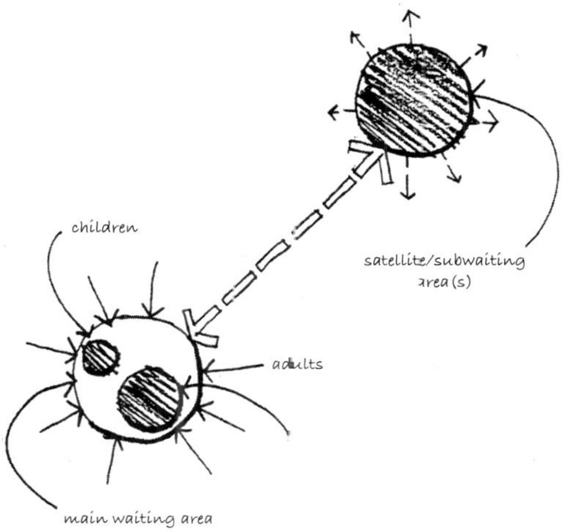

A large main waiting room, situated in the front, adjacent to the main entrance and the registration-intake desk, is assumed to be a core requirement for all outpatient clinics designed in the United States. It is not necessary for it to be the sole waiting area. It is much better for the patient to relocate to a smaller waiting room. The patient advances to the sub-waiting room, or second-stage waiting area, prior to the exam room consultation, to await the results of a lab test, or to wait for another family member. Advantages include closer contact between parent and child, less congestion in the main waiting area, and significantly less foot traffic in corridors, which can interrupt staff work flow, cause stress, and diminish the quality of care rendered. Satellite waiting areas should therefore include comfortable furnishings, adequate ceiling and wall-mounted fluorescent and incandescent light fixtures, carpeting where feasible to reduce sound transmission, and pleasant colors. Locate this space within the heart of the clinic, near exam and counseling rooms without sacrificing privacy and confidentiality. Do not design a sub-waiting area that encourages children to race up and down the corridors.

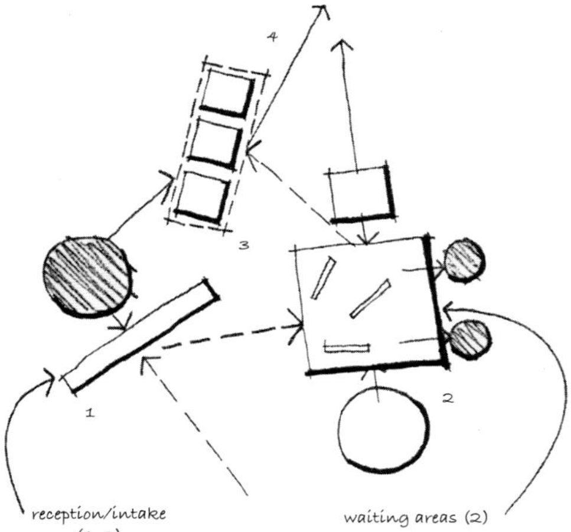

ENTRY—INTAKE

4.3 THE RECEPTION AND WAITING MILIEU SHOULD SUPPORT MULTIPLE FUNCTIONS

The reception-intake area is a nucleus of activity. It is typically the center of administrative operations and the initial point of contact for the patient. It should be a welcoming place as well as a screening and control point—the gateway to the clinic. Staffing limitations may necessitate that a staff person must assume multiple roles, particularly in small facilities in rural settings. By the same token, the waiting area may have to double function as a seminar room for community health education or a prescreening area in addition to its basic function as the place where one waits before the examination. Clear signage at the entry and intake reception will direct people to the sign in, waiting area, counseling, treatment, and administrative areas. Seating in the waiting area should be flexible to allow rearrangement in response to these changing uses. The waiting area should be large enough to allow for movable partitions to subdivide the space as warranted, particularly on days of peak utilization.

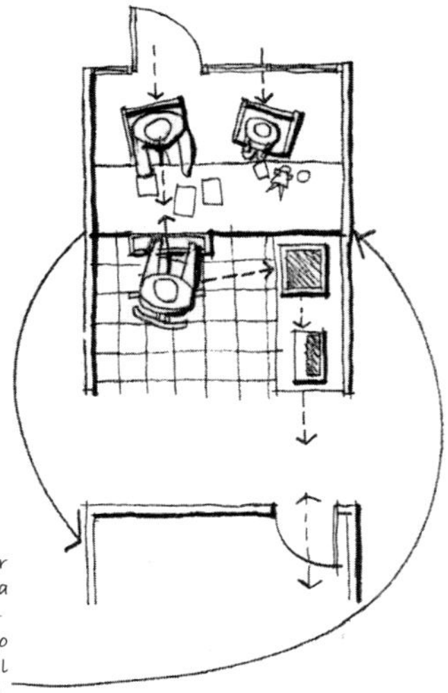

ENTRY—INTAKE

4.4 COMPUTERS FOR MEDICAL RECORDS DATA ENTRY, STORAGE, AND RETRIEVAL SHOULD BE UNOBTRUSIVE

The administrative area is a hub for the counseling and treatment functions. Direct access should be provided to the medical records data entry system. The major advantages of computerized data base systems for medical records, in theory, include the ability to retrieve data relatively quickly without perusing large quantities of files stored conventionally on shelves, requiring fewer personnel than in the past, and comparative ease in updating records compared to the longhand methods of recordkeeping. Transparency should be of high priority in the size and positioning of computer hardware. Greater spatial efficiency should occur as a by-product but this is not possible if the intake room is too small to meet the requirements of the staff person. The biggest problem is usually lack of a side credenza, or a desktop that is too narrow. The optimal width of these intake rooms is 5′6″ to 6′ x 11′ in their depth. The server unit should be located unobtrusively nearby, preferably in a small room.

ENTRY—INTAKE

4.5 TO MAXIMIZE PATIENT CONFIDENTIALITY, DESIGN AN INTAKE INTERVIEW ROOM INSTEAD OF AN ALCOVE

Patients are afforded the least privacy where they need it most—during registration and intake. The most effective way to provide confidentiality for patients during intake is to conduct the interview in a semi-private room, acoustically isolated from the constant buzz of the adjacent waiting room. Wing walls with open backsides to the waiting room are totally unacceptable. This has become even more important since the enactment of Health Information and Privacy Act (HIPA). Provide a full-height glass door and an adjacent floor-to-ceiling window in each intake room. No more than six intake rooms should be aligned in a row. More than six become too oppressive for the patient from a wayfinding perspective. These rooms should be configured so its door opens onto either an adjoining waiting room, or a corridor. The desktop should have a rounded, raised edge to discourage children from climbing over onto the staff side. Provide space for two chairs for patients to sit comfortably. The intake office should be 5′6″ wide at minimum. Do not install glass or Plexiglas between the staff person and patient. These rooms should open directly on their backsides to a "back of the house" workspace.

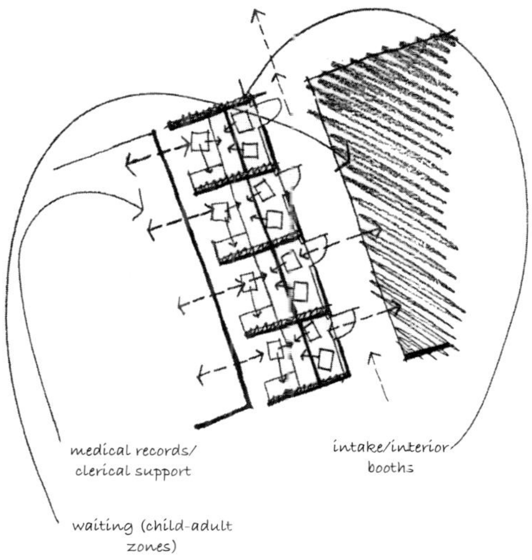

ENTRY—INTAKE

4.6 COMPUTER WORKSTATIONS SHOULD REPRESENT A BALANCE BETWEEN TECHNOLOGY AND THE HUMANE DIMENSIONS OF HEALTH CARE

The use of information technology in the management of large, continually changing data sets is a major aid as well as challenge to the health care provider. Computer technology and software exists to facilitate data management and interactive dialogues between user (patient) and the individuals who operates the informational database. This relationship vis-a-vis paperless medical information records systems is therefore mediated by an administrative staff person. At the present time, the operating software and hardware is accessible only to staff persons. In situations where paper-based records systems are still in use, provide direct access between the intake office and the medical records storage area. Minimize unnecessary walking distances where possible. It is hoped in the near future that the patient will be able to access one's medical history oneself at a private workstation provided in an alcove adjacent to either the main waiting room or the sub-waiting room.

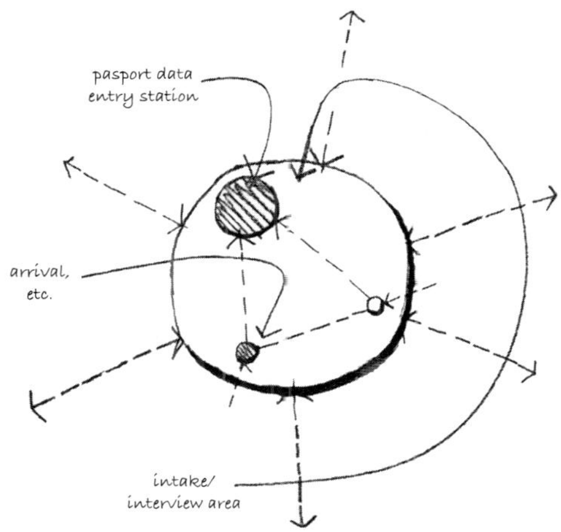

ENTRY—INTAKE

4.7 PROVIDE ERGONOMICALLY DESIGNED WORKSPACE IN THE INTAKE ROOM

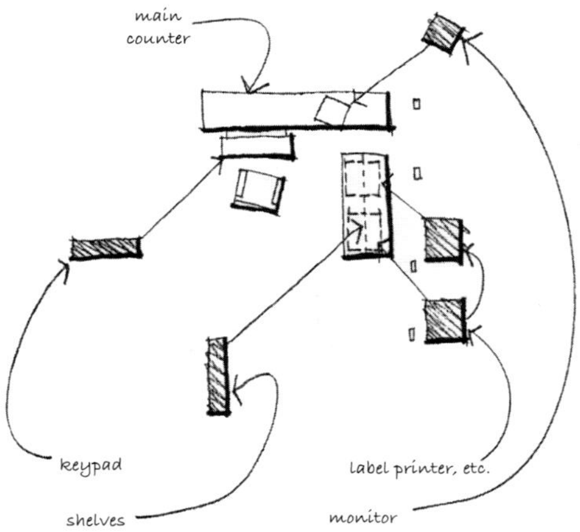

Too often, staff complained of workspaces in their intake rooms that were too narrow and therefore awkward to use by staff and patient. The most complaints centered on countertops too narrow to accommodate computer hardware. The hardware typically consists of the keypad, monitor screen, and label printer. This makes it impossible to have adequate countertop workspace for paperwork, or a place for one to comfortably sit during conversation with the patient. In response, provide front as well as side desktops to house the monitor, keypad, and printer, and create an open uncluttered countertop between the clerk and the patient. The printer can also be stored above the countertop level on a shelf above to conserve space. These ergonomic measures can significantly improve the management and flow of information. In addition, electrical outlets need to be adequate in number and close to the primary work area to allow the proper set up of the equipment, and to provide a supportive person-machine relationship.

ENTRY—PATIENT SUPPORT

4.8 PATIENT SUPPORT AMENITIES SHOULD BE NEAR THE MAIN ENTRANCE

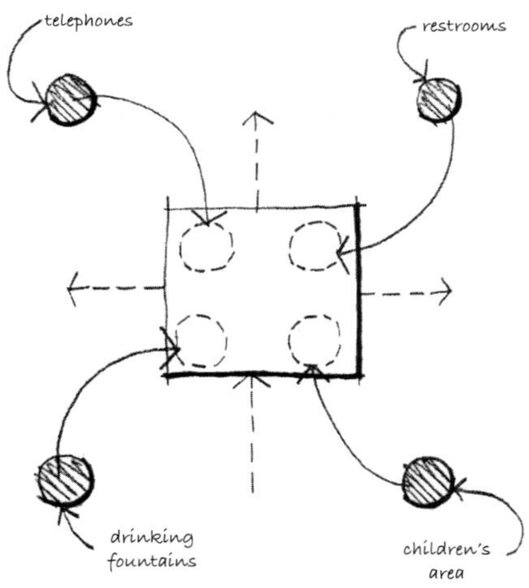

The intake-reception area functions as the first point of contact for the patient with regard to the administrative functions of the health center. Easy access to the waiting room is of necessity, in addition to close proximity to restrooms, telephones, and drinking fountains. Nutritionists generally do not recommend vending machines in these areas due to nutritional health concerns. Directional signage should promote wayfinding. The telephone should not be located in a highly public area, such as immediately next to the main intake counter or window, as this violates patient confidentiality. The telephone is best located either in a remote corner of the waiting room, or, preferably, in an alcove adjacent to the main waiting room. Locate the phone for maximum privacy for patients while allowing mothers to observe their children while speaking on the phone. For this reason, the alcove should not have a door, as it would be difficult to hear one's child in the adjacent waiting area. These amenities should be universally accessible to all.

WAITING ROOM—SUPPORT

4.9 DEDICATE AN INTAKE-INTERVIEW ROOM FOR DETERMINATION OF PATIENT ELIGIBILITY, AND VITAL RECORDS SERVICES

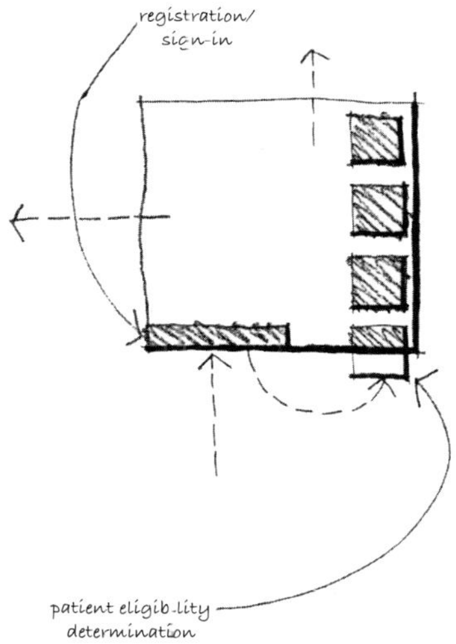

In facilities which experience a consistently high level of patient utilization, it is prudent to ease the patient flow at and near the main desk if a separate space is created for determination of patient eligibility. This negates the need to house this function at the main desk. It also lessens the chance of tedious bottlenecks which often occur during clinics. This is particularly the case on days when more than one clinic occurs simultaneously. This space should be a semi-private alcove or small room adjacent to the main waiting room, not far from the main entrance. This space should be marked with effective signage to identify it as eligibility determination and/or vital records services. Provide space for two chairs on the patient side of this semi-private alcove; countertop height should be 30 inches. See above for additional information on the design of intake spaces.

EDUCATION—SUPPORT

4.10 PROVIDE HEALTH EDUCATION INFORMATION FOR PATIENTS IN WAITING AREAS

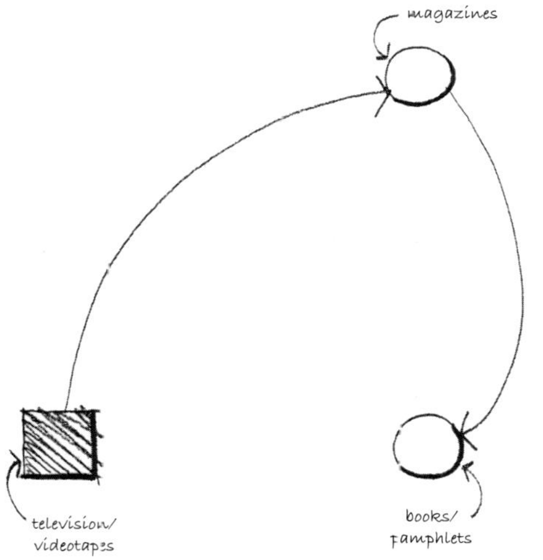

Upon arrival at the clinic and after signing in, time is spent in the waiting room prior to the intake interview, the initial exam, or while waiting for the results of tests or other follow-up procedures. On days when more than one clinic is running concurrently, the waiting room can become quite crowded. Magazines are typically present in the waiting areas of health care clinics and physicians' offices and, sometimes, a television. Videotapes and DVDs can be effective health educational tools—adjuncts to the clinic experience—when shown in waiting areas. Typically, these tapes may last 15 minutes with a continuous loop for automatic playback. They can be shown on conventional TV monitors. These monitors can be housed in laminated wood cabinets to soften the appearance of the waiting room or suspended from wall brackets or ceiling brackets to enable the maximum amount of floor area to remain free and unobstructed.

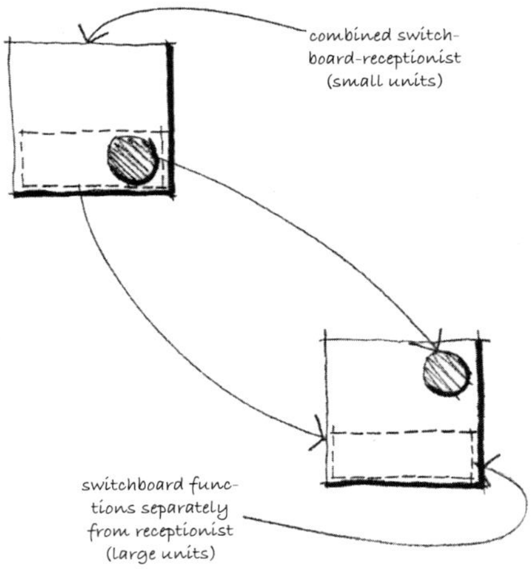

RECEPTION—SWITCHBOARD

4.11 LOCATE THE CENTRAL RECEPTION COUNTER AT OR NEAR THE MAIN ENTRANCE

Incoming calls should be received at a central point at or near the main reception desk. In small health centers, the receptionist usually doubles as the person responsible for handling incoming calls; this person may also periodically visually survey the main entry area and immediate outdoor environs, such as the parking lot. In the larger clinics, this role is specialized to the point where the central reception station is in a separate room adjacent to the clerical area. Provide a roll down screen to lock this space at night and to secure the medical records area from the main lobby and adjacent waiting room.

WAITING ROOM—SUPPORT

4.12 BALANCE HARD AND SOFT SURFACES, OPEN AND SCREENED VIEWS, AND PUBLIC AND SEMI-PRIVATE ZONES

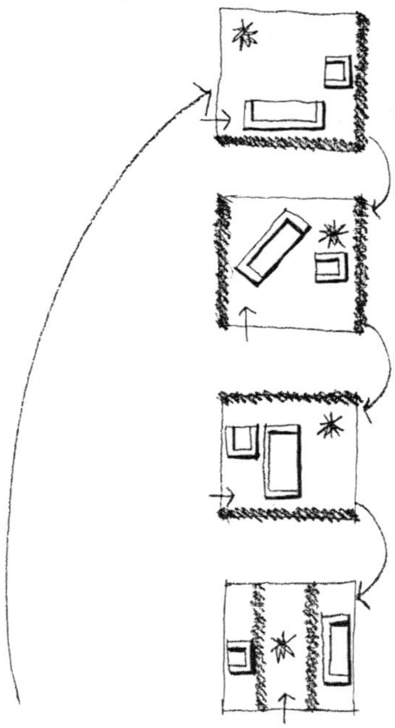

Spaces that receive particularly high use need to be designed for ease of maintenance. Wall surfaces, floors, and furnishings must be durable and able to be cleaned without undue effort or expense. Yet, if this goal becomes singular, the end result will likely be banal, harsh, and institutional. A balance must be attained between ease of maintenance and upkeep via the proper design of hard surfaces yet layered with softer surfaces, i.e. carpeted floors and wall tapestries, if warranted. Similarly, a waiting room can be separated from an adjoining hallway with a half-height wall or an open grid screen. Room-to-room glass walls in waiting areas can result in a loss of visual privacy and are a potential safety hazard to children, unless clearly marked, and safety glass is specified. The public zone between the main entrance, the sign-in desk, and the semi-private zone of the seating area should provide a balance in terms of materiality, room-to-room views, and the need for patient confidentiality.

VITAL RECORDS

4.13 VITAL RECORDS SERVICES SHOULD BE AUTONOMOUS FROM YET LOCATED WITHIN THE ADMINISTRATIVE REALM

The storage of vital records is an important service provided to the general public. These records include birth certificates, death certificates, and marriage certificates. It is important to separate these functions from other aspects of the administration, yet housed within the heart of this realm. A vital records office should, therefore, be somewhat autonomous with a separate window or door near the main waiting room to accommodate those who visit the health unit solely for the purpose of obtaining vital statistical data. This space need not be a completely separate office if located within a large open-plan office. The open-plan office, however, must be lockable. This space should contain one desk for each staff person (typically one or two persons), comfortable chairs (one to two per desk), vertical lockable file cabinets for records on one wall of the office and ample space for cabinets and shelves for forms used by staff. Include room-to-room glass between this workspace and the corridor. Provide visual and acoustical separation from the waiting room-entry area.

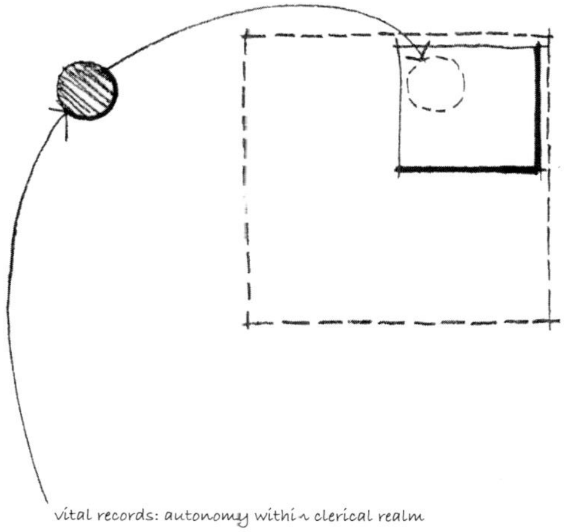

INFANTS—SUPPORT

4.14 PROVIDE A SEMI-PRIVATE SPACE FOR A MOTHER TO BREASTFEED HER INFANT

The large open waiting room typically is crowded during clinics, noisy and bustling with activity. People come and go continually. Whether the majority of persons are waiting to be called or merely passing through to have a set of plans checked by the parish sanitarian, privacy is at a minimum. Mothers who need to breastfeed their infant while in the clinic need a place where they can do so without going into a completely separate room. Therefore, create an alcove or a partitioned area separated from the main part of the waiting room for mothers to breastfeed infants. This space should not be adjacent to a busy corridor nor viewable from a highly public room. It must be relatively serene, equipped with comfortable seating, artwork, plants, carpet, direct and indirect lighting, and warm colors. Provide enough chairs for three to four mothers at a time, with their children, if the children cannot be monitored in the adjacent waiting room.

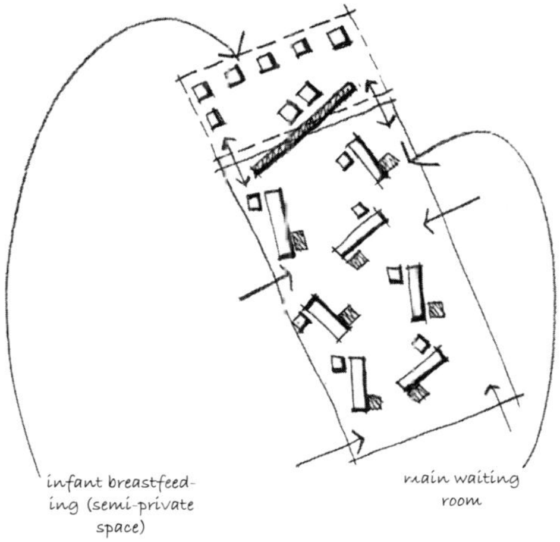

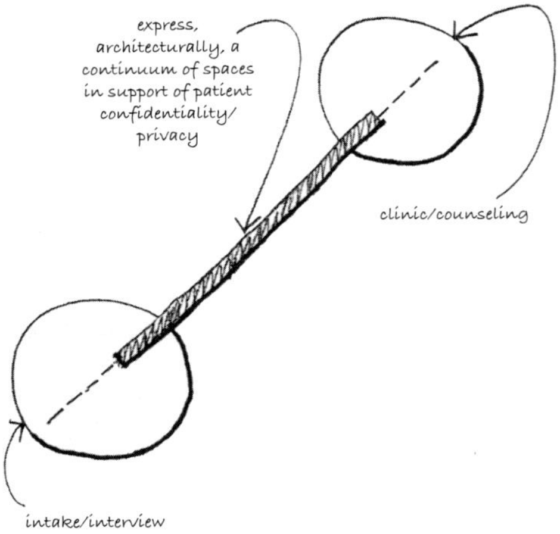

PATIENT CONFIDENTIALITY

4.15 PATIENT CONFIDENTIALITY SHOULD BE A HIGH PRIORITY

It was found that public areas on clinic days are nearly always noisy and filled with activity. This is entirely appropriate and as it should be, to a point. Too often missing, however, is a genuine sense of empathy with respect to honoring the right of the patient to the maximum privacy possible. This manifests in the concept of patient confidentiality. It is inappropriate for patients to be required to divulge personal data in a public area such as a busy hallway or through a small cutout in a glass window. Therefore, design spaces that satisfy the work needs of staff without sacrificing the privacy needs of patients. This applies to reception intake areas, waiting rooms, and exam rooms in particular. Establish neutral zones where, for instance, a nurse and patient can meet on common ground, as opposed to situations where the dignity of the patient and his or her family is compromised.

CIRCULATION—INFORMAL NICHES

4.16 DESIGN WINDOW SEATS AND ALCOVES FOR CONSULTATION WITHOUT FORCING RETREAT TO A PRIVATE OFFICE

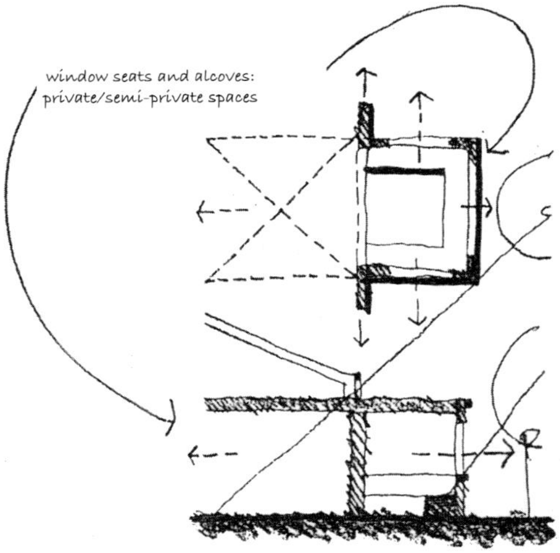

Many patients come from homes where, unfortunately, little privacy exists due to overcrowding or inadequate housing standards, particularly in large multi-unit complexes. These intrusive situations at home make it particularly important for patients to feel that their privacy needs will be respected while at the community public health center. However, it is not always possible to meet one-on-one with a staff clinician in a private office, particularly during busy clinics. In response, strategically located window seats and alcoves adjacent to the examination, immunization, and similar spaces provide opportunities for dialogue, a short conversation among a few staff persons, or a conversation among two or three patients who share a common health problem away from public areas.

CIRCULATION—PRIVACY

4.17 OFFSET ENTRANCES TO ROOMS TO PROMOTE PATIENT CONFIDENTIALITY

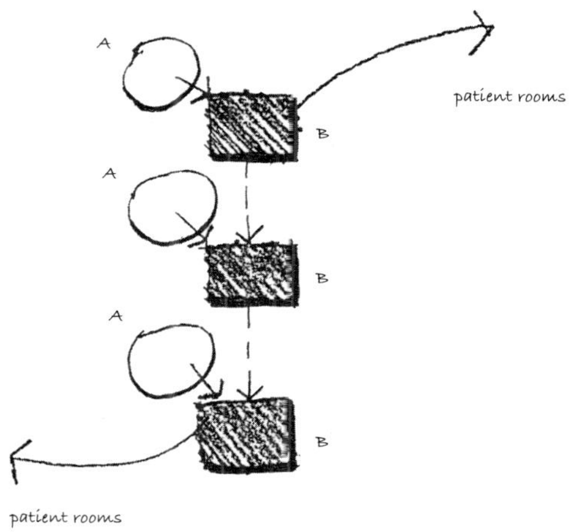

Entrances offset along a corridor or a court can promote privacy. Staggered entrances within a corridor allow a staff person to leave the door open without engaging in direct visual contact with those in the room across the hall. For nursing staff, this may allow for one to remain in contact with activity in other parts of the clinic while one completes paperwork. Also, in certain situations, mothers can still keep an eye on children without actually having them in the nurses' office. While it is desirable to offset entrances to exam and immunization rooms, the doors need to be closed during consultations and examinations. However, the staggered doorway concept offers flexibility in that the door to an exam room can be partially open to allow for some contact with the patient's children who may be in the nearby sub-waiting room, if necessary, during one's appointment.

CHILDREN—CENTRALIZED PLAY

4.18 PROVIDE A SAFE PLAY ZONE WITHIN THE MAIN WAITING AREA

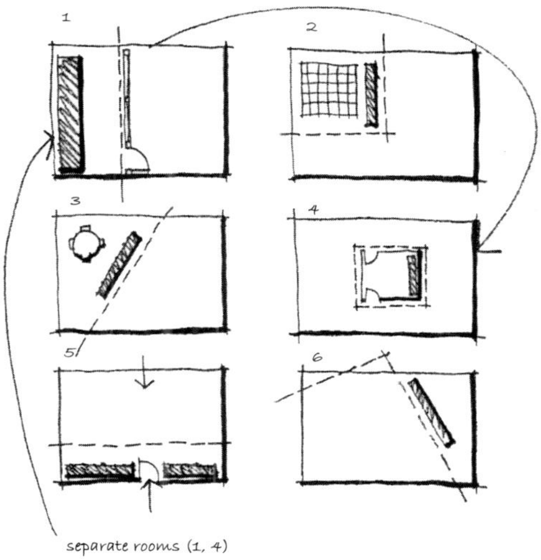

Waiting rooms and entrance foyers that do not accommodate the special needs of children cause an unnecessary burden on parents. Overcrowded conditions in waiting rooms become nearly unbearable when mothers must hold infants and toddlers on their laps due to a lack of chairs. The problem is typically twofold: 1) a waiting room that is too small, and 2) an absence of play amenities for children. Most survey respondents indicated that no designated play area exists in their facility. Create a place—be it a small, carpeted corner or a built-in desk workspace along a wall—for kids only. Locate this area within the waiting room or in an alcove immediately adjacent but do not provide a door. This space can decompress the waiting area by inducing a somewhat calming effect on parents and staff alike. The play zone can be acoustically separated through use of safety vision glass. Carefully encode the glass so children do not run into it thinking there is no glass, with an abstract pattern of colors, a stripe, or a translucent mural depicting people, places, or things.

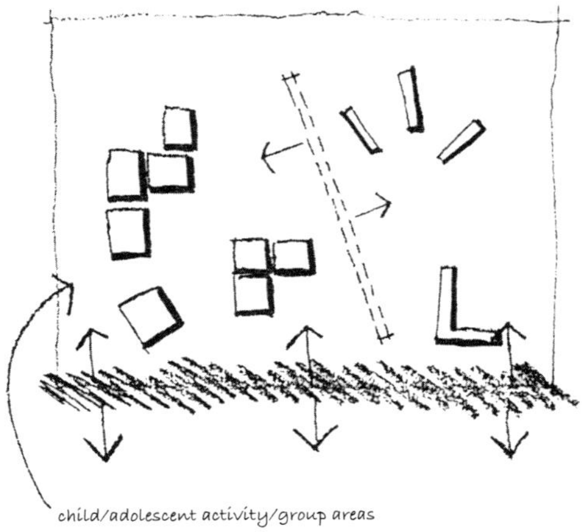

CHILDREN—PLAY OPTIONS

4.19 ENCOURAGE IMAGINATIVE OUTDOOR PLAY OPTIONS FOR CHILDREN WITHOUT DIMINISHING THE QUALITY OF CARE

Children need to play, for it is said that "play is the work of children." In an outdoor playroom for young children, provide safe, moveable play objects and fixed play objects to provide choices for a child. This is especially important if a number of children are using the outdoor "playroom" at once. This reduces the competition for scarce resources, i.e. too many children fighting over too few play options. These options should neither disrupt the quality of health care dispensed nor the rate at which it is delivered. Avoid loud toys or play equipment that squeaks or make other irritating noises. A squeaky sound from a toy can be an irritant to a nurse in an adjacent office. Provide a high level of acoustical separation between the outdoor playroom and interior zones where privacy and quiet is of utmost priority. For instance, locate a hallway or a medical records storage room next to this outdoor space as it creates a buffer between it and staff offices or exam rooms.

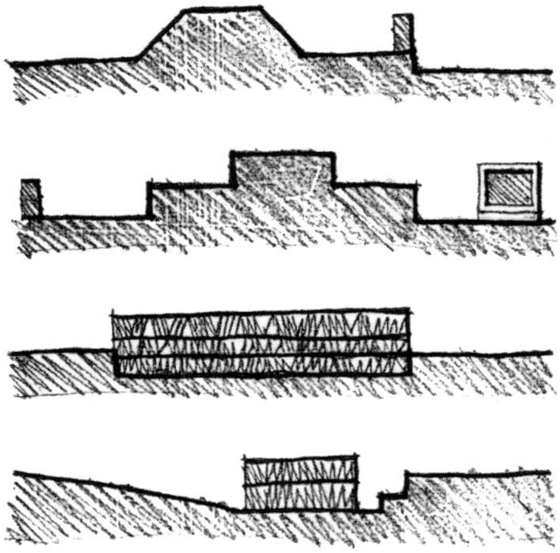

CHILDREN—SUPPORT

4.20 PROVIDE CARPETED LEVEL CHANGES WITHIN THE CHILDREN'S PLAY AREA

Multi-level environments can provide a variety of spaces for children. Carpeted elevations or depressions in the floor create new forms of seating for a variety of uses. These can be used as informal play spaces, retreats, or places for a quiet conversation. Elevated areas can be used as miniature stages, a raised writing or reading surface, or just a place to sit. Carpeted level changes with very low rises can stimulate imaginative play among children. It is recommended that: 1) these amenities only are incorporated in rooms that are designated for children's use; and 2) they be in rooms large enough to also have approximately 50 percent flat floor area for conventional activities. This space should be adjacent to the main waiting room and should be visually accessible (transparent) although acoustically buffered. Refer to other guidelines on the child's play zone.

CHILDREN—SUPPORT

4.21 PROVIDE READING AND AUDIOVISUAL MATERIALS FOR CHILDREN WITHIN THE CHILDREN'S PLAY ZONE

Magazines, books, and videotapes can keep children busy and engaged. These reading and audiovisual materials should be available in one corner of the main waiting room and, in larger health units, in the space designated for children's activity. These materials should be stored on low shelves along a wall or kept in a box in a corner. Pillows should be provided near the materials with lighting levels suitable for reading. In a designated play zone adjacent to the main waiting room, provide a table, chair, pillows, and carpeted level changes. Materials can be stored in recessed "shelves" within the backside of the raised steps, or conventionally in a large box or on open shelves. Perhaps provide a child's height ceiling (4 feet) in a cube for children to sit within and read, or watch a tape or a DVD on a nearby monitor.

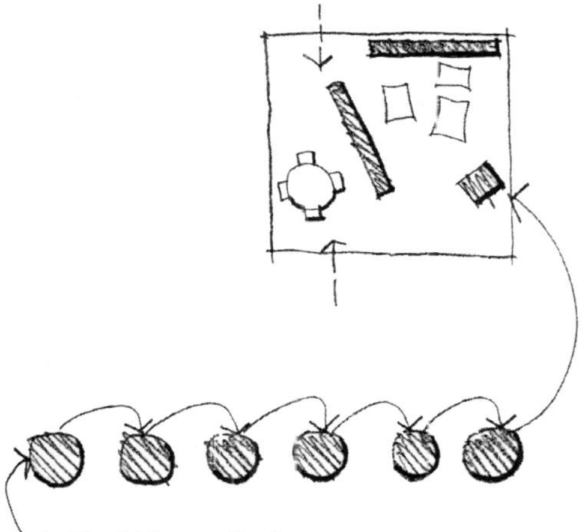

CHILDREN—OUTDOOR PLAY

4.22 PROVIDE AN OUTDOOR SPACE FOR OVERFLOW USE ADJACENT TO THE MAIN WAITING ROOM

The waiting room is typically overcrowded and noisy on most clinic days. A dedicated play zone for children within the waiting room can help. In addition, an outdoor room adjacent to the waiting room becomes an extension of the interior environment. It functions as a decompression space for young children to burn off energy under the watchful eye of parents or volunteer staff. Adults may also benefit from being able to sit outside. Provide for direct visual contact and acoustical separation. It is important for a mother to be able to see what is going on outside from within the waiting room. Enclose this space with walls on all sides with openings in them for light and view from the child's viewing height. This space must be safe and secure. Children cannot be able to leave this "outdoor room" except through the building. Provide benches for mothers and staff, shade, play amenities, soft ground surfaces, and a water fountain.

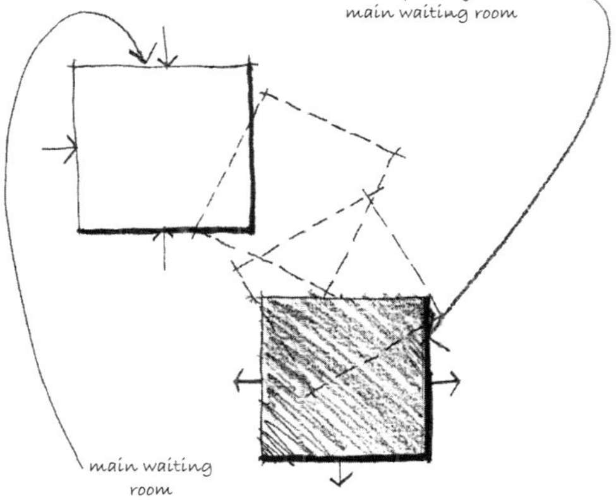

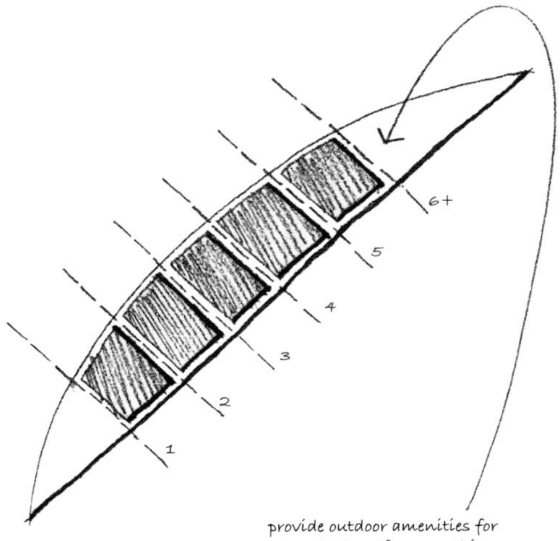

CHILDREN—PRESCHOOLER PLAY

4.23 FOCUS THE CHILDREN'S OUTDOOR PLAY SPACE ON THE ABILITIES AND NEEDS OF THE PRESCHOOLER

From the outset, a number of logistical constraints (such as a lack of funds or available space) will limit the size and design of the outdoor playroom. These factors, together with the fact most children who visit are infants, toddlers, or of early grammar school age, mandate that this space cannot be all things to all children. It is unrealistic to assume otherwise unless funds are earmarked, i.e. a playground onsite, without drawing away needed dollars for the building itself. Therefore, focus on the needs and abilities of the very young child, from about one year of age to kindergarten age. The preschooler age group can perhaps benefit most. Therefore, do not allow ball playing or games that require running. Provide multifunctional play equipment that afford options and are developmentally appropriate. Older children can observe their younger siblings or remain in the indoor realm, engaged in activities such as reading or tabletop games.

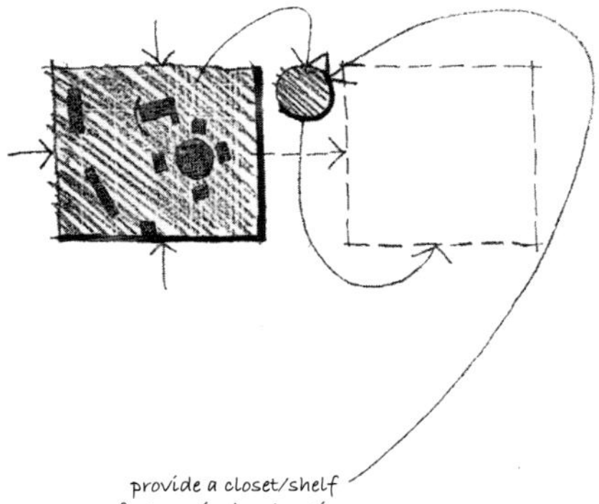

CHILDREN—SUPPORT

4.24 STORE PLAY OBJECTS USED IN THE CHILDREN'S OUTDOOR PLAY SPACE IN AN ACCESSIBLE LOCATION

The play space, if included, should be equipped with a small table and chairs. Objects such as a jump rope and building blocks need to be stored indoors. If exposed to the elements, these toys are subject to damage over time. Provide a storage closet in the portion of the main waiting room nearest the door to this outdoor space. The play objects should be stored in the closet at the end of each day.

CHILDREN—SAFETY

4.25 PROVIDE ABSORPTIVE SURFACES TO PROTECT THE CHILD IN THE OUTDOOR PLAY SPACE

Safety and cleanliness are major concerns in the design of outdoor play areas. The space should restrict the range of activities. Protection from liability as the result of personal injury has become a serious concern among health care organizations in the United States. This type of space for children will, therefore, only succeed if it restricts the range of activities and hence the probability for personal injury. The play space should be supervised by mothers and volunteers. The recommended size of the outdoor play space (approximately 250-350 square feet) precludes multiple play surfaces, such as grass, dirt, sand, or Astroturf. These surfaces may pose safety and cleanliness problems. Therefore, provide a soft outdoor grade mat over most or all of the space, and consider padding walls and/or fences to absorb the impact of falls. Carefully select the doors and windows opening onto this space so children do not mistakenly try to run through them.

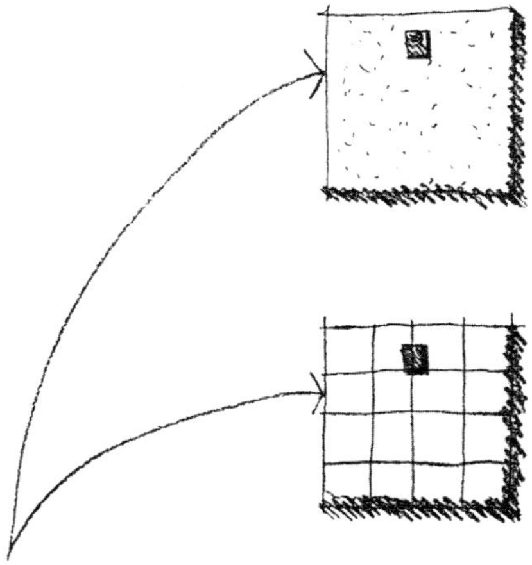

select durable, 'non-institutional' materials and finishes

CHILDREN—SAFETY

4.26 PROVIDE A NON-MOVEABLE PLAY OBJECT OUTDOORS THAT ENSURES SAFE CLIMBING AND MOVEMENT

Climbing is an important aspect of child development. Hand-eye coordination and muscular development is enhanced and this is most evident in situations where the child is presented with more than one climbing option. Allow for imaginative play to occur: fantasy and imitation. Include in the outdoor space area a timber (or similar) flexible play device that includes a ladder, climbing net, slide, or tunnel tube which presents options to the child. This will make the most efficient use of limited space and preclude the need for more than one play object for climbing. Locate this device so mothers and staff can directly view the children from elsewhere in the outdoor space and from the main waiting room indoors.

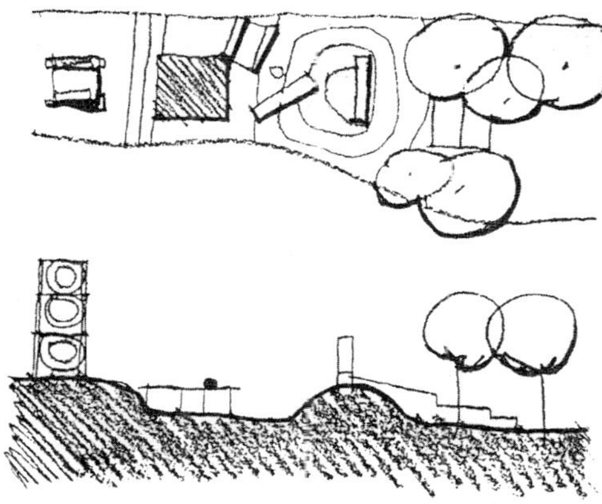

create a stimulating but controlled play setting

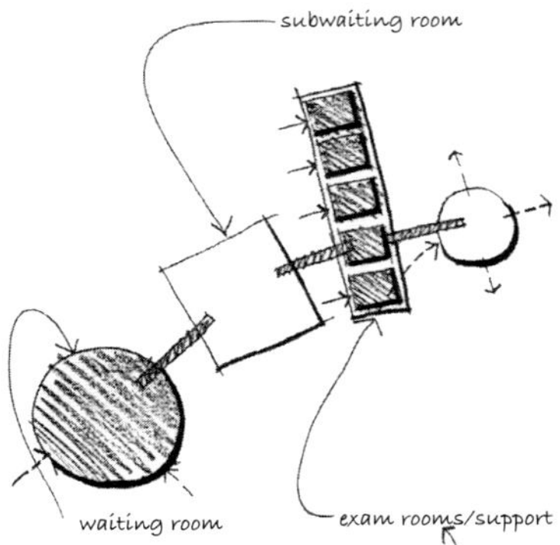

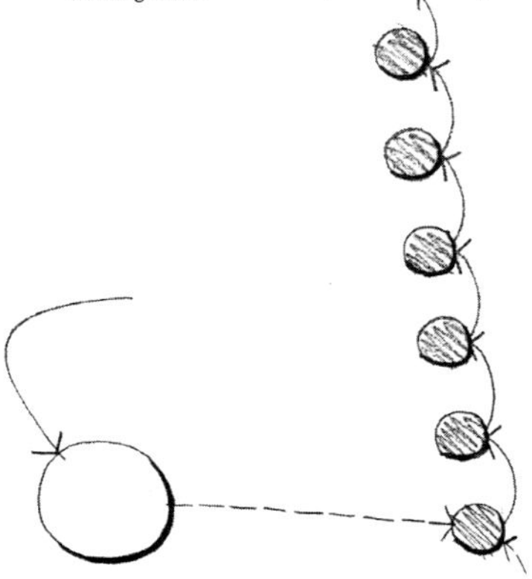

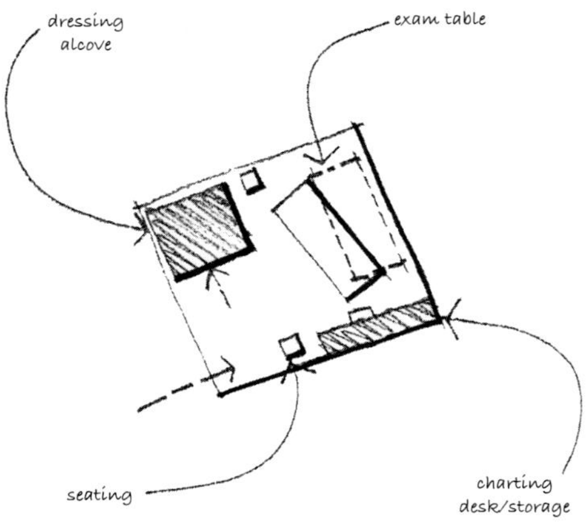

EXAMINATION—TREATMENT

4.27 THE EXAMINATION ROOM SYMBOLIZES THE HEART OF THE CLINIC ENVIRONMENT

The exam room must support a high degree of fit between staff and patient needs, in addition to needs unique to each constituency. The exam room should be located at the heart of the clinic and easily accessible to staff and patient support spaces as well as waiting areas. Provide wall and ceiling mounted artificial lighting fixtures. Allow natural daylight to bathe the room vis-a-vis windows whose sill height is high enough to not compromise the confidentiality of occupants. Do not provide carpet. Accent colors on framing, doors, and walls can achieve an uplifting ambiance. Include plants and artwork. Door placement and directional swing should not compromise patient privacy. Include an intercom system and wireless telecommunications system. Provide a clean, dignified appearance, an area for infants, space for two chairs for patients, and a comfortable exam table. The dressing alcove should be included within the exam room with a wing wall or draw curtain. The recommended size for the examination room is 125-130 square feet, including the dressing area. Include wood moldings or Plexiglas chair rails to protect walls.

EXAMINATION—FURNISHINGS

4.28 SELECT AN EXAM TABLE COMPATIBLE WITH THE DESIGN AND LAYOUT OF THE EXAMINATION ROOM

In a pre-SFI replacement facility, the staff was rather surprised to find that the exam table cabinet doors opened on the wrong side in relation to the window, the door, and the fixed countertop work area. The table then had to be awkwardly relocated, or "floated," away from the wall in order to provide the needed access for staff to be able to get to the adjacent amenities. This problem can be entirely avoided by selecting an exam table compatible with the layout of the exam room. In addition, the exam table drawers should be easily accessed by staff and locked when not in use in order to keep inquiring children from opening them while adults are looking away or are not in the room.

CLINIC—FIRST AID

4.29 THE LOCATION OF THE FIRST AID STATION SHOULD BE CLEARLY MARKED WITHIN THE CLINIC

The treatment of cuts, bruises, and fractures typically does not fall within the scope of services provided at a community public health center. Outpatient medi-centers, hospitals, and the like exist to provide emergency health care. Nonetheless, the staff must be equipped to treat persons who may get hurt while on site. This usually applies to children: a child may accidentally trip down a flight of stairs or get a hand caught in a doorjamb. In these situations, a first aid station should be established on-site to preclude the need for persons with minor cuts and bruises to have to be treated elsewhere. This first aid station should be incorporated in one of the examination rooms. Reference books and online emergency medicine databases should be immediately accessible.

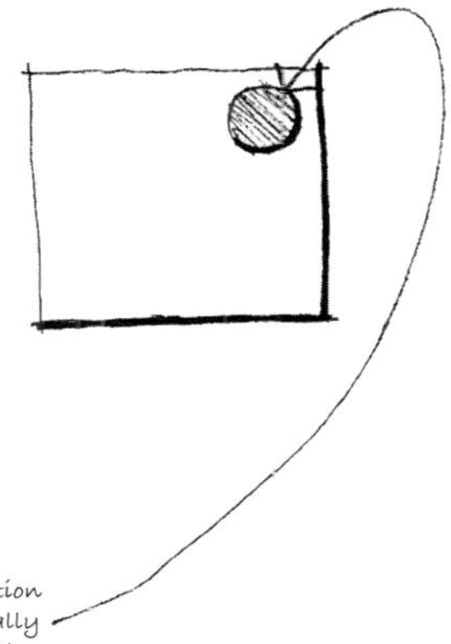

NUTRITIONAL EDUCATION

4.30 DESIGN MULTI-PURPOSE ROOMS AS A SINGLE SPACE WITH FLEXIBLE PARTITIONS TO CREATE SMALLER ROOMS

It does not make sense to design a separate room for each and every function, as this results in excessive construction costs and adds an unnecessary burden to building maintenance and upkeep responsibilities. Such strategies often result in room underutilization, i.e. a designated vision screening room used only for one purpose two days out of the month would be idle nearly 90 percent of the time. For these reasons, it is important to explore the double and perhaps even triple-functioning of rooms in a manner that does not decrease the quality of health care delivered to constituents, i.e. WIC kitchen, conference rooms, family planning education. A large room, perhaps near the center of the health unit, can serve as a combination meeting room and kitchen if carefully zoned. This room should seat a maximum seventy-five people, equipped with flexible furnishings. Provide a projection booth, screen, and movable partitions on a ceiling track to subdivide the room into two or more smaller rooms. This allows for small group activities to occur simultaneously.

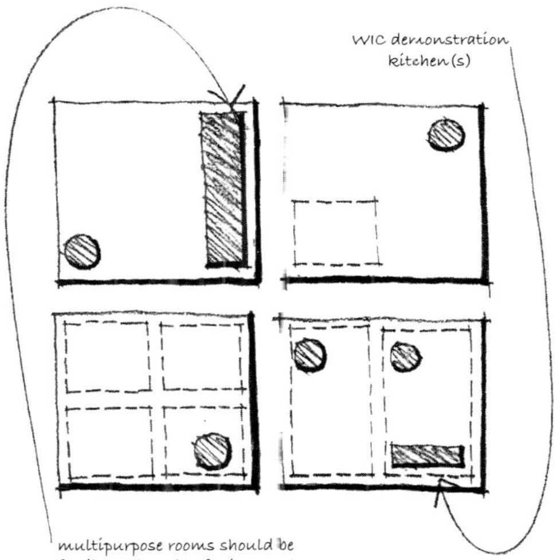

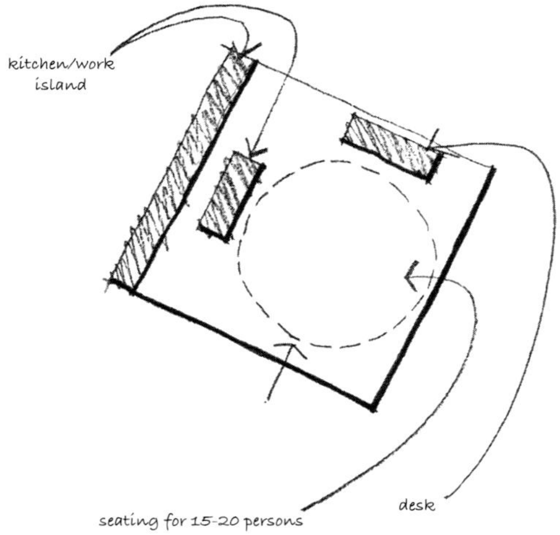

NUTRITIONAL EDUCATION

4.31 NUTRITIONAL EDUCATION KITCHENS SHOULD BE FLEXIBLE TO ACCOMMODATE MULTIPLE INSTRUCTIONAL PROGRAMS

Nutritional education, as presently structured, is based on a combination of hands-on demonstration with more traditional classroom instruction. Unfortunately, too often the kitchen is not designed to allow its use for both purposes due to lack of space, poor layout, or inadequate seating. In order to allow the kitchen to double-function, design it for use as a food preparation area complete with triple sinks, as mandated by state health guidelines, an oven, refrigerator, cabinets, dishwasher, a microwave oven, adequate countertop area, and audiovisual equipment. Design this space for use by groups of four to ten persons; include a work island situated between the oven-sink and the large open portion of the room, and a workstation for the nutritionist. Equip the island with an overhead mirror. Folding partitions subdivide this room into two smaller rooms without sacrificing the functional integrity of either. Explore the possibility of a folding wall between the kitchen and an adjacent sub-waiting room so this space can double as a viewing area.

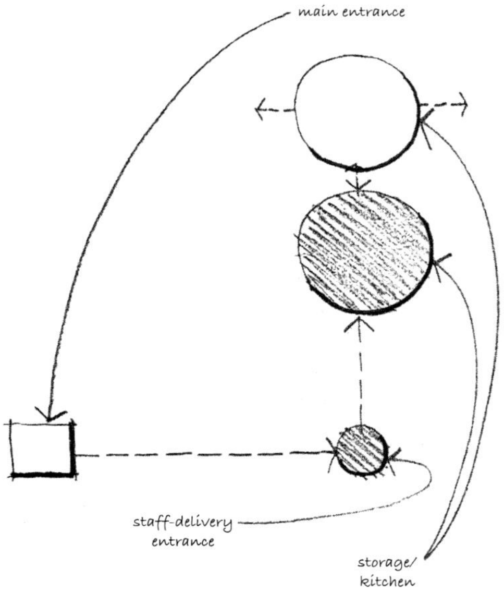

NUTRITIONAL EDUCATION

4.32 PROVIDE A PANTRY WITHIN THE NUTRITIONAL EDUCATION KITCHEN AND DIRECT ACCESS TO A SERVICE ENTRANCE

Deliveries of food supplies to the nutritional education kitchen should be possible without requiring that supplies be brought through the main entrance used by patients and others during normal hours of operation, for this sacrifices patient confidentiality and can be disruptive. Establish a logical flow of goods from the parking lot-delivery area to a side or secondary entrance that is not used by the public and is accessible to the kitchen. Provide adequate storage within the kitchen or in a small adjoining lockable room for storage of supplies such as dry bulk goods and stacked folding chairs for use in classroom instruction. This room must be secure at all times. Avoid situations where nutritional education supplies and equipment is kept in rooms too distant from the kitchen except, perhaps, for equipment seldom or infrequently used.

NUTRITIONAL EDUCATION

4.33 NUTRITIONAL EDUCATION KITCHENS MUST PROVIDE SPECIAL SINKS AND COMMERCIAL-GRADE OVEN HOODS

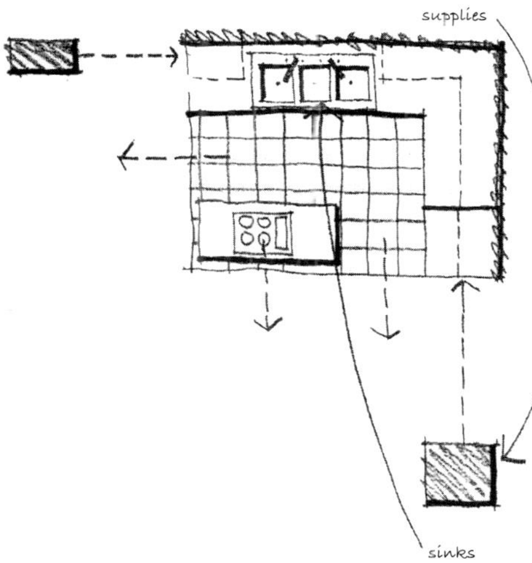

The kitchen should be residential in character and in amenity in order to approximate the kitchen in one's home or apartment. This includes wood cabinets, conventional appliances and countertops, and conventional lighting, both from lighting fixture and daylight transmitted through one or more windows. Storage for equipment, eating and cooking utensils, and food supplies is required. However, health regulations require that all nutritional education kitchens be equipped with triple sinks to allow for the separation of hand washing from food prep activities and a commercial grade exhaust hood above the cooking island. The sink should be located between zones of countertop workspace and fully accessible to the handicapped. The space beneath the sink must allow space for a wheelchair-bound person's use. Provide a space for refuse and chair storage.

NUTRITIONAL EDUCATION

4.34 EQUIP THE KITCHEN WITH AMPLE COUNTERTOPS AND ISLANDS FOR FOOD PREPARATION DEMONSTRATIONS

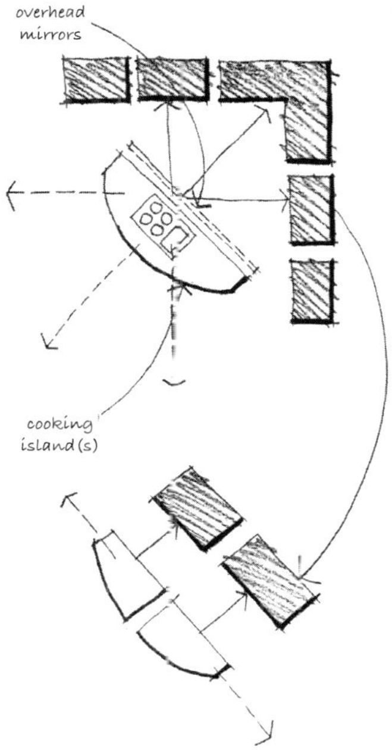

The arrangements of the countertops and islands are important for food preparation in the nutritional education kitchen—whether for small groups or larger classroom instruction. It is prudent to design work island counters that are forty inches wide minimum. The 2000 SFI survey did not focus on this degree of detail within room types, but it was found during the course of the twenty-five case studies that many otherwise functional kitchens are limited in their flexibility due to a lack of countertop space and work islands. In addition, arrange the island(s) to allow access by many at the same time. Perhaps separate the island into two to allow for additional movement for demonstrations, if warranted, due to high use or more than one demonstration occurring at once. This configuration allows for the direct participation of clients and an opportunity for social interaction. Provide an overhead mirror for cooking demonstrations. Do not include ovens that can be easily touched by children. Therefore, include vertical ovens with doors and controls above the reach of small children.

PASS-THROUGH PORTALS

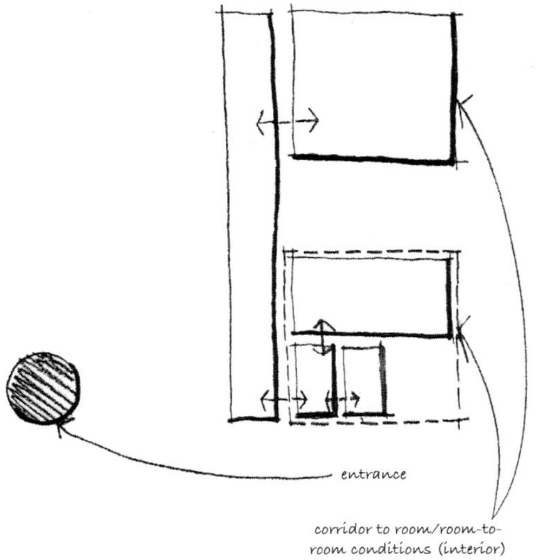

4.35 IMPROVE THE TRANSPORT OF FORMS, RECORDS, AND SPECIMENS WITH PASS-THROUGH WALL OPENINGS

Typically, the staff has to walk down hallways or enter the offices of others in order to deliver or retrieve forms of one sort or another. Forms and medical records are frequently stored in wall-mounted chart racks. This can be effective in the clinic when combined with an interoffice intercom although vertical slotted portal openings in walls along corridors and between clerical offices can further improve the flow of these vital materials. Do not, however, locate these wall openings in areas adjacent to noisy waiting rooms or busy hallways if privacy and sound control is required. In the field research it was found that patients, after being interviewed, often had to return to the public restroom in the most public portion of the facility in order to extract a urine specimen for lab testing back in the clinic. This room should be adjacent to the laboratory, connected via a pass through stainless steel portal (actually a small door 12" x 12" in size equipped with a handle).

CLINIC—ADJACENCIES

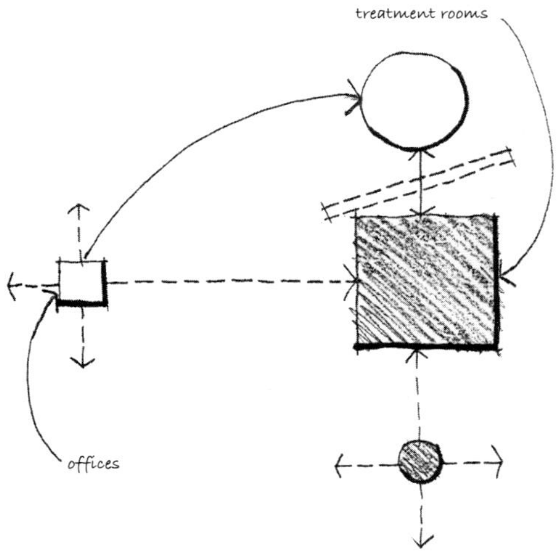

4.36 CLUSTER NURSING STAFF OFFICES APART FROM YET NEAR DIAGNOSTIC AND TREATMENT ROOMS

The nursing staff is extremely busy much of the time on hectic clinic days; they must cope with back-to-back appointments with few breaks, particularly on the days with major clinics, i.e. WIC/Child Health, Family Planning, and STD clinics. Although the staff lounge should be located away from the main hub of activity in the clinic, it is desirable to locate nursing staff offices adjacent to examination and consultation rooms. Explore the use of a door to connect the nurse's office with the adjoining exam rooms in a manner that makes it possible to move from office to exam room without entering the corridor. The office should include a desk, storage space, shelving for supplies, perhaps an exam table, and chairs. An alternative in small-scale care settings is to make the nursing office and the exam room one and the same, with a desktop for charting space, computer, exam table, supply cabinets and sinks, with a dressing alcove or in-room pull curtain device.

CLINIC—TRANSFORMATIONAL ROOMS

4.37 EXPLORE THE CREATION OF INTERCHANGEABLE TREATMENT AND SEMINAR ROOMS

In the institutional structure of a hospital the care provider's office is too often in a completely different part of the building, or in a different building, far from the exam room where one's patients are seen. In an outpatient clinic this need not be the case. Small scale is an advantage as this facilitates greater provider-recipient contact. Clinical staff offices and exam treatment rooms should be viewed as symbolic: strong proximal linkages result in less time spent moving through corridors and more time in contact with the patient. Avoid situations where patient space or "turf" is too isolated from staff turf. Develop a layering of staff and patient space. The nurse's office may double as the exam room. A flexible strategy is to create a cluster of transformational exam-seminar rooms connected to adjoining staff offices, minimizing the need for lengthy double-loaded corridors where staff offices are on one side and exam rooms on the other.

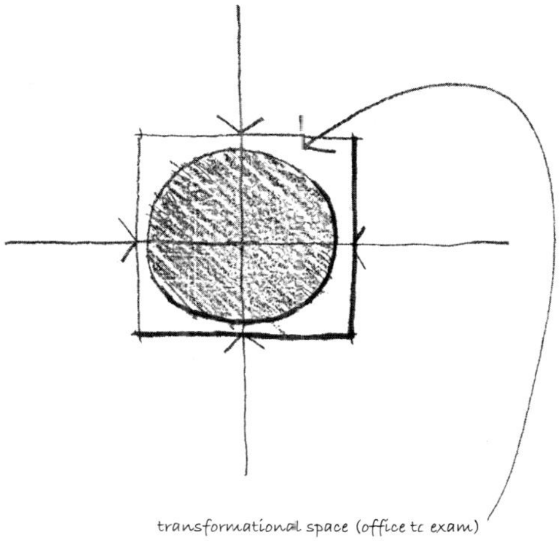

transformational space (office to exam)

STAFF OFFICES

4.38 PROVIDE A MIX OF PRIVATE AND SEMI–AUTONOMOUS OFFICES FOR STAFF

Specialized workspaces are essential to day-to-day operations. Clerical functions associated with general recordkeeping can be performed in an open-plan office setting. This work area should be adjacent to the main reception-intake area, near the facility manager's office and the medical records room. Open-plan spaces allow staff to perform tasks that require precision and concentration while at the same time requiring contact with coworkers. Spaces able to be semi-private include but are not limited to clerical functions and nursing administrative workspace. Therefore, provide a mix of open-plan semi-private and closed private work areas in response to the organization's culture, communication styles, and individual duties and responsibilities.

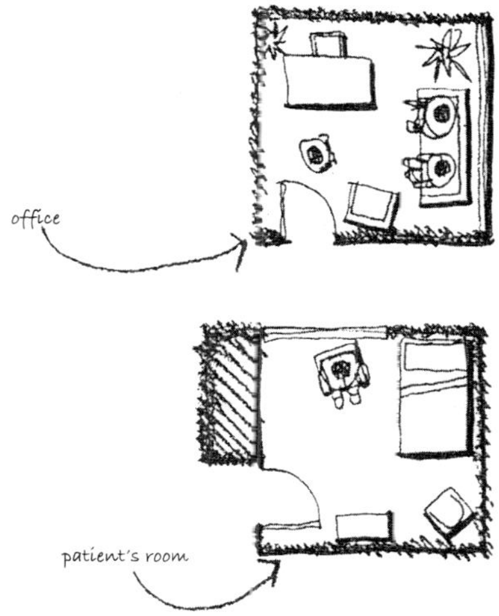

allow for personalization (within cost parameters)

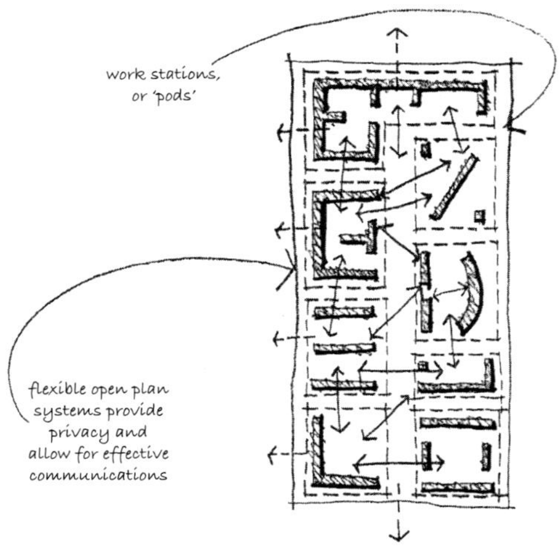

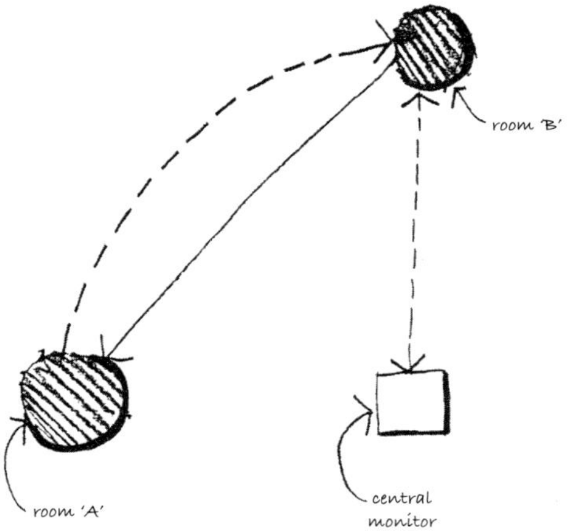

STAFF OFFICES

4.39 DESIGN OPEN-PLAN OFFICES FOR NURSING STAFF WITHOUT SACRIFICING PERSONAL SPACE

Open-plan offices, such as Steelcase systems or Herman Miller systems, for nurses allow for individual work spaces with five-foot-high partitions, shelves which house desktop lighting, ample space for a desk, chair(s), and cabinets, and above all, sufficient privacy while allowing for flexibility. Provide windows that yield full views, carpet, places for plants, closets for coats and personal artifacts, and insure that the overall workspace is lockable. Provide separate pods within staff work areas, such as in the nurses' open-plan workspaces with components constructed of a flexible, interchangeable kit of parts in order to respond to changing requirements.

STAFF—WIRELESS INFORMATION TECHNOLOGY

4.40 PROVIDE WIRELESS TELECOMMUNICATIONS SYSTEMS

In more than one case study, patients were beckoned through an intrusive overhead public address system. This unnecessary situation may create indignation on the part of the patient, as well as staff, with negative consequences accumulating over time. The patient is treated with indifference and disrespect in such situations. The clinic staff should be able to communicate with each other anyplace, anytime within the facility via a wireless communications system. It increases efficiency when the staff has the option to call one another while away from the hard wire phone line in one's office. In addition, a hand-held device can be given to the patient—just as it is used in restaurants—to relay nurses' requests from the receptionist to the patient that it is his/her turn to proceed to the sub-waiting room or a specific examination room.

RESPITE

4.41 PROVIDE A STAFF LOUNGE TO FUNCTION AS A RESPITE

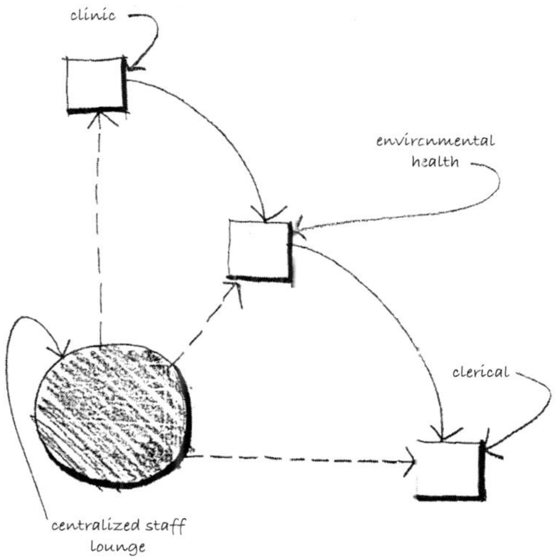

The provision of a respite within the facility for staff is important. Staff should have a room away from the hub of the clinic's stressful conditions, a place where one can take breaks, yet remain not too distant. Create a room that will provide a sense of retreat, convenience, and comfort. In virtually all case study site visits, staff expressed a strong desire for a space strictly for their use. Ideally, this space should have a staff-only restroom, kitchen area, refrigerator, microwave, couches and/or chairs, counter(s) and cabinets, and acoustical separation from other parts of the building. In settings with small in-unit staff lounges, it was learned that staff routinely have to leave the building to achieve a sufficient sense of respite. Provide an adjacent outdoor shaded patio with a fence. These amenities can improve morale, productivity, recruitment, and retention.

RESPITE

4.42 PROVIDE SEPARATE BREAK AREAS FOR CLINIC AND NON-CLINIC STAFF BASED ON THE SIZE OF THE HEALTH CENTER

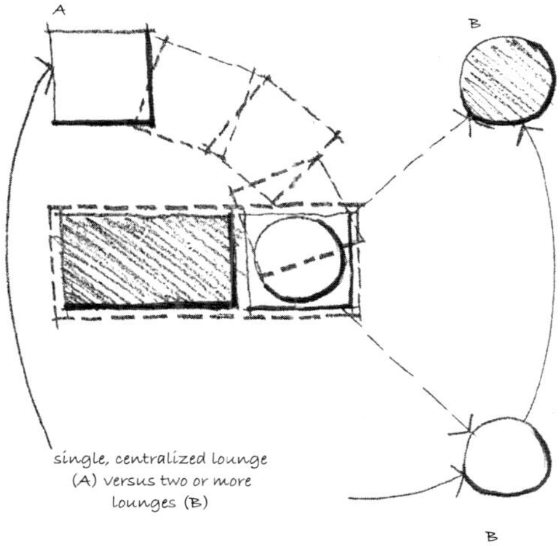

In urban settings with high levels of utilization, the degree of specialized services may dictate separate lounges for clinical staff apart from the non-clinical staff. In larger facilities multiple staff lounges allow for decentralization and more personal space to obtain needed respite. These break rooms should be designed to convey their importance to well being. Second, location is an important factor because these spaces should not be too close to or distant from the hub of activity in the event of emergencies or unusually heavy patient case loads which tend to necessitate short breaks. Key determinants in assessing the need for multiple staff lounges include the size of the facility, range of programs offered, staffing patterns, and the degree of emphasis on improving staff morale, productivity, recruitment, and retention.

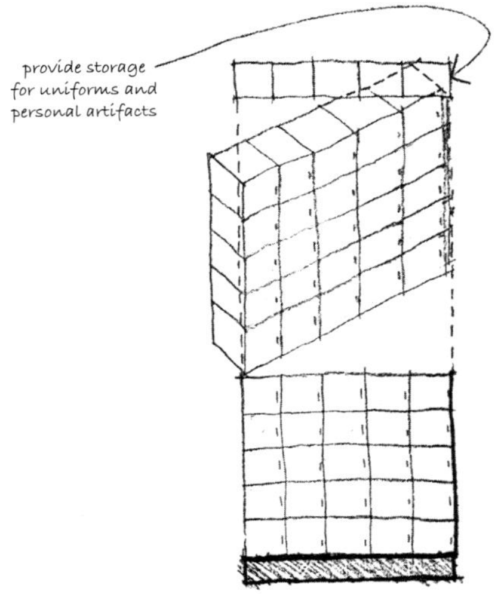

STAFF—PERSONAL SPACE

4.43 INCLUDE PRIVATE LOCKERS FOR STAFF IN OR NEAR THE STAFF BREAK ROOM

In a number of SFI case study facilities, little or no provision was made for closets or other places for the storage of personal items such as coats, umbrellas, a portable radio, and so on. This is a constant irritant for staff, particularly for those who do not have private offices. Every individual should have some lockable space for personal items, and additionally, lockers should be provided for the storage of larger items. This space should be located in or near the staff lounge. Each locker should be no larger than 1′ x 1′ x 1′ and stacked as a grid along one wall of the staff lounge or in a separate alcove space adjacent to the break room. All such devices should be safe and secure.

COMMUNICATIONS

4.44 PATIENT AND STAFF INFORMATION WALLS PROVIDE MEDICAL, LEGAL, AND RESOURCE INFORMATION

An information wall should be provided for patients for the posting of memos, news items, schedules, descriptions of new medical procedures, and so on. This board should be located in or near the waiting room. The same should be done for staff information, and this space should be located in or near the staff break room. In areas where more than one language is spoken, provide this information in a multi-lingual format, perhaps supplemented with a taped narrative via a TV monitor/VCR unit. Locate these information walls in spaces that are visible to the intended readers, but not in a way that makes it easy for children to remove or damage the posted materials.

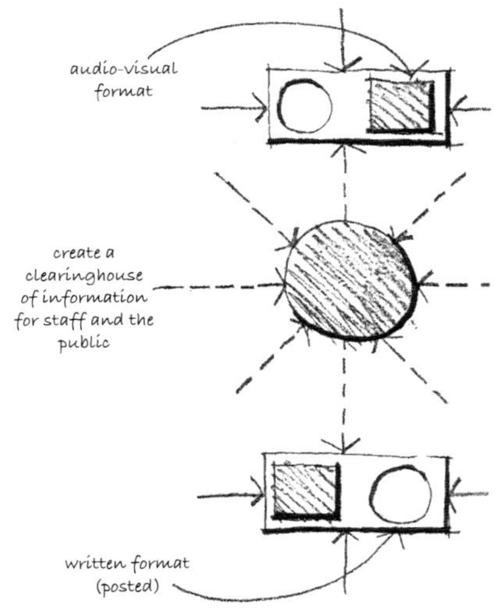

PAMPHLETS

4.45 PROVIDE A PAMPHLET DISPLAY RACK OR SHELF IN THE EXAMINATION ROOM

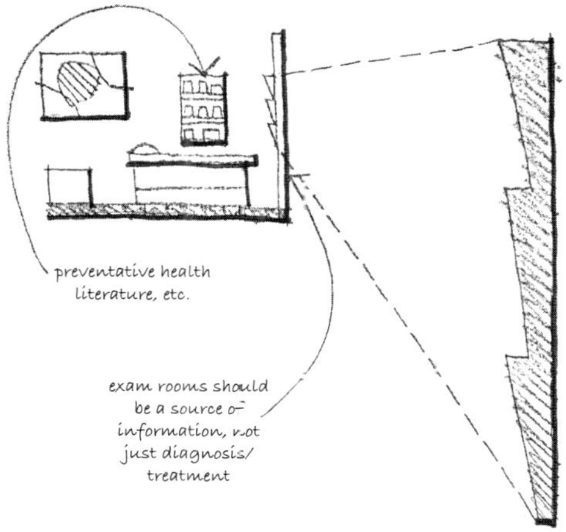

Often, pamphlets are poorly displayed or kept in closets, away form the main flow of patients. Even for staff, the adage "out of sight, out of mind" applies because they are less prone to disseminate health education literature if it is not immediately available at their fingertips. In response, decentralize the placement of this literature. Place it in the exam rooms and in the waiting rooms on racks hung on the wall. These racks can be made of transparent Plexiglas so that they are visually unobtrusive elements within the room. An appropriate size is 24" x 24" with three or four shelves mounted on the wall above the reach of small children.

ENTRY—SANITARIANS

4.46 PROVIDE AN ENTRY VESTIBULE AND CLOSET AT THE SANITARIAN'S ENTRANCE

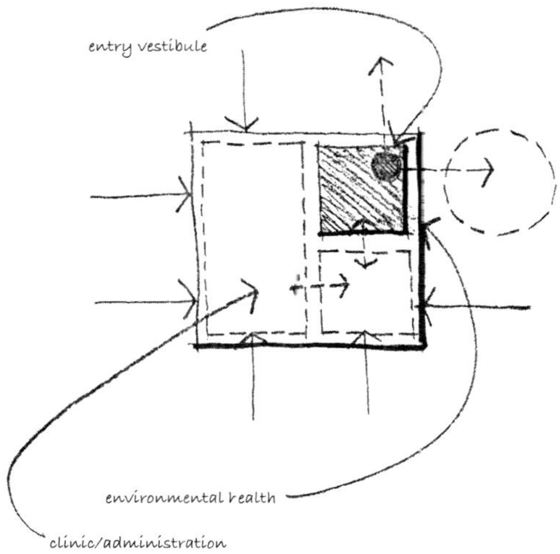

The sanitarian is continually coming and going. They spend much of their time in the field, making frequent inspections at construction sites and returning to the home base of the community public health center after field inspections. This calls for a dedicated entry for sanitarians, in order to separate this foot traffic from that of the clinic. Provide an entry vestibule as a transition zone between indoors and out, a place for storage and concealment of boots and other equipment used in the field, and a coat closet. This area is to house ice chests, land leveler, tripods, etc. Do not install carpet or seating in this space. It need not look like a mudroom at home, as this entry vestibule may be used by the public as well if it is not feasible to create a staff-only entry for the environmental health program staff.

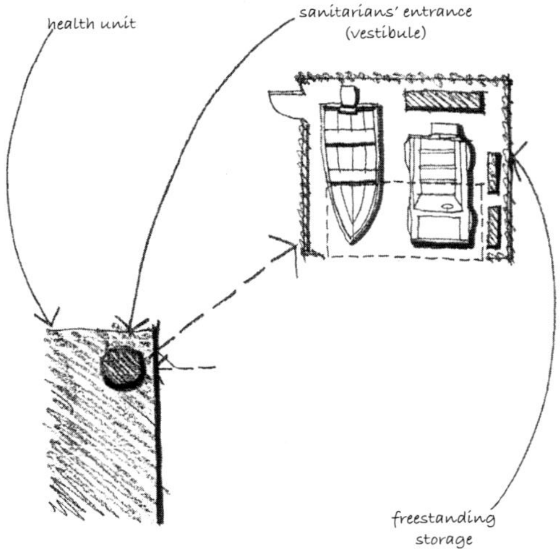

EQUIPMENT

4.47 SANITARIANS SHOULD HAVE A FREE-STANDING OR ATTACHED GARAGE/STORAGE AREA FOR THEIR USE

The sanitarian's work may require trekking through water, mud, and forested areas. One gets dirty when involved in these tasks and must change clothes during the day when moving from field to office and vice versa. In terms of equipment, a garage storage space is needed either within the building, or a freestanding shed provided for the storage of perhaps a boat, a four-wheel drive vehicle, shovels and other tools, and work clothes. It is recommended that this space be a freestanding garage with a steel or aluminum roll-up door. Provide a place for the boat to be washed, whether in the garage or outdoors. Alternatively, a carport may be appropriate. Provide one or two designated parking spaces.

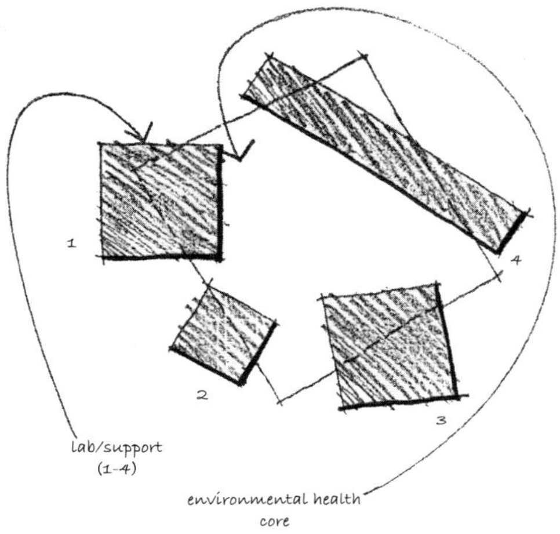

LAB SUPPORT

4.48 AN ENVIRONMENTAL HEALTH LAB AND SUPPORT SPACE IS REQUIRED IN THE DAILY WORK OF THE SANITARIAN

A laboratory is needed for use by the environmental health staff. This room should be located adjacent to the dedicated staff entry, separate from the clinic entry. This room should house a refrigerator (half height minimum: thirty inches) and a freezer for the storage of water samples, dog vaccines, ice packs and dog and cat heads prior to transportation to the main laboratory for analysis. Provide ample cabinets and a sink with soap, towel dispensers, and durable countertop area for preparation of specimens for storage and transportation. Adjacent to the lab, provide a space for the review of new construction drawings. A closet or storage room large enough for bulky blueprints, various reports, and documents is needed. Provide privacy, as well as a table and chairs for gatherings for up to six people. This room should be next to the waiting area. In addition, a storage closet or fixed wall-mounted cabinet should be placed next to the receptionist/secretary's desk.

SPEECH AND HEARING

4.49 SPEECH AND HEARING ASSESSMENT SHOULD BE BUFFERED FROM THE MAIN FLOW OF ACTIVITY

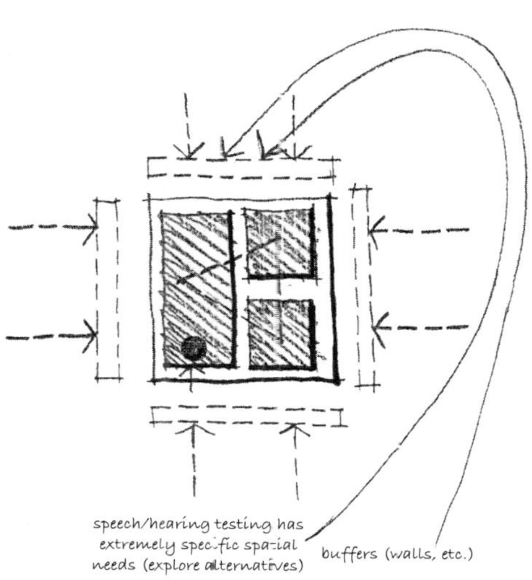

Speech and hearing evaluation requires specialized testing equipment, ambient air quality levels, acoustical levels, seating, and lighting. For audiology equipment, provide privacy, no light leaks from the hallway, no windows, universal design access to and from the sound booth, a sufficiently large work area for a desk, equipment storage, control console, one chair for the staff specialist, and two chairs for patients. Lighting levels on both sides of the glass wall of the booth must be equivalent to preclude distracting glare on only one side or the other. Provide a phone and intercom, acoustical tiles on the walls and ceiling, a lockable, blind door to the hallway, and artwork. The recommended booth (Tracor or equivalent) is a double-walled steel booth with two chairs, acoustical tile, and two speakers. Avoid fluorescent lighting, as it emits a distracting hum. Provide space for a portable audiometer.

VISION SCREENING

4.50 VISION TESTING EQUIPMENT SHOULD BE PROVIDED IN EACH EXAM ROOM

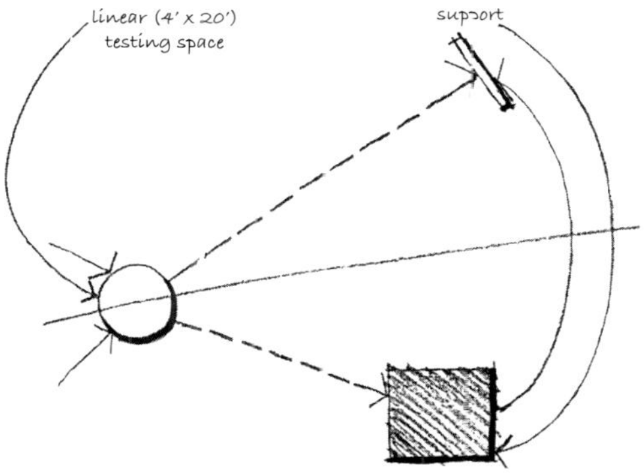

It was a surprise to learn, during the early phase of fieldwork, that so many facilities still used separate rooms dedicated for testing patients' vision and hearing. In the older clinics of the 1950s this was understandable, as the equipment was so bulky. In the majority of clinics documented as case studies, vision testing occurred in inappropriate spaces, i.e. in corridors, the staff kitchen, or in the nutritional education kitchen. Due to new countertop vision testing equipment there is no longer the need for twenty feet between the eye chart and the patient. This work is now best done in the examination room. It is recommended that the windows are so they do not cause excessive glare in relation to the positioning of the vision testing equipment. For patients with acute light sensitivity, the exam room should be able to be darkened with 100 percent blackout shades.

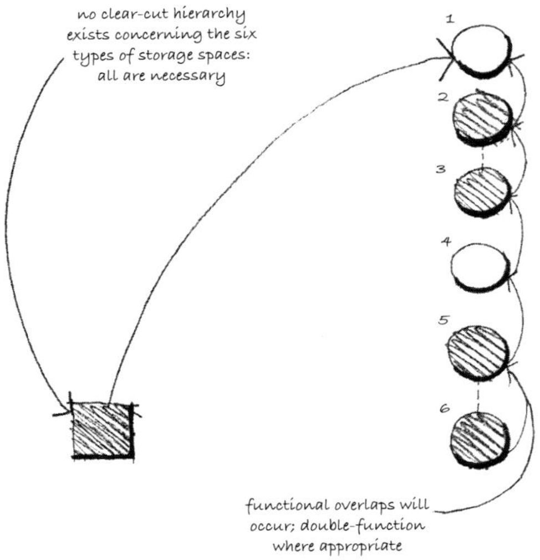

STORAGE

4.51 CAREFULLY ADDRESS THE MULTIPLE STORAGE REQUIREMENTS OF THE HEALTH CENTER

Storage space seems too be the first item to be cut from a building project that is over budget. This is because no one occupies these spaces, and therefore it has no advocates per se. Regardless, storage is required for six basic types of items: 1) clerical forms and office supplies; 2) medical records; 3) medication and drugs; and 4) bulk storage for furniture, custodial supplies, etc; 5) environmental health storage for samples and blueprints; and 6) personal items such as coats. Neglect of the importance of storage usually results in inadequately sized rooms, poor locations in terms of functional adjacencies, or worse, the absence of one or more of the six types of storage spaces entirely, as the research team learned during the case studies. In short, these are "stepchild" spaces, considered of low priority compared to examination rooms, offices, and laboratories.

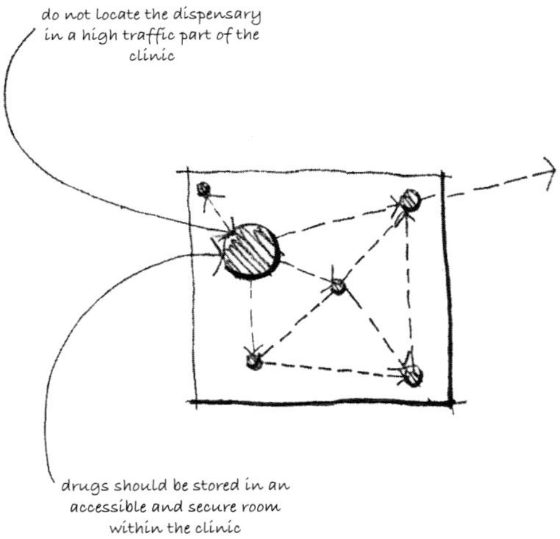

MEDICATIONS

4.52 PHARMACEUTICALS MUST BE STORED AND DISPENSED FROM A SECURE LOCKABLE SPACE WITHIN THE CLINIC

Medications, birth control pills and devices, and immunization paraphernalia must be stored and dispensed from a secure, lockable room to maximize staff control. The room should be located as near as possible to both the clinic and the nursing director's/unit director's office. This helps to ensure routine surveillance as well as to minimize nursing staff travel distances. This room should not be located adjacent to or within the public realm, i.e. waiting rooms, restrooms, vending areas, or other highly trafficked paths. The door should not face these areas either. It is recommended that a "blind" door (without windows) be specified in order to deter potential onlookers. Within the room, provide built in shelves on one or more walls, each with a fourteen-inch depth minimum and fifteen-inch clearance height from shelf to shelf. Provide a built-in desk for recordkeeping and a computer workstation.

CLINIC—SUPPLIES

4.53 ACCESSIBLE STORAGE MUST BE PROVIDED WITHIN THE CLINIC FOR MEDICAL SUPPLIES

The storage of medical supplies in the clinic must facilitate direct access by nursing and medical staff throughout the day. This lockable space should be a small walk-in room with shelves on three sides, floor to ceiling, with good lighting, and shelves that are no deeper than twenty-four inches. This room should be windowless since daylight is not required and as a security precaution. In larger units, more than one room may be required, although it is recommended that a main medical supply room be supported by a satellite medical supply closet at the opposite end of the clinic, adjacent to the nurse's office(s). A strong argument can be made, however, for storing all medical supplies in a single, lockable, centralized room at the heart of the clinic, on an inner hallway in a staff only work zone, or along a main hallway if this is deemed more workable.

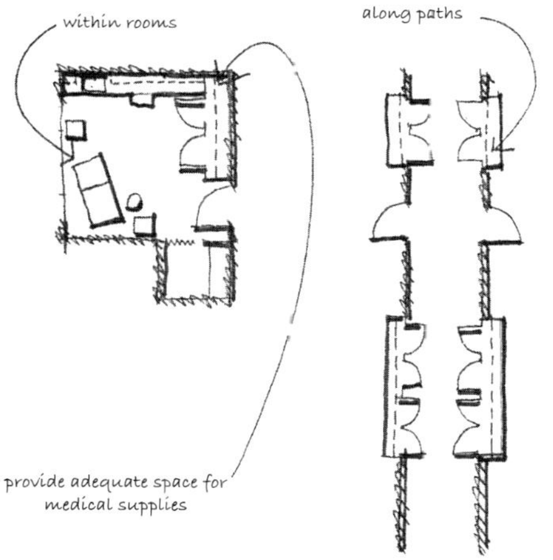

CLERICAL SUPPLIES

4.54 STORE ADMINISTRATIVE OFFICE SUPPLIES IN A SECURE AND ACCESSIBLE LOCATION

The clerical staff must have direct access to the dozens of standardized forms which must be filled out each day. These forms provide necessary documentation and become part of the permanent file for each patient. In the case study of parish health units analyzed, it was found that the staff devised ingenious methods for open shelf forms storage in order to make them easier to retrieve. The key determinants of file storage and retrieval are that forms have to be in a centralized location, such as immediately behind the reception desk or in a hall behind the reception desk, they must be easily scanned to make it virtually impossible to overlook anything, and they must be out of the reach of children such as in a staff-only area.

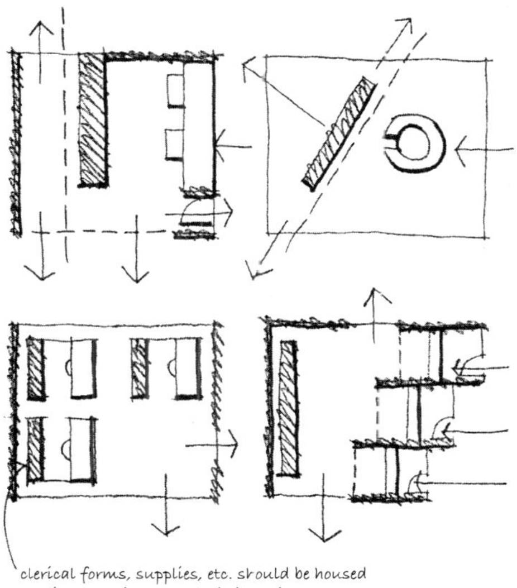

5. REGIONAL SUPPORT

RECEPTION

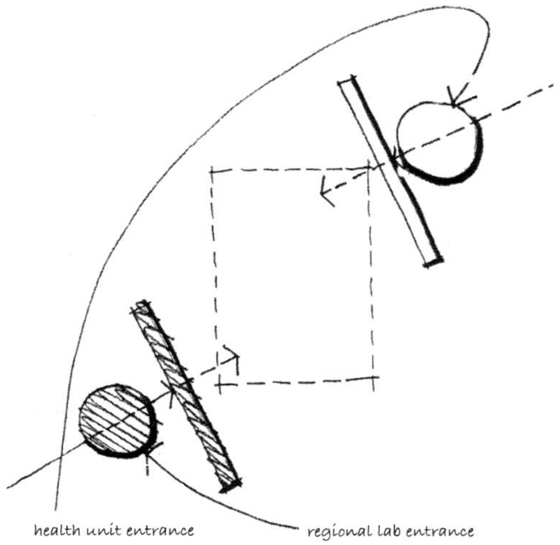

5.1 PROVIDE A SEPARATE ENTRANCE, FOYER, AND RECEPTION DESK AT THE ENTRANCE TO THE REGION LABORATORY

Laboratory staff should have a public entrance and reception area to receive visitors and which functions as a connecting thread to the general public. This entrance should be easy to identify from the exterior, with a glass outer door. The foyer should connect to a small waiting area with chairs adjacent to a reception counter. The reception desk should be adjacent to the main office. This portion of the lab must be secure at all times. It is imperative that access to the lab be strictly controlled: only authorized personnel are allowed in the work area. Consider the installation of key card door access systems. The lab consultant and/or the architect should provide "tear sheets" of specific equipment options for review by the client. Provide a duplicate set of final, appraised lab equipment and systems for the client and the contractor.

REGION STAFF

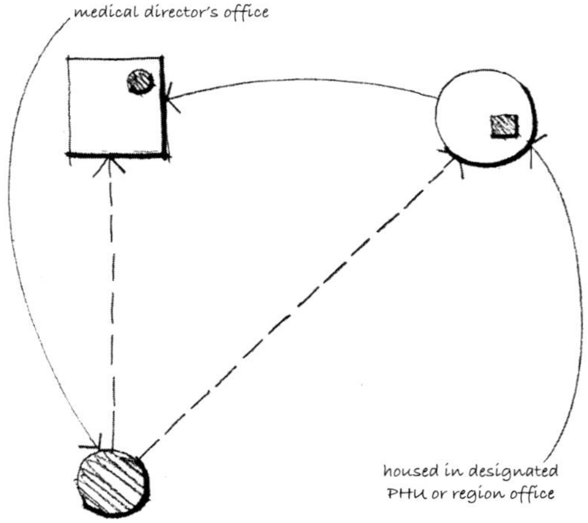

5.2 HOUSE THE REGION ADMINISTRATIVE OFFICE IN A FREESTANDING BUILDING IN A HEALTH CENTER WITHIN A SHARED BUILDING

This is desirable from an administrative standpoint. While it is preferable for many reasons to have a separate facility for the region office, this is not always practical due to staffing shortages, travel distances, and the like. Provide an office for the medical director. If this is not possible, combine these functions in a single building alongside a clinic and there include a satellite office for the medical director. This office should be of sufficient size to conduct staff meetings and patient consultation and amenities, such as built-in shelves, a desk, four chairs minimum, and a small conference table. If budget and space permits, provide space for a sofa. Whenever possible, provide a parking area designated only for "region staff" and spaces for state vehicles.

LABORATORY SUPPORT

5.3 PROVIDE BUFFERED WORK SPACES IN REGION LABORATORIES

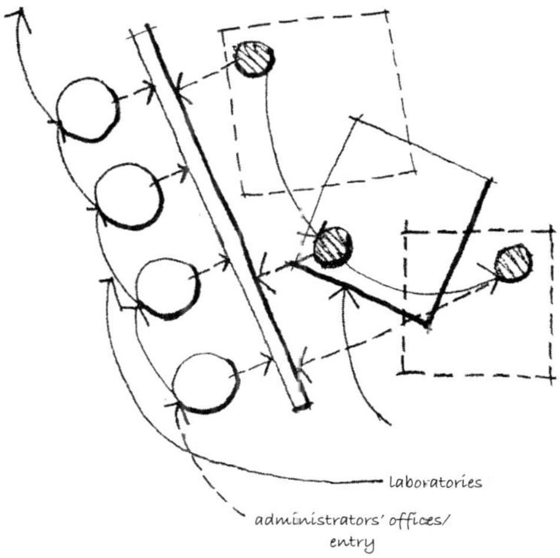

A parallel exists between the regional lab administrative and clerical staff and their counterparts at the health center: neither group is well suited to individual compartmentalized offices nor completely open partition-less workrooms. In offices, if a midpoint exists, it is represented by the landscaped, flexible partition concept where five-foot high wall/shelving component systems are arranged into office pods with work support amenities such as tables and built-in lighting. In labs, the selection furniture is more than a matter of personal aesthetic choice. Wood casework has a pleasant appearance, is less noisy, and can be repaired or refinished in places. On the other hand, drawers in steel casework slide easily and interior dimensions are slightly greater. The casework should be ordered from the same manufacturer since there are different tolerances among various manufacturers.

WORKSTATIONS

5.4 PROVIDE WORK ISLANDS WITH HANDICAP-ACCESSIBLE LAB BENCH COUNTERTOPS IN LABORATORIES

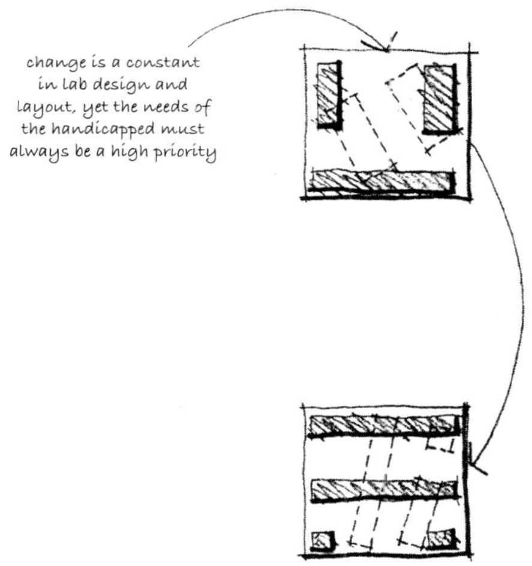

The traditional layout of labs has been characterized by long rows of workstations, with staff facing one another in double rows. An alternative lab layout, particularly in specialized labs supporting the work of ten or fewer persons, is to provide a work island in the center of the room, or multiple work islands depending on the number of staff. This provides a place for staging, testing, and evaluation of work. It also provides space for informal interaction. All workstations in the lab should be universal in design, allowing for wheelchair access. Adjustable lab benches are useful in this context because they can be raised or lowered based on users' capabilities. All materials for countertops and floors must be resistant to acids, bases, and organic solvents. Furniture systems range from the fixed base cabinets at fixed bench top heights to modular systems.

EQUIPMENT

5.5 CLUSTER LABORATORY TESTING EQUIPMENT WITH SIMILAR SPATIAL, STRUCTURAL, AND ENVIRONMENTAL CONTROL REQUIREMENTS

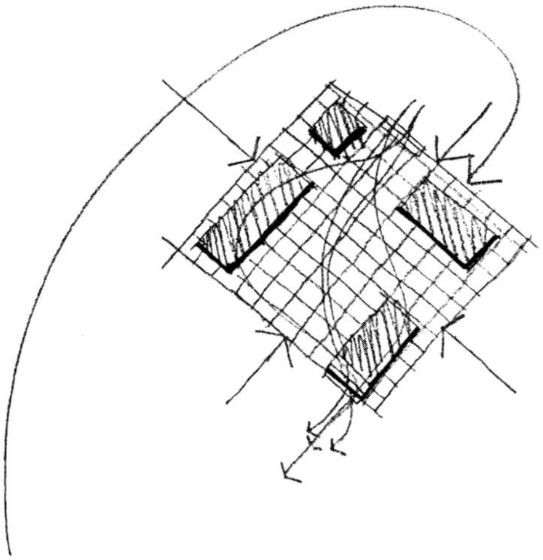

house equipment with similar HVAC needs in a centralized location in lab

It was learned during the case study fieldwork that on evenings, weekends, and over long holiday breaks when the HVAC systems are shut down to conserve energy costs, testing equipment has been damaged because highly sensitive gauge settings become dislodged due to excessive cold, heat, or high humidity levels in the laboratory. The purpose of the air-handling system is to provide environmental control to prevent airborne contamination. This is best achieved with proper microbial filtration and air pressure differentials to direct the airflow from clean to less clean areas. Store valuable testing tools in one or more rooms where the HVAC can remain on at all time, without sacrificing work productivity or efficiency. Zone these spaces so that temperature and humidity can be controlled independent of the rest of the building. This measure can save equipment repair and replacement costs, which in the long run can amount to greater savings compared to the short-sighted policy of weekend and evening HVAC shutdowns in the laboratory.

REGIONAL LABORATORY—DAYLIGHT

5.6 CONTROL THE AMOUNT OF DAYLIGHT SOLAR GAIN IN LABORATORIES WITH BLACKOUT SHADES THAT CAN BE ACTIVATED AS NEEDED, PRECLUDING THE NEED FOR WINDOWLESS ROOMS

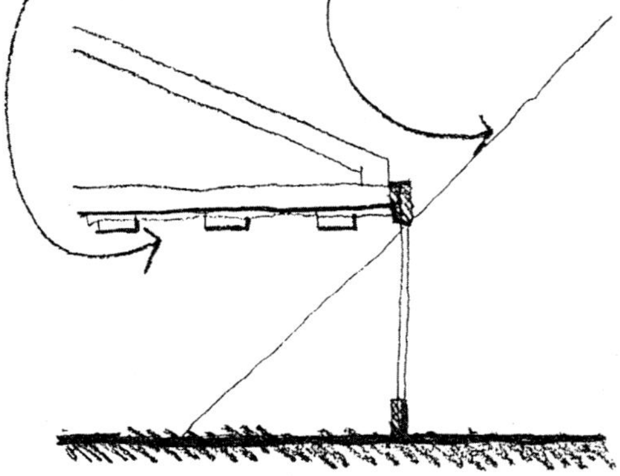

incorporate multiple types of lighting throughout the facility

A frequent compliant voiced by staff in region lab facilities is at times the excessive transmission of sunlight into the testing area, causing contamination of experiments. This is a difficult situation in older laboratories, which often have continuous windows along the perimeter walls. Rather than overreact by calling for windowless labs, as this cuts off view amenity and useful information about the world beyond the lab, include blackout shades or curtains that can be activated as warranted. These can be electronically or manually operated. New types of glazing provide UV protection.

LAB—CAMPUS

5.7 IN URBAN AREAS IT IS EFFECTIVE TO HOUSE THE REGIONAL LAB ON A SHARED SITE WITH THE HEALTH CENTER

In the urban areas of the state where the community public health center is located on the same site adjacent to a regional lab, a number of advantages are accrued. This allows for the convenient transfer of expertise, specimens for testing, savings in land costs, transportation costs, and a more focused presence in the community. A potential problem is that the state agency is responsible for upkeep of the lab, whereas the local parish government is responsible for upkeep of the health center. A dual stewardship therefore must be carefully worked out. Explore the availability of federal grants related to environmental protection, coastal zone management programs, and other grant funding sources when planning new or renovated laboratory facilities on shared sites.

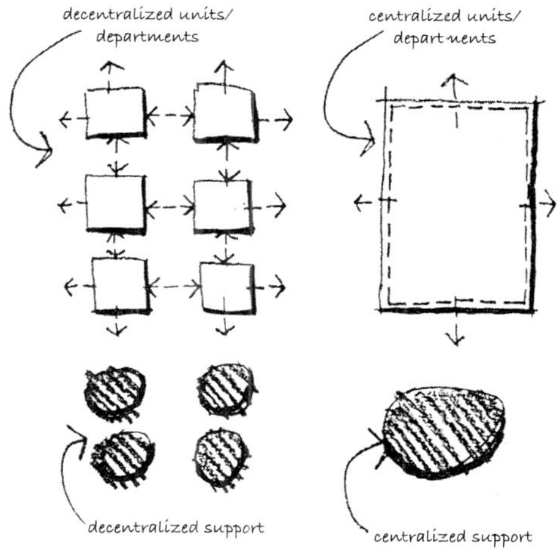

ELECTRICAL

5.8 SPECIFY FULL SPECTRUM ILLUMINATION AND ADEQUATE HVAC SUPPORT IN REGION LABORATORIES

In recent years significant advancements have been made in artificial illumination. These new light fixtures and lighting elements afford much more accurate spectral distribution compared to traditional fluorescent tube lighting. Fluorescent lighting only provides partial spectral distribution: colors are rendered in hues of orange, green, or blue, giving an unnatural appearance to skin tones. The trend in labs is toward the use of more high-powered equipment yet electricity is usually the most underestimated service. Some laboratories built in recent years have soon run short of power and are having to revise their electrical systems. A 200-ampere panel per every 400 square feet is considered acceptable; 25 to 30 percent of panel capacity should be reserved for the future expansion of the system.

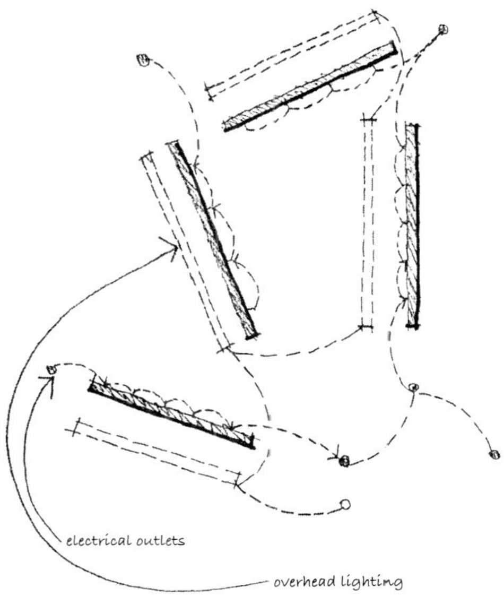

EQUIPMENT

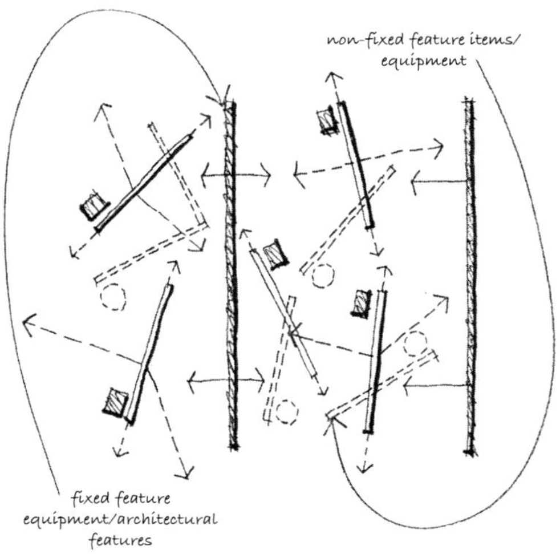

5.9 CONSIDER NUMEROUS POWER, FIXED EQUIPMENT, AND GENERAL SERVICING SYSTEMS IN LABORATORIES

Each lab workroom has highly specific functional requirements. A laboratory planning specialist should be consulted early on in the facility planning process to discuss and evaluate various support systems, including the provision of electrical supply, natural gasses (nitrogen, carbon dioxide, hydrogen, etc.), water purification systems, hot air ovens, autoclaves, prefabricated walk-in coolers, vacuum and steam systems, air exchange rates, ducts for hoods, and ceiling systems. At least one double sink should be provided for each laboratory, with ends of a peninsula or regular workbench satisfactory locations for sinks. If sinks are near the back of the laboratory, they tend to become collecting points for items which are used infrequently. Options for finishes within a laboratory allow a variety of materials and their selection is an important part of laboratory planning.

EMERGENCY POWER

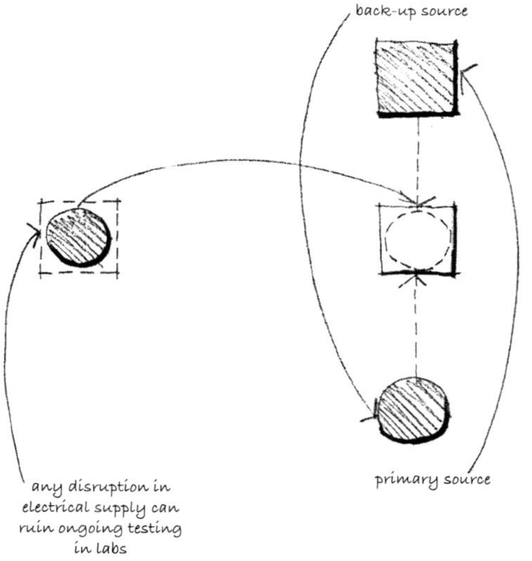

5.10 PROVIDE AN EMERGENCY BACKUP SYSTEM FOR ELECTRICAL POWER IN LABORATORIES AND CLINICS

A determination must be made as to which equipment must be on emergency backup power in the event of system failure. Items such as refrigerators, incubators, minimum lighting, hoods, animal room air conditioning, fire alarms, and security systems should be considered. A decision must also be made as to the desired length of continued operation. A region laboratory requires more emergency power if normal operations are expected to continue unaffected. Normally, the prime objectives are: 1) to assure continued operation of safety equipment, minimum lighting, ventilation, etc, at least long enough to terminate any procedures that may have been in progress at the time of failure; 2) to prevent loss of specimens due to insufficient refrigeration or incubation; and 3) to assure proper ventilation in animal holding areas in labs. Similarly, determine the rooms in a health unit to be connected to the backup generator.

6. TOTAL ENVIRONMENT

IMAGE

6.1 THE FACADE AND ENTRY SHOULD REFLECT THE IDEALS AND VISION OF THE HEALTH CENTER

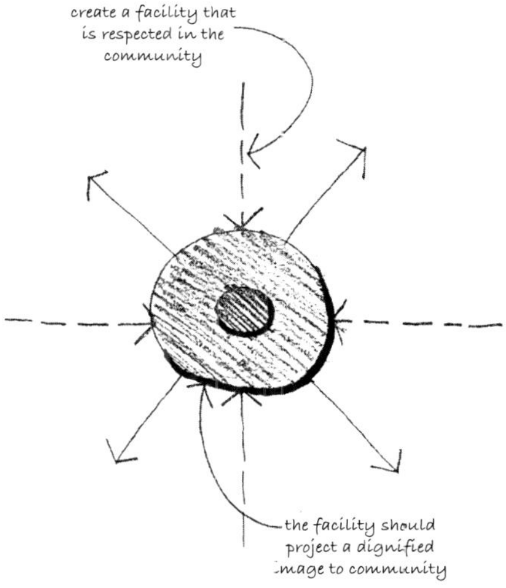

The entry sequence should be clearly identified within the context of the neighborhood, the surrounding buildings, and the facility itself. The symbolic messages conveyed by the entrance and facade should focus on an inviting a residential aesthetic. The modernist clinic-as-miniature hospital ethos must give way to the residential scale of the neighborhood. Restated, a comforting, inviting image is to be sought which is a synthesis of home and clinic. The architecture should be geared, above all, to the family unit and to the individual, not to technology per se nor to external determinants that would significantly compromise the mission of community-based care.

IMAGE

6.2 DEVELOP AN INVITING, DIGNIFIED MAIN LOBBY AND WAITING AREA

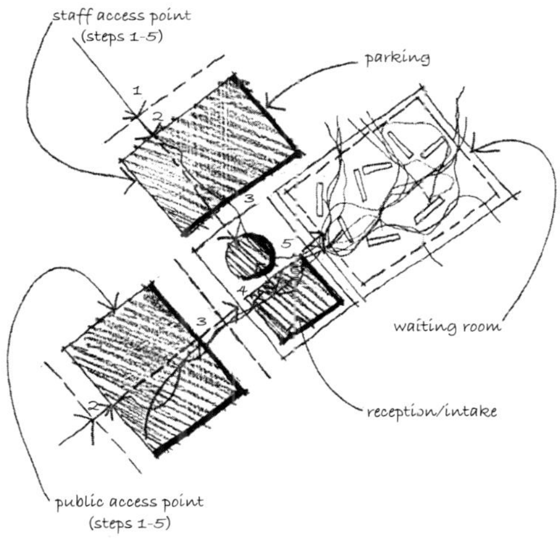

The spatial sequence from exterior to interior typically consists of arrival on the site, parking, arrival at the main entrance, and entry to the main waiting room. The entry and waiting area represent a significant percentage of the total floor area of the building, and yet these spaces too often project the image and ambiance of a bus station. The message appears to be one of institutional indifference: rows of rigid, plastic seats, bland, harsh wall and floor surfaces, and drab colors. The link between the quality of the health center, the quality of care, and its utilization by patients is deep rooted. Therefore, create an inviting, pleasant, person-focused lobby and waiting area through the use of plants, daylight, windows which yield interesting views, interesting ceilings, comfortable seating, and a warm color scheme with textured wall and floor surfaces.

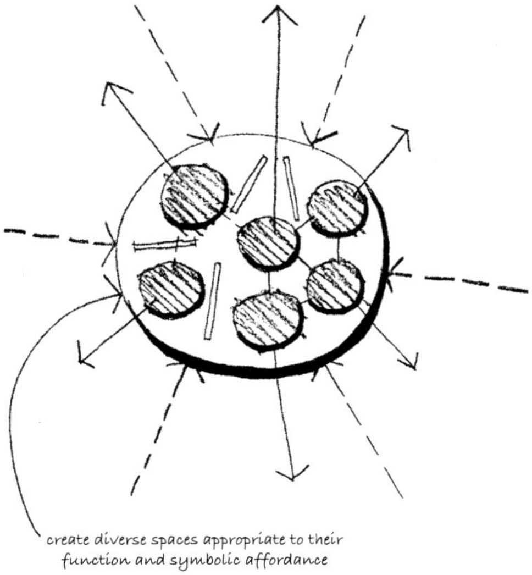

CONFIGURATION

6.3 EXPRESS FUNCTIONAL AND SYMBOLIC REALMS IN THE DESIGN OF THE HEALTH CENTER

It has been argued the hospital, along with the industrial-age factory, is among the earliest modernist building types. The roots of modernist hospital design date from the work of Florence Nightingale in her emphasis on strict functionality, cleanliness, and the critical importance of an uplifting, bright treatment environment in contrast to the dark, drab hospitals and clinics common up to that point in time. Her two landmark books were *Notes on Hospitals* (1858) and *Notes on Nursing* (1859). With the advent of modern technology the hospital became a testing ground for the marriage of architectural functionalism (form follows function) with emergent machine-based technologies (x-ray technologies and new advanced surgical procedures). The hospital itself came to be known as a machine for healing. Eberhard Zeildler's book *Healing the Hospital McMaster Health Science Centre, Its Conception and Evolution* (Toronto, 1978) and the late Roslyn Lindheim's seminal article "How Modern Hospitals Got That Way" (*Environments for Humanized Health Care: Proceedings of the Symposium, March 8-9, 1979, Berkeley, California* [Berkeley,CA, 1979]) paved the way for the reappraisal of the viability of minimalist modernism in health care architecture.

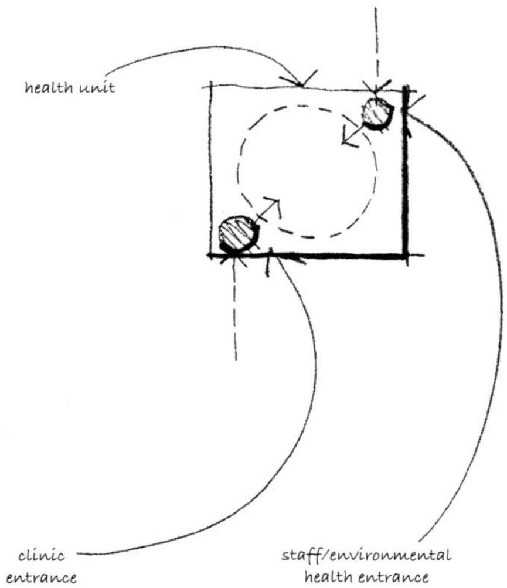

ENTRY SEQUENCE

6.4 PROVIDE SEPARATE ENTRANCES FOR CLINICAL AND NON-CLINICAL FUNCTIONS WHICH SHARE THE SAME BUILDING

Community health centers house environmental health functions in addition to the outpatient health clinic. Many contain meeting rooms or an auditorium for use by community groups on a weekly or monthly basis in the evenings. It is inappropriate from the standpoint of staff workflow and patient confidentiality for someone seeking a plan review or sewage permit to have to enter the clinic waiting area. Wherever possible, create a separate entrance or at the very least a single shared entrance with separate hallways to provide separation between clinical versus non-clinical functions. Each entrance to the facility should be clearly identified and located adjacent to the parking area.

ENTRY SEQUENCE

6.5 THE ENTRY SHOULD BE A SECURE BUFFER ZONE

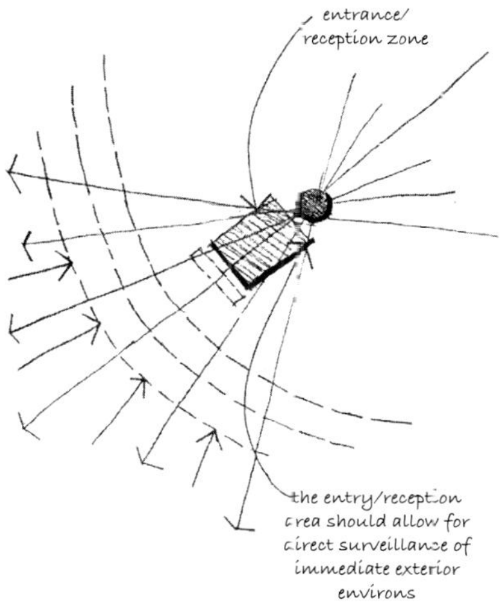

The entry to the facility should be clearly marked from the exterior for easy access, yet access should be controllable to an appropriate extent as dictated by the neighborhood context and the amount of crime in the immediate area. A buffer zone should be created between the door threshold and the reception-intake desk/counter. This zone is to allow unwanted intruders to be screened prior to getting too far into the facility. The vantage point can also take the form of a window or one way mirror, and might include a buzzer system for the exterior doors as well. On the exterior, an additional buffer zone could be established by a low wall or screen, vegetation, wood concrete, or lattice grid without blocking the view to the outside or diminishing its identifiably from the exterior. This element can be incorporated into a vehicular drop off area, or porte cochère.

CIRCULATION

6.6 CORRIDOR CIRCULATION SHOULD CONNECT WITH BUT NOT BISECT POCKET SPACES

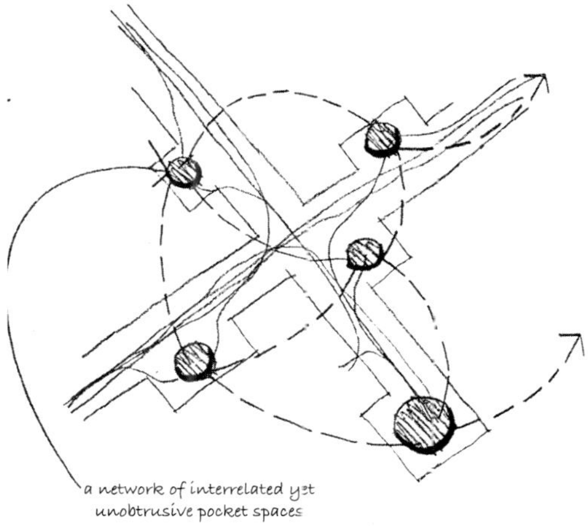

Traditionally, double-loaded clinic configurations with five or six-foot width hallways were designed as conduits for people and supplies moving from room to room. These paths were not designed to accommodate seating or such equipment as weight and measurement scales, although both functions were found to commonly occur out of necessity in many health units. Provide alcoves or pockets of space adjacent to the hallway, whether single or double-loaded, which makes it possible for the movement of people, supplies, and equipment to not cut through, or bisect, these pockets of space. Therefore, circulation occurs along the side, not through the middle. Use screens, recesses, window seats, differentiated ceiling height, and floor texture changes occurring at intervals along the length of a hallway, in order to signify changes in path direction and the intersection of hallways.

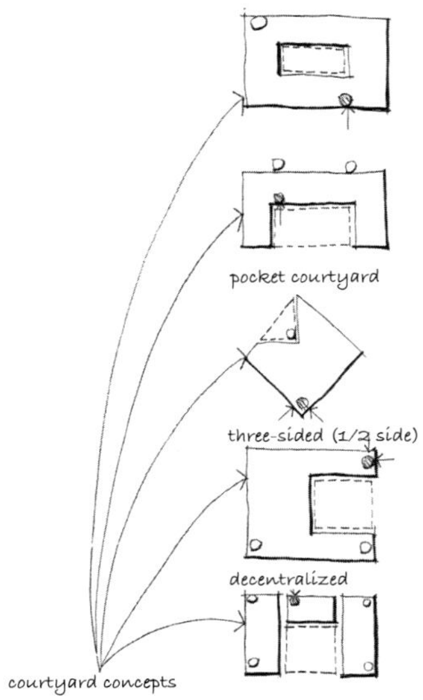

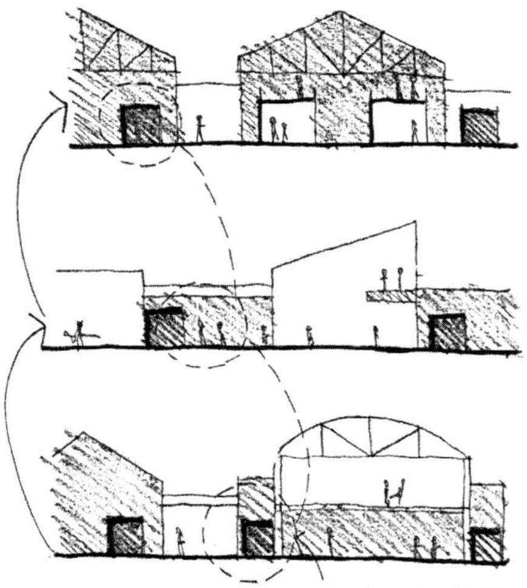

create a hierarchy of ceiling/ roof forms and heights

COURTYARDS

6.7 CREATE AN OUTDOOR COURTYARD WHICH FUNCTIONS AS AN EXTENSION OF THE INTERIOR REALM

The 1950s "shoebox clinics" did not provide adequate windows, and views, let alone adequate access to outdoor spaces for use by staff and patients. The resultant effect is as if one is inside a shoebox. You are either inside or out—no midpoint exists. This has had an unfortunate effect on staff morale and work effectiveness through the years, and has been at the core of why these clinics are unyieldingly institutional. Provide a semi-private courtyard. This space should have a gate for staff-only use, a separate door into the sanitarians' entry vestibule and wing, and an entrance into the nursing wing. The staff lounge should overlook this landscaped space and the nutritional education kitchen. Provide spotlights and an electronic security system to protect it at night.

CEILINGS

6.8 DIFFERENTIATED CEILING HEIGHTS EXPRESS DIFFERENCES IN FUNCTION

The "shoebox clinics" of the 1950s were housed in rectangular boxes with flat roofs. Differences in ceiling heights were unacceptable. The unfortunate result was that it was impossible to accentuate a particular room, i.e. the main entrance versus the waiting room. It has become acceptable to design the ceilings and the roof of a health care facility in a much more expressive manner than was possible before. Ceilings and roof forms should express a hierarchy of functions. In hallways and at the main entry the ceilings should differ from those in the clinic. Each realm should be designed in this manner, thus making the care environment easier to locate and navigate, as ceiling heights and roof forms such as open trusses, vaulted ceilings, and varied horizontal heights help people form memorable, concrete images of key spaces.

FENESTRATION

6.9 CAREFULLY DESIGNED AND POSITIONED WINDOWS, CLERESTORIES, AND SKYLIGHTS CONTRIBUTE TO A DYNAMIC ENVIRONMENT

Windows not only provide one with a means to look in and out, they also provide a natural light source. Natural daylight establishes visual interest and the highlighting and shadows needed for visual relief. Maximize functional and aesthetic amenity through the provision of windows and skylights. Adequately sized and positioned windows can extend the interior space and a meaningful link between indoors and outdoors. Psychologically, people tend to experience an oppressive sense of over-enclosure, isolation, and confinement in windowless environments. Beyond, rooms that are minimally windowed with small apertures, poor proximity to the occupant, opaqueness, poor screening, or poor views have been perceived by both staff and patients as the equivalent of architecturally windowless conditions. Unfortunately, minimum building code requirements may be met although such windows are psychologically dysfunctional.

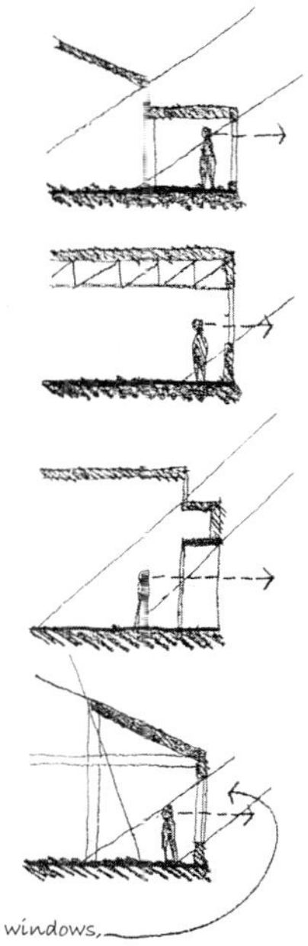

ROOM-TO-ROOM WINDOWS

6.10 INTERIOR GLASS CONTROLS NOISE WHILE PROVIDING VISUAL STIMULATION AND DAYLIGHT AMENITY

A wall between two rooms is merely that—an absolute divider that isolates two spaces from one another in terms of view, sound, light, and function. This is extreme, a condition that precludes the potential for functional separation and the accommodation of far more subtle spatial co-variances. For instance, room-to-room glass walls between the main waiting room and the reception desk and interview stations can provide visual access and sound separation while creating an open, deinstitutionalized atmosphere. Similarly, glass walls along corridors and at the entrance to the major domains of a community health center foster spaciousness and the activation of what would otherwise be drab spaces, monotonous and under-stimulating to the human senses. Explore applications of liquid crystal technology to partially obscure or completely darken such windows with the flip of a switch or dimmer.

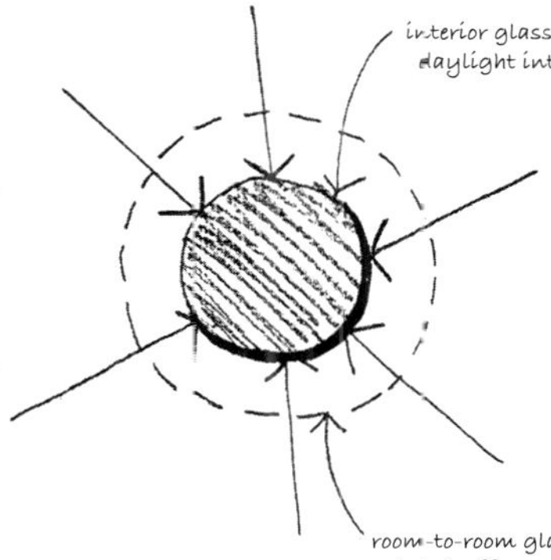

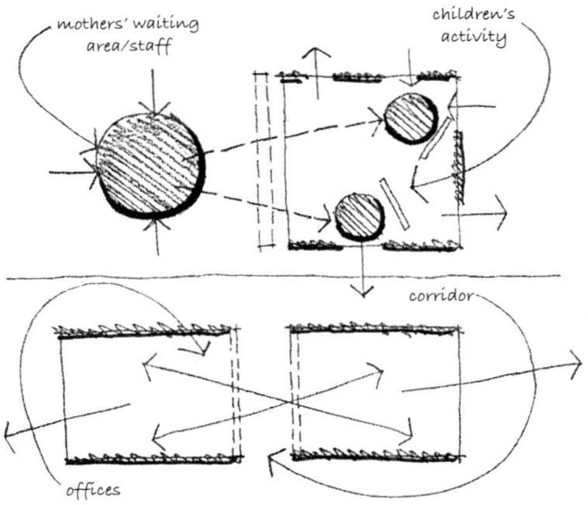

INTERIOR WINDOWS

6.11 PROVIDE INTERIOR WINDOWS WHICH AFFORD VISUAL SURVEILLANCE

There are numerous trade-offs in weighing the benefits of including room-to-room interior windows. Advantages include the ability to observe the flow of events in the public realm, to observe patients unobtrusively through one-way mirror glass, or to increase security through visual surveillance of an adjacent space. Further, interior office windows allow patients and staff the opportunity to have a private session while keeping an eye on children in the adjacent space. As stated above, recent advances in interior window technology includes liquid crystal technology applied to "read-out" windows. The provision of a window offers the choice to the user to keep it open or closed, therefore adding to its adaptability. Include operable window blinds as these allow the occupant far greater personalization.

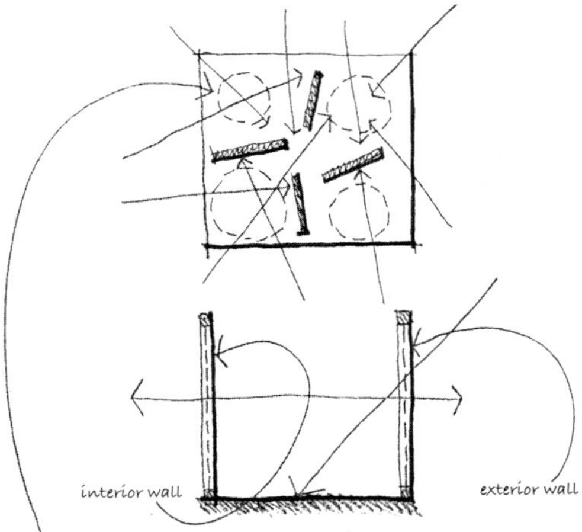

create a semi-transparent interior through use of glazed partitions

INTERIOR WINDOWS—SAFETY

6.12 FLOOR-TO-CEILING VISION GLASS WALLS HAVE ADVANTAGES AS WELL AS DISADVANTAGES

An interior glass wall between two or more spaces can create a sense of transparency and spaciousness in opposition to the tendency observed in the case study fieldwork to over-compartmentalize with too many small spaces separated by opaque traditional walls. Glass partitions can allow for increased transmission of daylight into interior reaches of a unit, i.e. from a kitchen unit on adjoining corridor. This can also aid in wayfinding among patients because the glass can break up the monotony of an unbroken corridor with its row of blind doors arrayed on either side. On the other hand, safety measures must be taken so children do not run into transparent glass walls. This can be accomplished with a pair of carefully horizontally positioned hand railings, perhaps at eighteen inches and thirty-six inches above the floor, or brightly colored tape or graphics to signify that this wall is not a doorway or open passage. Second, as previously stated, glass walls may sacrifice patient and staff privacy unless curtains or screens are provided.

LIGHTING

6.13 LIGHTING SHOULD BE FLEXIBLE TO RESPOND TO THE NEEDS OF MULTIPLE-USER CONSTITUENCIES

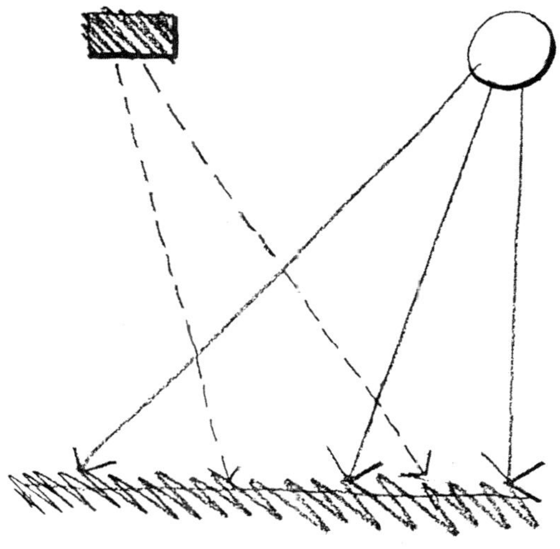

The lighting conditions within health care facilities tend to be extreme: either too bright (fluorescent ceiling grid fixtures), too harsh (overhead lighting only without a blend of fluorescent and incandescent fixtures) or too low (only one overhead light in an exam room augmented by a poorly located light over the desk). As such, the needs of persons with significant visual impairments remain unmet. The Illuminating Engineering Society recommends that, for people sixty-five years of age (who have normal vision for their age) about twice the level of illumination should be provided as would be required for normal twenty-year-olds. However, such standards must be guided by the specific task being performed and aesthetic considerations. For the aged, avoid use of highly reflective-glare causing surfaces. Be certain that light fixtures cannot be used as toys or weapons. Increase illumination levels at key intervals at entrances, in large rooms, and along corridors to increase legibility of signage.

TASK LIGHTING

6.14 PROVIDE DESKTOP TASK LIGHTING COMBINED WITH FLUORESCENT LIGHTING

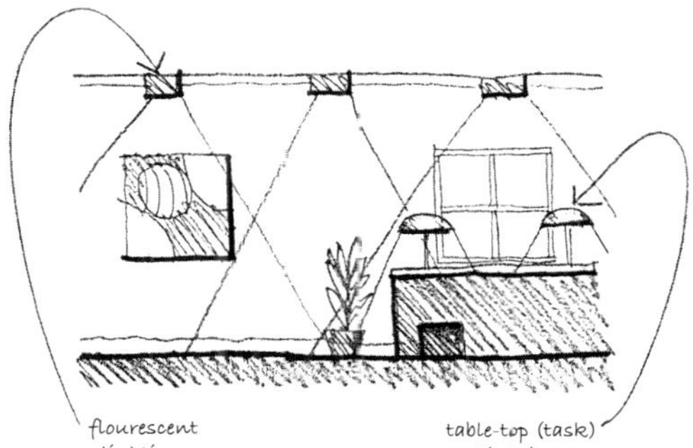

Fluorescent lights are a major contributor to the institutional ambiance often associated with health care facilities. It is not a coincidence that fluorescent lights are rarely found in residential environments. The light is harsh and artificial: the light spectrum is only partially represented. Certain colors take on an eerie hue and skin tones are distorted. Beyond these reasons, largely aesthetic, are functional justifications for achieving a balance between fluorescent lighting, task ambient incandescent lighting on desktops or recesses, and natural daylight. This provides the most options for work needs. In offices, encourage desktop incandescent lamps or lighting elements mounted on the underside of wall-mounted or partition-mounted shelves. This allows for maximum flexibility in light sources. Provide dimmer switches where appropriate to help staff blend multiple types of light sources each with its unique attributes that can contribute to a supportive work and treatment environment.

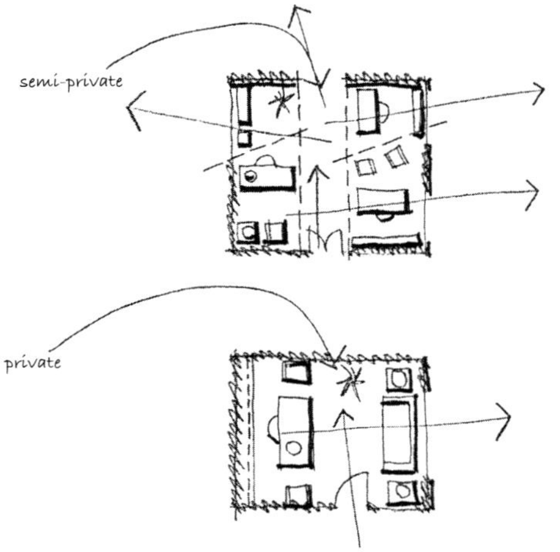

FURNISHINGS

6.15 FURNISH EACH STAFF WORKSPACE WITH SUPPORT AMENITIES

Staff express a preference to have their offices furnished with the typical office features such as wall tack space, a desk, lockable file cabinets, bookshelves, adequate overhead and possibly desktop lighting, windows and "good" views, a pleasant color scheme and carpet, if feasible. Nurses' offices should be large enough for three or four chairs and a sofa to accommodate a mother and small child. Some staff expressed the need for at least a small area rug where infant and latency-age children might sit on the floor and entertain themselves with toys while staff is interviewing/treating the mother. Open-plan (semi-private) work areas, in addition to the above mentioned amenities, should be adjacent to clerical support spaces, i.e. supply room, records room, and photocopy room.

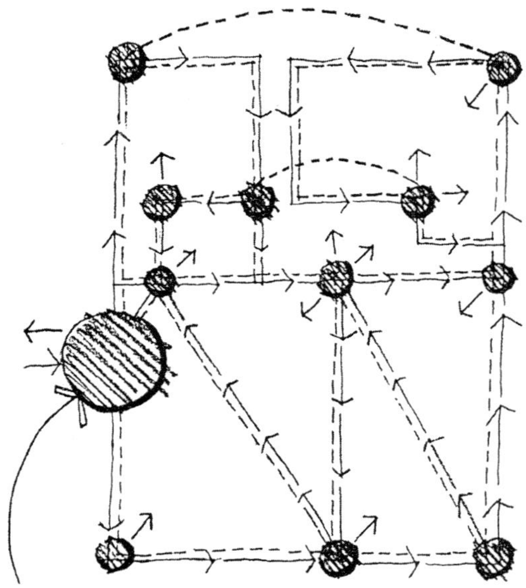

SEMI-PRIVATE SPACES

6.16 LOCATE ALCOVES THROUGHOUT THE HEALTH CENTER TO PROVIDE PLACES FOR INFORMAL CONVERSATION

Niches located along circulation paths provide opportunities for use as overflow waiting areas during busy clinics, and places for less formal contact between staff and patients. These spaces should not, however, be used for weight and measurement functions, sign-in and intake procedures during peak utilization periods, and other overflow functions due to bottlenecks, congestion, and overcrowded corridors, all of which are in violation of state fire codes that prohibit the blockage or impediment the building's points of egress and ingress. Locate these niche spaces along perimeter walls to allow for windows and daylight without sacrificing the privacy of patients. In windowless conditions, if unavoidable, provide adequate artificial lighting or incorporate clerestories and skylights to activate these spaces.

RESOURCE LIBRARY

6.17 PROVIDE A RESOURCE LIBRARY AS A PLACE TO PERUSE NEWSLETTERS AND LITERATURE ON RECENT MEDICAL ADVANCEMENTS

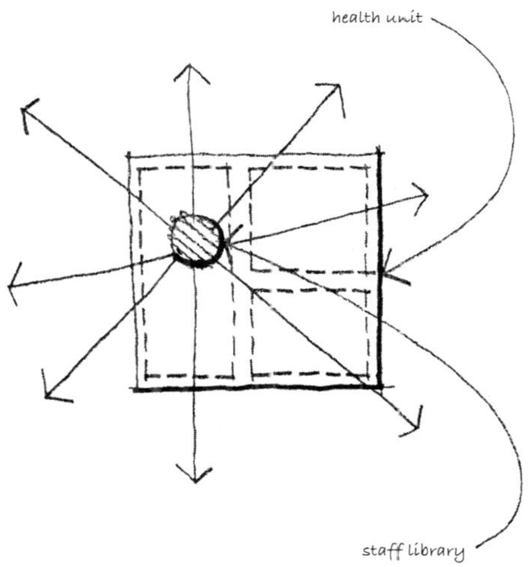

The responsibilities involved in performing one's job can make it difficult to stand back and regain perspective. This can be achieved if staff is provided with information of value to them. It can be a form of stress reduction as well as continuing education to be able to seek refuge in a room that allows one both respite and a learning experience. The problem of combining a learning-research library within the staff break room is that those who want to talk dominate the ambiance of the room. Therefore, provide magazines, newsletters, organizational correspondence, journals, and books in a resource room near to the staff break room or connected by a common entrance. Provide residential furnishings, area rugs, hardwood floors, windows, task lighting, and fixed incandescent lighting.

CHILDREN

6.18 FURNISHINGS AND EQUIPMENT FOR CHILDREN SHOULD BE SELECTED FOR FLEXIBILITY AND PORTABILITY

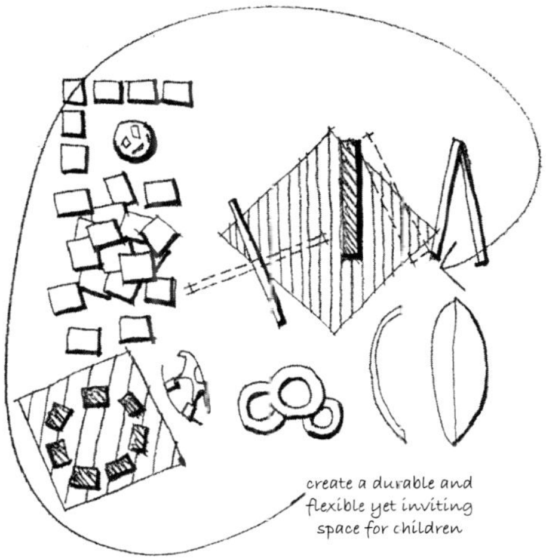

The selection and arrangement of the furnishings and equipment in the children's play zone is of high priority. Items should include a variable stimulating blend of furnishings and equipment to create a warm inviting space. Provide a combination of smooth non-slip interior tile on the floor and a durable grade of carpet. Movable lightweight furnishings encourage children to rearrange their surroundings to suit their particular interests and abilities. In the children's play zone design custom items, or purchase manufactured whimsical or themed furniture, such as elephant chairs, goose lamps, etc.

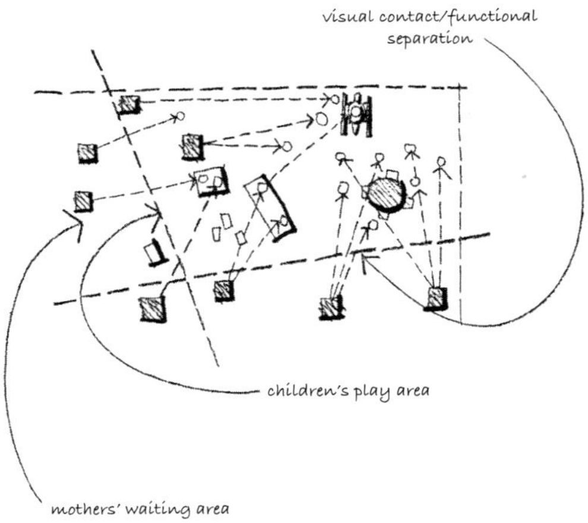

CHILDREN

6.19 EASE OF SUPERVISION OF CHILDREN BY MOTHERS IS OF HIGH PRIORITY IN THE HEALTH CARE ENVIRONMENT

To minimize disruptions inadvertently caused by children, design the facility to clearly structure the boundaries and limits of children's spatial movement and activity. In poorly designed outpatient health care settings, staff and mothers spend an undue amount of time verbally reprimanding their children. A visual link between the mother's space and places where children are likely to be is essential. A window in the interview room, can, for example, insure visual contact while allowing for brief functional separation. This can be particularly effective when an older child looks after a younger sibling in the waiting room.

UNIVERSAL DESIGN

6.20 THE HEALTH CARE ENVIRONMENT SHOULD BE DESIGNED TO ACCOMMODATE CHILDREN OF VARIOUS AGES

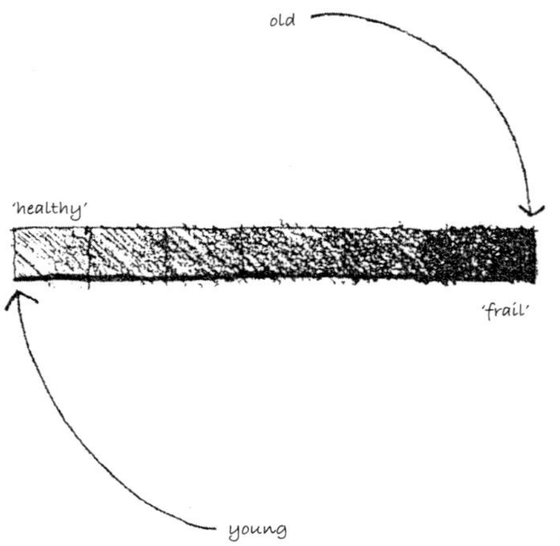

Design to achieve the goal of being universally responsive to the full range of human functional and cognitive capabilities. Sinks, toilets, fountains, and faucets must be designed so children, and persons with disabilities, can easily reach them. A high percentage of patients are mothers who may have an infant, a toddler, and a small school-age child with them. Therefore, it is necessary to design for multiple age groups. In a number of case studies it was found that there are no toys or child-dedicated play spaces for infants and toddlers. Few older children reading were observed, and a few facilities did not even have a TV in the main waiting room. In short, design for multiple levels of age-appropriateness.

WAYFINDING

6.21 INCORPORATE REDUNDANT CUEING TO DECREASE STRESS BY MAXIMIZING ENVIRONMENTAL LEGIBILITY

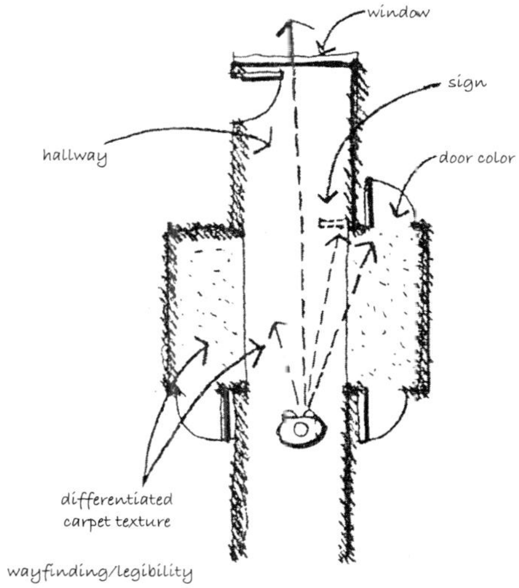

Redundant cueing is a design strategy to make it easier for persons with physical and sensory limitations, particularly elderly persons, to navigate and negotiate the built environment. It has been proven most useful to persons with visual, mobility, and cognitive impairments. Information in the physical setting is communicated to, and hence interpreted by, the user through its presentation in more than one mode. The same message is conveyed in more than one way. Some examples: one sees the emergency exit sign at the end of a hallway and a corresponding directional sign immediately across from one's door with an arrow pointing to the sign at the end of the hall; a change in floor texture corresponds to a change in wall or handrail texture, signaling that one has entered another portion of the building; alarms that emit visual as well as audible signals.

WAYFINDING

6.22 INCORPORATE "NON-SIGN" MARKERS TO ENHANCE WAYFINDING IN THE HEALTH CARE ENVIRONMENT

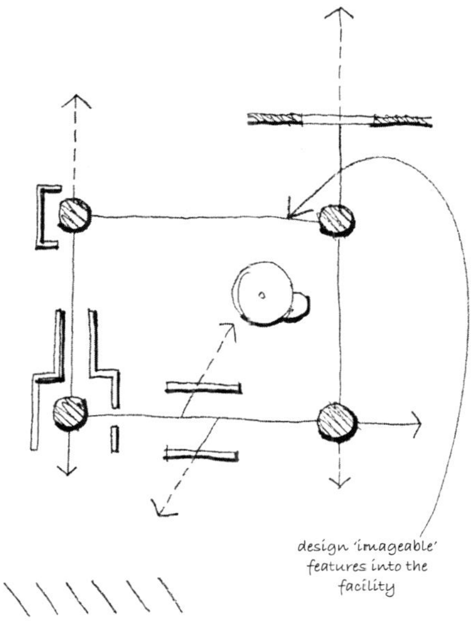

In addition to legible and easily understandable directional and informational signage, various types of non-verbal markers can aid in wayfinding in ambulatory health care settings. A more easily navigated environment can be created via landmarks, plants, pictures, changes in color schemes, strategically placed windows, doors, and the development of variations of major architectural features or concepts: corridor configuration, room shape, natural daylight vis-a-vis clerestories, skylights, doorway threshold design, floor patterns, and so on. The use of identifiable fixed and non-fixed elements within the building(s) and on the grounds to supplement written signage systems is a form of redundant cueing. Too many ineffective signage systems result from their being an afterthought or otherwise installed after the facility has been built.

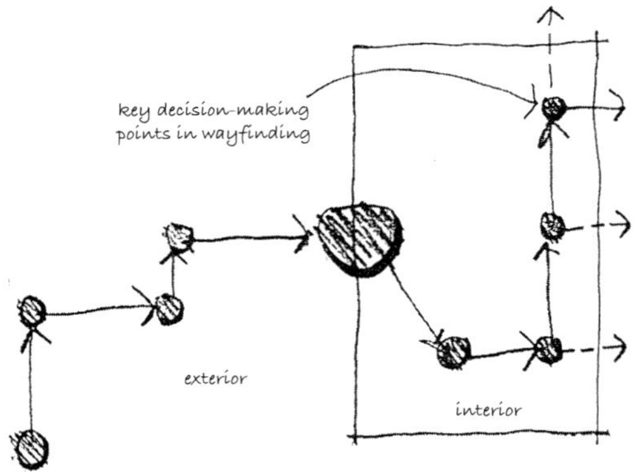

SAFETY—WAYFINDING

6.23 DIRECTIONAL SIGNAGE SYSTEMS SHOULD BE ATTUNED TO THE NEEDS OF THE SENSORY IMPAIRED

Well-designed health care facilities have identifying, directional, and informational signs attuned to the specialized needs of patients, staff, and visitors. The results of the 2000 SFI survey indicated that 83 percent of respondents were no more than "somewhat" satisfied with the signage in their facility. Poor signage is a source of confusion and disorientation. Very negative first impressions are likely if one cannot find the main entry, reception desk, or the exam room. Signs should be color contrasted to their backgrounds and feature clearly identifiable letters and symbols. Non-glare accent lighting and backlit signs aid legibility. Room numbers and descriptions along corridors should not be flush mounted on doors or walls. This makes it difficult to see them unless one is almost directly in front of them. Room ID signage and directional signs should in most cases project from the wall or from the ceiling above at a 90-degree angle to the path of circulation.

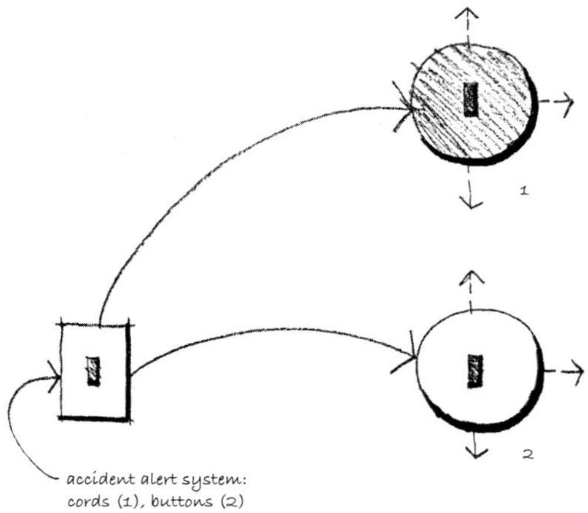

EMERGENCIES

6.24 EMERGENCY CALL BUTTONS AND PULL CORDS IN HALLWAYS ARE THERAPEUTIC ASSISTIVE DEVICES

The Americans with Disabilities Act of 1990 (ADA) called for all public accommodations to be accessible to all persons who are physically or developmentally disabled, regardless of race, color, creed, age, or occupation. Call buttons and pull cords have become standard items in environments for the aged. These facility types include housing, institutional settings, and recreational settings for the elderly. In the 1990s, this became increasingly common in other building types not only for use by the aged but for all whose disabilities are within the legislative parameters of the ADA. Therefore, include pull cords or call buttons, clearly marked in key public circulation routes and in rooms such as exam rooms and restrooms. Locate these assistive devices to make them un-accessible as play objects for children.

EMERGENCIES—WAYFINDING

6.25 DESIGN INNOVATIVE "YOU ARE HERE" LOCATIONAL MAPS

A detailed floor plan of the facility, indicating all means of egress in the event of fire, is required by code. All too often, however, a poorly drawn plan is thrown together by a staff person and crudely taped to the wall. This can cause problems if hallway widths and distances to exits are inaccurate, or worse, if critical information is unknowingly omitted, i.e. doors, stairways, or breakout windows. A related problem exists when the fire exit plan is poorly located, illegible, or if one is unable to orient oneself. Therefore, give great attention to the provision of a scale drawing; reproduce it at a size large enough for individual rooms to be seen from five or more feet away and by persons with impaired vision, i.e. the aged. Always provide a "You are here" indicator marked in red or another easily seen color. This floor plan should be a wayfinding aid as well as emergency egress assistance device.

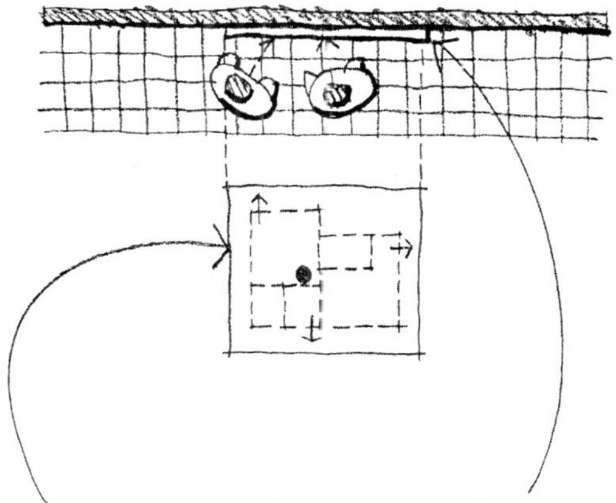

emergency evacuation plan (wall-mounted)

CORRIDORS—DAYLIGHTING

6.26 AVOID BLIND CORRIDORS THAT ARE INSTITUTIONAL, DEVOID OF DAYLIGHT OR VIEWS TO THE OUTDOORS

One of the main characteristics of institutional architecture is the long double-loaded windowless corridor. It is little more than a bleak space for all who must use the building. The lack of daylight or view precludes the type of spatial punctuation so essential within buildings. In a health care facility, it is particularly important to break up the corridor with "events" of this type. Therefore, create open corridors with visual connections to the exterior, such as a view at the end of a corridor, a clerestory above, and windows (room to room or to the exterior). This will help to animate and enliven the facility for all its inhabitants, especially when emphasized with varying ceiling heights, spatial configurations, color schemes, and floor patterning.

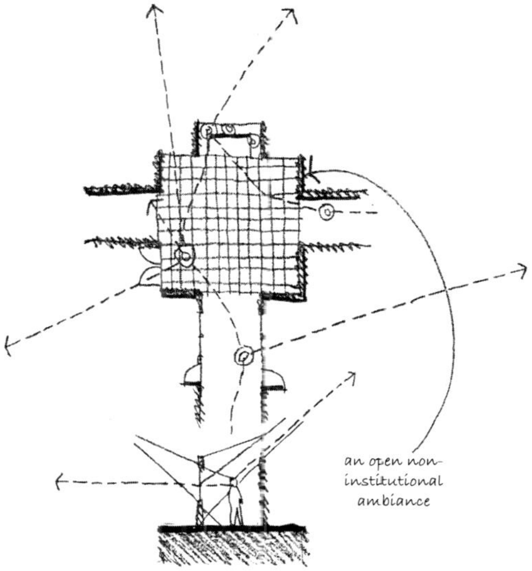

MAINTENANCE AND UPKEEP

6.27 INCORPORATE DURABLE WALL SURFACES, DOORS, AND WINDOWS WITHOUT CREATING AN INSTITUTIONAL IMAGE

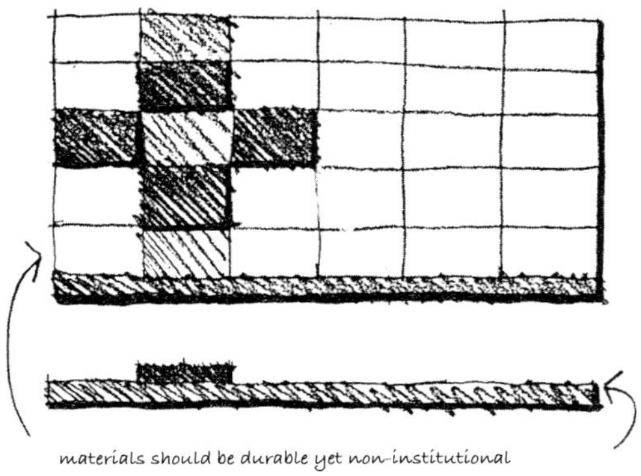

materials should be durable yet non-institutional

To avoid broken windows an efficient solution in some situations is to install windows of shatterproof glass or a polycarbonate resin sheet such as Lexan rather than breakable glass. This is particularly important for doors and in waiting areas if sells are low to the floor. All doors, screens, fasteners, and locks must be durable. Avoid corner moldings which project and can be easily torn off if knocked. All countertops must have rounded corners. Do not locate sharp, projecting surfaces or hardware at the eye level of a child. Materials of construction and interior finish materials must be highly durable and yet non-institutional in aesthetic appearance. Avoid concrete block walls, steel industrial-grade doors, and harsh overhead fluorescent light fixture-trays. These and similar conditions may only provoke resentment and create a dreary, uninspiring, harsh appearance.

UNIVERSAL DESIGN

6.28 PROVIDE ACCESSIBLE DOOR HARDWARE, SWITCHES, OPERABLE WINDOWS, DRINKING FOUNTAINS, AND TELEPHONES

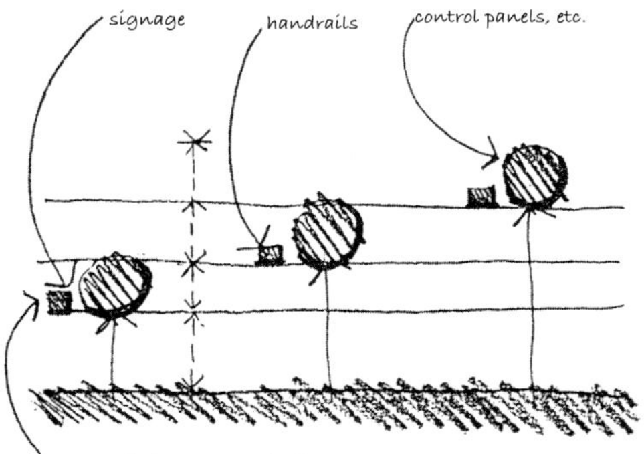

the specialized needs of children and the elderly warrant close attention to planning and design

The ADA and its subsequent legal interpretations mandated for the first time that all public facilities must be accessible to the disabled. The phase in period for retrofitting existing facilities varied by type (up to twenty years in some cases) but it would appear to be logical that a community health center must be retrofitted to be made accessible as soon as possible, if it is not already in compliance. The numerous items which must comply include drinking fountains, directional graphics, ramps, rails, wall switches for elevators and lights, telephones, and all doors. Although the ADA does not include window hardware, this should also be incorporated in the universal design of an accessible health unit. The facility must accommodate the needs of those in wheelchairs, the visually impaired, hearing impaired, cognitively impaired, developmentally disabled, and special user constituencies.

CARPET

6.29 CARPETING SHOULD BE USED IN SOME AREAS TO CREATE A SOUND BUFFER AND TO DE-INSTITUTIONALIZE

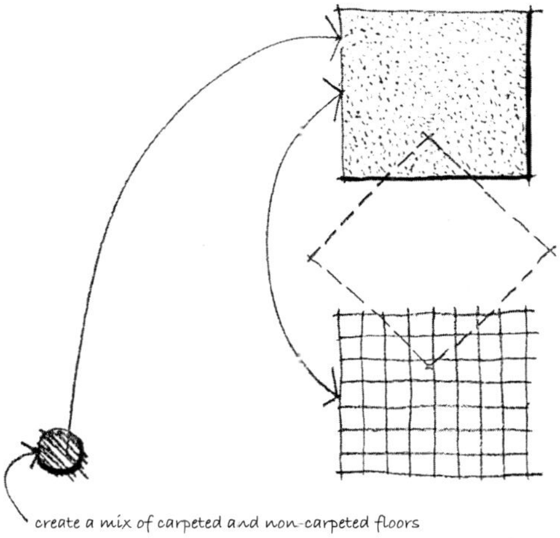

The SFI team made a special point to question the staff at all twenty-five case study locations as to their views on carpet. It was found that people were either strongly pro or con. The most consensuses occurred on the benefits of carpet in terms of a means to reduce ambient noise. Second, it can help to soften an otherwise unyielding institutional ambiance. Too many hard, reflective surfaces in a space—be it a corridor or an office—can cause intensification of relatively minor sounds like footsteps, conversations, doors opening and closing. Over time these irritants become environmental stressors. However, do not place carpet in chronically wet areas, near sinks, or in high traffic areas.

ACOUSTICS

6.30 CONSIDER TILING OR CARPETING ONE WALL OF THE ROOM AS A MEANS OF NOISE ABATEMENT

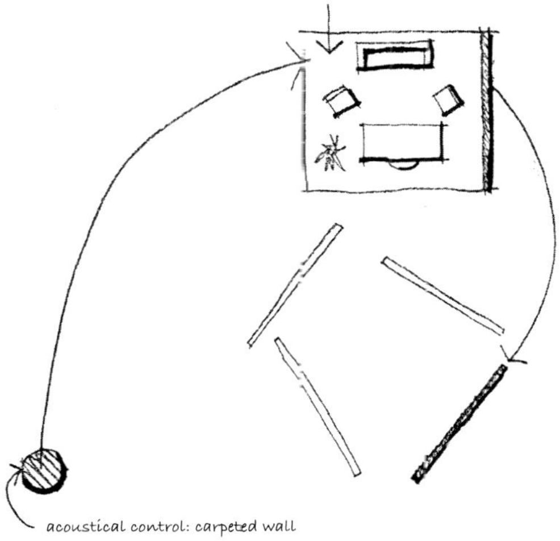

The traditional exam room is comprised of entirely hard, non-absorptive surfaces: floors, walls, windows (if present), and ceilings reflect and amplify sounds. Additionally, unless one wall is painted in an accent hue, or the floor or ceiling is of a different color, the space is visually monotonous. Therefore, explore ways to create a more interesting room aesthetically while at the same time providing acoustical amenity. This can be achieved by carpeting or tiling an accent wall; this can add a bit of diversity to the room, increased room-to-room privacy can be achieved, and this wall can double as a pin-up surface in some instances.

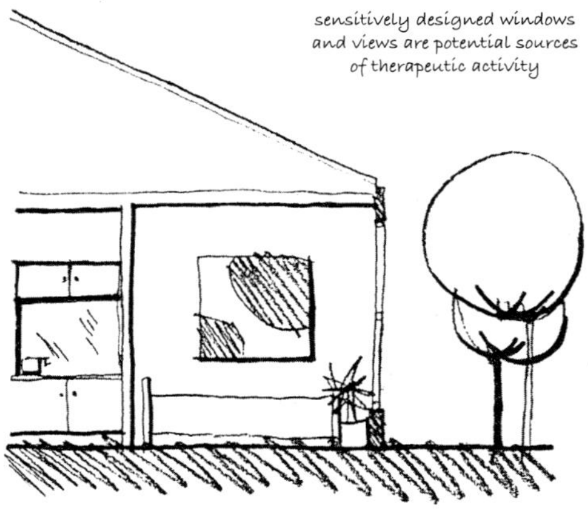

SEPARATIONS

6.31 PARTITIONS OF VARYING TYPES CAN CONTRIBUTE TO THE CREATION OF FLEXIBLE ZONES

A low partition wall or screen wall can contribute to a hierarchy of public and semi-public zones. A half-height wall partition can be positioned to visually separate a main entry foyer from the main waiting area, and office work areas, such as the sanitarian's plan review room can be separated from adjacent offices without creating completely separate rooms. A partial height wall partition (forty-two inches) should be of durable surface materials, made to withstand considerable wear. More elaborate partitions to subdivide a room include five-foot high wood cabinets on wheels or fixed cabinets with countertops, thus creating multiple zones. The partitions themselves must be designed and installed for ease of operation. Folding screens and accordion partitions should be mounted on tracks, perhaps operated electronically. In some situations, an overhead lockable sliding garage door may be appropriate, as it also provides security.

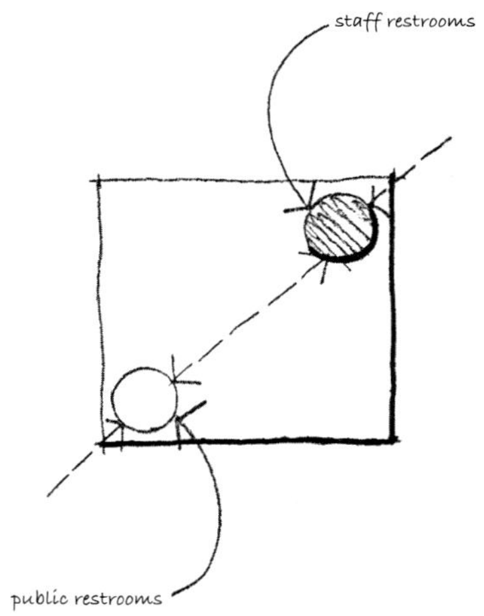

RESTROOMS—ACCESS

6.32 PROVIDE PUBLIC RESTROOMS IN THE MAIN RECEPTION/WAITING REALM, APART FROM STAFF RESTROOMS

The public restrooms are key support amenities because mothers need to be able to change a child's diaper on a moment's notice, or must remain near the restroom due to the nature on one's illness. Immediate access is of high priority, as is of course separate women's and men's restrooms. Provide visual separation by means of a wall or by recessing the doors within a wall so they do not directly face the waiting room or other public area. Do not require staff and the public to share the same restrooms—provide separation in order for the staff restrooms to be properly located within the core of the clinic, separate from the highly public realm of the facility. In small units, in contrast to the public restrooms, a single restroom for staff can be shared by men and women. In large units provide separate staff restrooms for men and women which are conveniently located, preferably near the staff workroom.

RESTROOMS—UNIVERSAL DESIGN

6.33 RESTROOMS MUST BE DESIGNED TO ACCOMMODATE THE NEEDS OF ALL RANGES OF PHYSICAL ABILITIES AND AGES

In order to provide a supportive environment for the disabled, equip restrooms with wheelchair accessible toilets, sinks with grab bars, and adequate seating areas to facilitate transference from wheelchair to toilet. Allow for a wheelchair to have full access to sinks equipped with handicap accessible hardware. This also applies to all doors, lighting switches, trash receptacles, etc. All portions of the health unit should be accessible to the handicapped, i.e. Braille coded hallways, entrances, wheelchair height telephones and fountains, ramps, chair lifts, elevators, accessible door threshold widths, and pull cords.

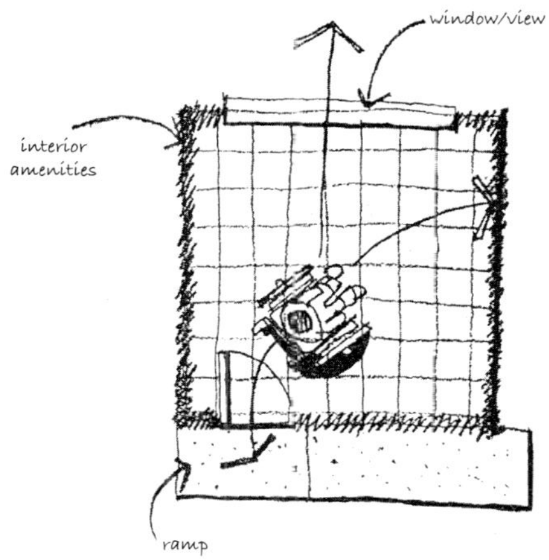

RESTROOMS—INTERNAL ZONES

6.34 RESTROOMS SHOULD BE COMPARTMENTALIZED WHENEVER POSSIBLE

Conflicts are minimized when compartmentalized restrooms allow for more than one person to use the restroom at the same time. Sinks, lavatories, changing table alcoves for infants and an entry foyer should be designed to accommodate functional separation. These spaces should be able to be closed off vis-a-vis swing doors or pull curtains. Budget limitations may in some cases limit the number of restrooms, thereby necessitating that the patient urine specimen washroom double for use with the general public, although this is not recommended. Above all, provide for basic personal hygiene needs and privacy within the restrooms. This applies to public as well as staff restrooms, regardless of their location within the facility.

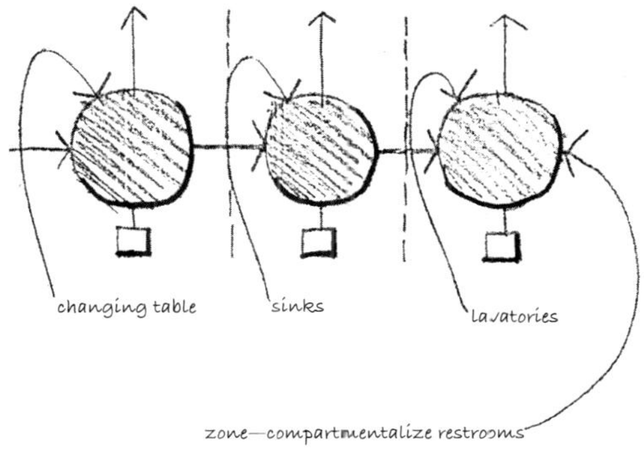

COLOR

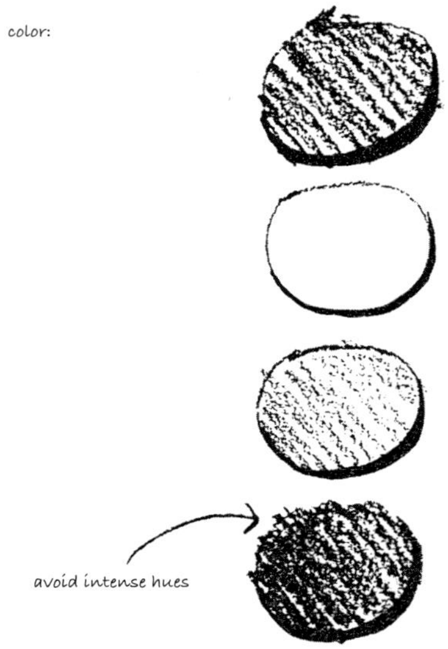

6.35 COLORS FOR WALLS, CEILINGS, FLOORING, FURNISHINGS AND CARPETING AFFORD AMENITY

Architects, interior designers, and environmental psychologists have researched color palettes and their affect on human behavior in a number of institutional building types, including schools, libraries, museums, hospitals, prisons, and various public buildings. In health care facilities too much of any one color is to be avoided. Avoid at all costs the image of the sterile white ward. Avoid dreary green and grays. Also avoid excessive use of excitable colors such as hues of red, orange, and purple. Warm color palettes are suggested for public spaces to encourage social interaction; cool tones and pastels have been found to be of soothing effect on patients. Hues of pink and complementary hues are of therapeutic effect. It is best to develop a multi-faceted color scheme that coordinates the color of furnishings, carpet, wall and ceiling surfaces, doors, and details such as window frames.

ENVIRONMENTAL CONTROL

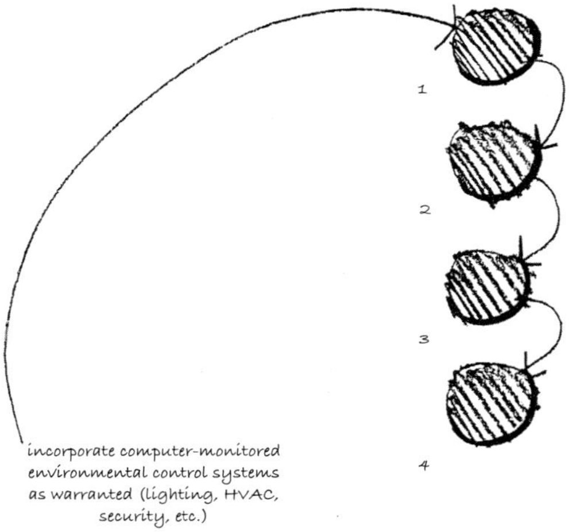

6.36 INCORPORATE COMPUTER–MONITORED ENVIRONMENTAL CONTROL SYSTEMS TO REDUCE OPERATIONAL COSTS

Recent advancements in "intelligent building" research and development have resulted in new systems to reduce overall building performance costs. The following systems can be monitored by these computer-based devices: lighting, heating, air conditioning and humidity control, and daylight control screens. Perhaps the most successful of these systems are those that automatically turn off lights at a predetermined interval of time after occupants have left the room. When properly specified and maintained, these systems have been shown to reduce annual energy consumption operating costs by as much as 40 percent. Coordinate this with LEED criteria. Also, tie in the emergency backup power generator.

ENVIRONMENTAL CONTROL

6.37 HEATING, VENTILATING, AND AIR CONDITIONING SYSTEMS SHOULD BE FLEXIBLE TO SUPPORT THE NEEDS OF MULTIPLE-USER CONSTITUENCIES

Older patients and staff members are less active and more susceptible to respiratory ailments and colds than younger people, and therefore require HVAC systems designed for narrower ranges of comfort. Many elderly people are so susceptible to loss of body heat they risk hypothermia. Pay particular attention to exhaust systems, filters, and air re-circulation in rooms, particularly where odor control and air quality must be controlled. Heating and cooling in areas normally occupied by older people provide a design capacity for a temperature of 75 degrees (see applicable codes and standards). Provide operable windows because occupants prefer to have a choice between mechanical and natural ventilation. Avoid drafts, especially at floor level. Proper maintenance of HVAC systems is essential. Incorporate passive solar design strategies.

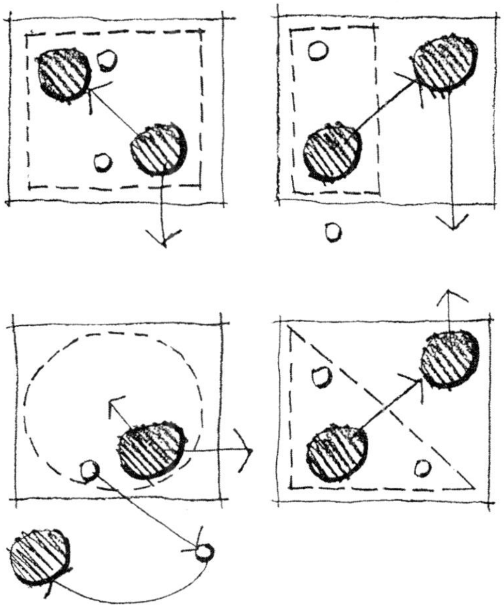

incorporate flexible HVAC systems—decentralized zoning

7. COST CONTAINMENT

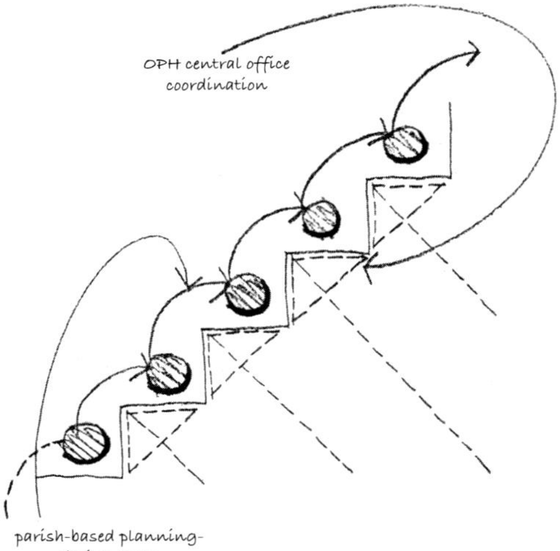

COORDINATION

7.1 ENHANCE AND UPGRADE THE HEALTH CARE NETWORKS WITHIN REALISTIC COST CONSTRAINTS

Before embarking on a major elective renovation and facility redevelopment program, priorities must be clearly established. Arrive at a set dollar amount for capital improvements to the physical plant after analyzing realistic design options and running preliminary cost analyses on one or more of the strongest planning and architectural strategies. Additionally, obtain input from department and program heads. All key members of the organization must realize, however, that interdepartmental "turf wars" often occur in health care organizations when the words "improvement," "expansion," and "renovation" come to the fore. The organizations must compete with one another for extremely limited resources. It is the responsibility of the administration and its designee to oversee the implementation of a strategic plan for coordinated facility improvements.

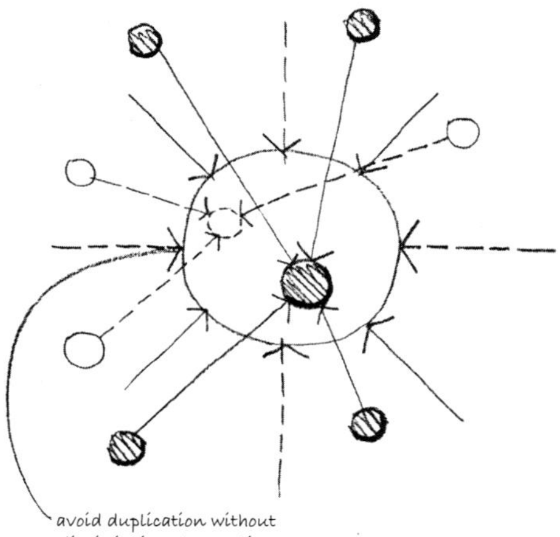

COORDINATION

7.2 REDUCE CURRENT OPERATING COSTS THROUGH CENTRALIZATION OF SUPPORT FUNCTIONS

Trade-offs between centralized versus decentralized support services and treatment strategies must be carefully weighed. Decentralized staff support services afford the opportunity to create smaller pockets of support for treatment programs, and help promote a sense of unity among staff and patients, but may incur higher per-patient costs. Conversely, large centralized health units can become alienating for staff and patient, although they may be less costly to operate. Bigger is not necessarily better with respect to the quality of patient care. The major challenge is to determine, on a regional basis, what should and should not be centralized within a health care network.

FEASIBILITY

7.3 EMPLOY POST-OCCUPANCY EVALUATION PERFORMANCE ASSESSMENT TO IDENTIFY UNNEEDED FACILITIES

All public health agency programs should be periodically evaluated in terms of the needs of the local community. Specific architectural criteria include four major areas: 1) patterns of occupant use (How well does the unit serve the needs of the users?); 2) environmental control (are the HVAC systems effective? Is it too hot or cold? Do occupants have the ability to regulate room temperature, for instance?); 3) maintenance and upkeep (Can this building or unit be maintained at a reasonable cost?); and 4) aesthetics and image of the facility (Is the exterior and interior appearance of the facility commensurate with the goals and philosophy of the organization?). Systematic post-occupancy evaluations can yield an overall picture of facility performance. A unit or building too small or outdated from a clinical or aesthetic standpoint should be assessed for sale or retrofitted to a new use.

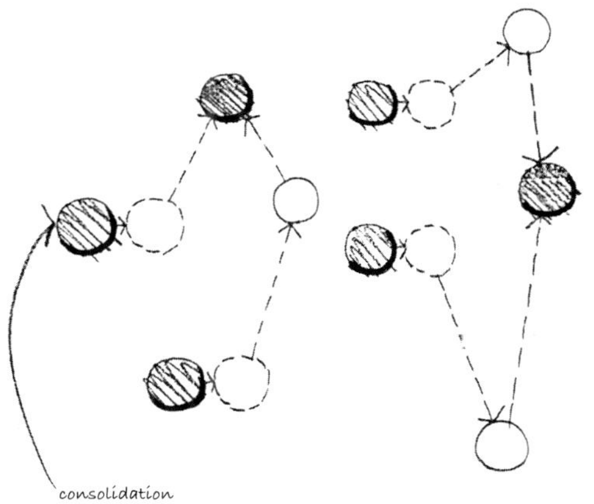

consolidation

FEASIBILITY

7.4 A WELL-PLANNED AND DESIGNED HEALTH CARE ENVIRONMENT REDUCES LIFE CYCLE EXPENDITURES

The recent and ongoing upheaval in the health care industry is directly reflected in the architectural settings which house these programs. The present climate of cost-containment, alternatives to hospitalization, the rise of home and community health care, increased competition among providers, facility obsolescence, and an undersupply of skilled nursing staff and allied support staff has a continuing impact. Therefore, the architectural environment must continue to be comforting and therapeutic, but highly adaptable to changing needs. Flexible facilities will yield cost savings down the road. In fact, the term "renovation" needs redefinition. In the past, it has implied moving "permanent" walls, electrical, heating, air conditioning connections, and such built-in items as cabinets and nursing station fixtures. Whenever possible, design units and building support systems that can be retained and relocated, enlarged or reduced without requiring the purchase of new equipment.

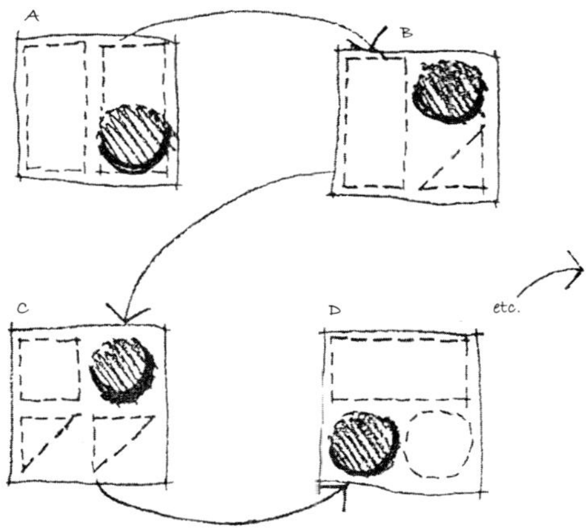

flexible health care facilities

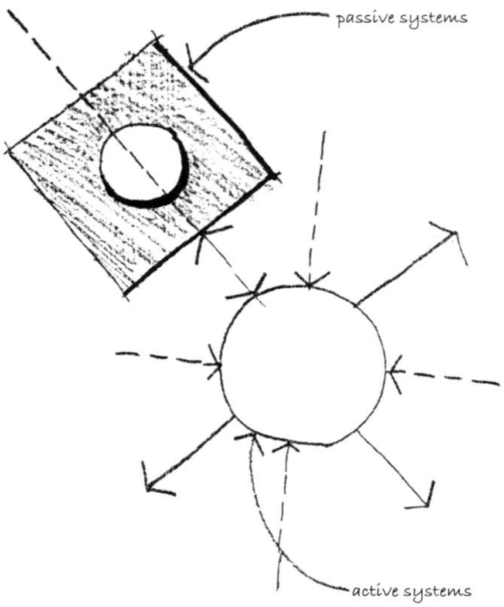

COST CONTAINMENT

7.5 PASSIVE SOLAR DAYLIGHT SYSTEMS ARE SOURCES OF OPERATIONAL COST SAVINGS

Passive systems can augment a baseline HVAC system in a health care facility. HVAC systems poorly fitted to client and occupant needs can result in even the most carefully developed annual operating cost projections, on paper, to be exceeded by as much as 40 percent in actual annual cost. Active solar technologies are expensive to install and have high initial operational cost, they require more maintenance, are less available, and generally not as aesthetically pleasing compared to passive solar design strategies. However, geothermal systems offer many advantages. Passive solar design techniques are cheaper initially and afford greater aesthetic latitude. These include Trombe walls (to maximize thermal mass), sun spaces that bathe reflected surfaces and solar optic-mirror systems, overhangs, shaded foyers, proper glazing, screenings, curtains, landscaping, proper building orientation on the site, and appropriate building massing and scale. Coordinate with LEED performance criteria during design.

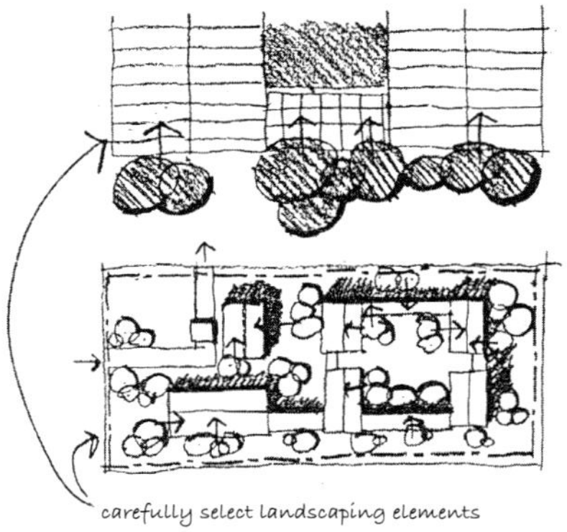

COST CONTAINMENT

7.6 USE ENERGY EFFICIENT LANDSCAPING AND BUILDING MATERIALS

The type and quality of landscaping elements around a health care facility, or the absence of landscaping, have a great deal to do with the energy costs of running the facility. Trees and bushes can screen the facility and outdoor spaces from direct exposure to the elements. Similarly, the materials of construction must be properly chosen and specialized to insure minimal operating costs. For example, in hot and humid regions like Louisiana, screen the facility from direct sunlight with deciduous (shade) trees relatively close to the perimeter walls of the building (particularly on the south and west faces); plant shrubs and trellises to help block sun and wind; avoid materials that absorb undue sunlight. A wide range of materials (wood, stone, brick, concrete, steel panel) are suitable if used appropriately. Coordinate with LEED criteria during design.

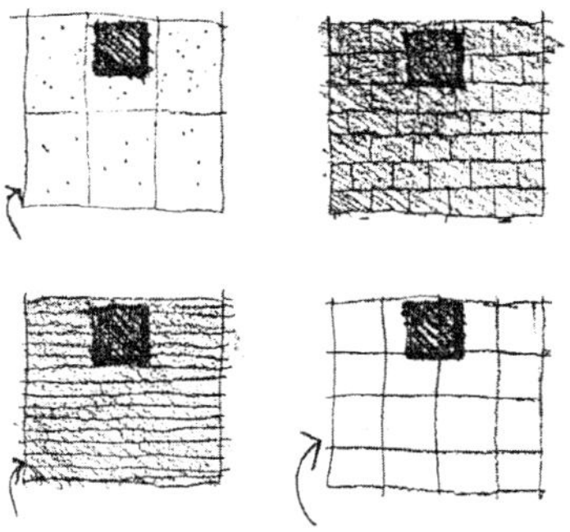

COST CONTAINMENT

7.7 CLIMATE IS A KEY DETERMINANT OF COST-EFFECTIVE HEALTH CARE ARCHITECTURE

Prior to the invention of air conditioning and mechanical heating, health care clinics were shaped far more profoundly that they are today by the need to regulate sun-daylight penetration during the summer months and the intrusion of cold air into the building envelope during the winter months. In the present era of advanced computerized HVAC systems the inherent benefits of certain pre-high-tech-design strategies for health care facilities must not be forgotten. The following architectural attributes are among those that should be interwoven with the benefits that result from appropriate use of high-tech HVAC systems in facilities: overhangs that shield direct sunlight from the building interior, operable windows and clerestories to facilitate cross-ventilation, protection from undue south exposure, courtyards, covered walkways, semi-linear configurations, pitched roofs to drain rainwater, and vestibules to control the flow of conditioned air. Coordinate with LEED criteria during design.

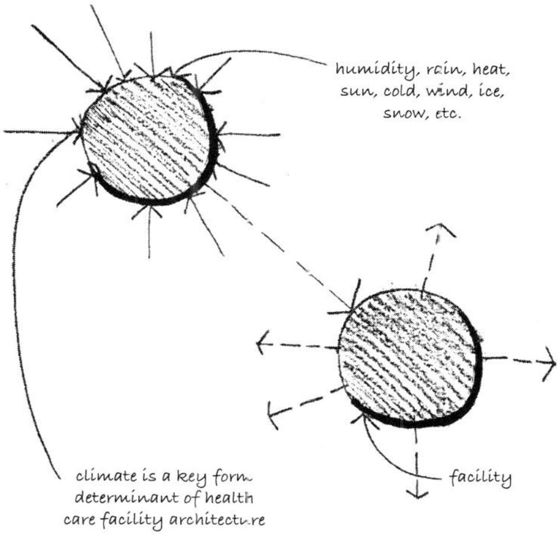

8. PHASED IMPLEMENTATION

RENOVATION AND EXPANSION

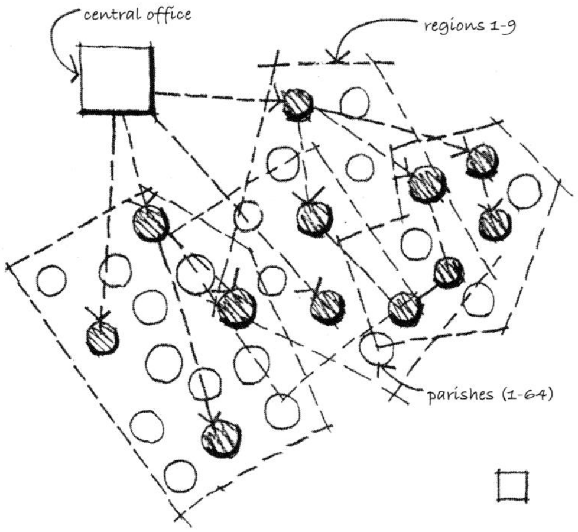

8.1 STRATEGICALLY PHASE IMPROVEMENTS TO HEALTH CARE NETWORKS OVER A MULTI-YEAR PERIOD

It is naive to assume that funds allocated for capital expenditures over the next ten years will be adequate to uniformly upgrade an entire statewide public health network of program sites. Major disparities in facility quality could still result between regions unless effective, enforceable, uniform standards are put in place. Third, gaps could exist resulting in a double standard by type of facility. As a result, regional offices, clinics, and labs may receive more or less funding that the parish health unit network. Therefore, it is essential that a funding allocation strategy be developed by the parent agency, providing each region and each community an assessment of what the agency believes should be done, identifies specific facilities earmarked for improvement, and establishes minimum standards of architectural quality and facility performance standards.

RENOVATION AND EXPANSION

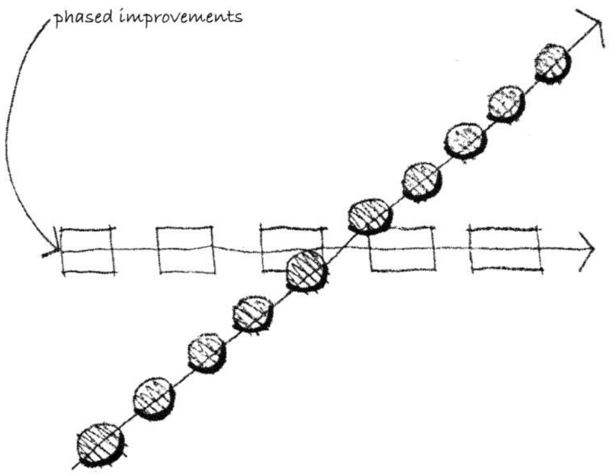

8.2 PHASE THE IMPROVEMENT OF EXISTING FACILITIES WITHOUT DIMINISHING THE QUALITY OF CARE

A carefully planned, orchestrated, and executed renovation or expansion can create a positive and progressive image. This requires the effective communication between staff working in tandem with the architectural and engineering team. The sequence of change should be mapped out in great detail. These events are line items, as are corresponding timetables for completion. Some programs or office functions may have to move out temporarily to trailers or another building to ensure their continued functioning during construction. The privacy needs of patients must be foremost. All construction activity must revolve around the patients: the quality of care must not diminish. Construct temporary wayfinding signage systems to minimize confusion, and schedule work at times least disruptive to patients and clinical staff.

SITE

8.3 DEVELOP LIMITED SITE ACCESS FOR CONSTRUCTION VEHICLES

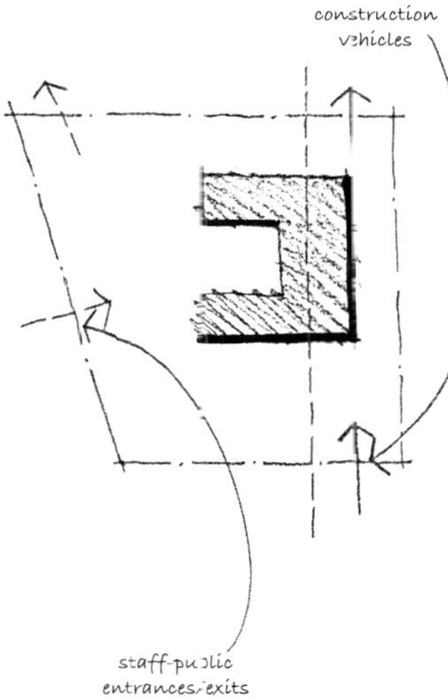

Noise is a major source of environmental pollution in health care facilities. Internally generated noise is disruptive and becomes a stressor to patients, staff, and visitors if experienced for prolonged periods of time. Groups of children in the waiting room can be a cause of noise. The problem is magnified exponentially when considering the noise generated during a facility renovation or expansion construction project. Trucks, in particular, can have a particularly disturbing effect on patients, staff, and visitors. Negative factors, besides noise, include rattled foundations as trucks pass by, the smell of exhaust, and an overall unaesthetic visual appearance. Therefore, limit the number of truck ingress-egress points to as few as possible—preferably only one access point.

SITE

8.4 DEVELOP SEPARATE VEHICULAR ACCESS ROUTES FOR CONSTRUCTION AND NON-CONSTRUCTION VEHICLES

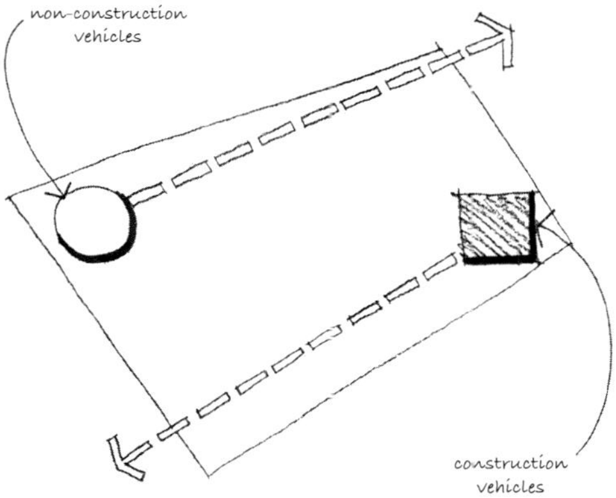

Create access points and routes for visitors, staff, and patients that are different from those provided for construction workers and vehicles. This can reduce noise levels and create a more favorable image in the eyes of the public, staff, and patients. The need for separation of construction-related patterns of site use and user constituencies becomes even more critical during periods of change in a health care facility. Due to the need to provide a supportive, reassuring environment for patients, poorly conceived and implemented strategies are counter-therapeutic.

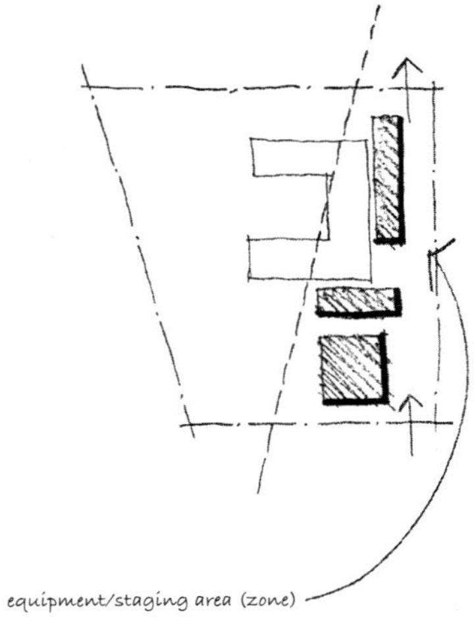

SITE

8.5 CONSTRUCTION EQUIPMENT AND STAGING AREAS MUST NOT IMPEDE USE OF THE FACILITY DURING CONSTRUCTION

Construction equipment requires overnight storage space when not in use. Fenced-off construction areas (hard hat-only spaces) are common in health care facility projects. These areas may contain equipment, materials, as well as on-site trailer offices of the foreman and project superintendent. These areas should be visually screened to block out unsightly views, but not become barriers. Most importantly, construction-related activity and the aforementioned spaces of construction support must not interfere significantly with the delivery of services. Specifically, outdoor courtyards and other kept landscaped areas should be preserved for patient and staff access and use during construction. Failure to provide functional separation hinders delivery of services.

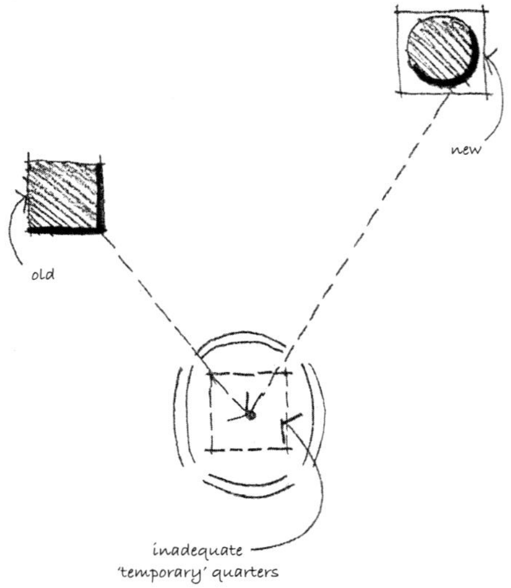

FORCED RELOCATION

8.6 AVOID TEMPORARY RELOCATION TO AN INAPPROPRIATE FACILITY WHILE AWAITING THE CONSTRUCTION OF A REPLACEMENT FACILITY

At some point in time, the pressure may be a great reason to seize the opportunity to obtain a new or improved facility if temporary quarters can be found to house the health unit and a move is made under the assumption that it will be of short duration. Understandably, many decisions may have to be made quickly if this happens. It is recommended that whenever possible the health unit should remain located at its present location until the new replacement building is completed. On the other hand, when the existing health unit is being renovated or expanded, relocation to temporary quarters is recommended only if a detailed feasibility study has been conducted to compare alternate sites in terms of access to the community, cost, size, flexibility, function, parking, and image. More often than not, haste makes waste when relocation must occur quickly and due diligence does not occur.

IMPLEMENTATION

8.7 CREATE A COMMUNITY PUBLIC HEALTH CARE ENVIRONMENT THAT SYMBOLIZES DIGNITY, LIFE, AND HOPE

The imagery and activity in the total facility and the surrounding site can generate an atmosphere of nurturance, growth, and optimism. Community health care facilities with posters and artwork, appealing colors, and amenities symbolize and inspire hope. Allied facilities can also be supportive in these ways to further the achievements and aspirations of their occupants. Incorporate life-themes, positive experiences, metaphors to the personal successes of others, contact with nature and inspire the personal goals that can be achieved. Create, and then communicate to others the health center's successful experience in promoting community well being through its successful programs.

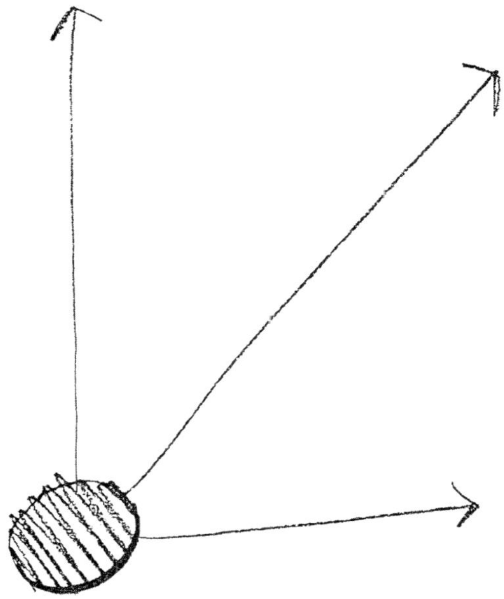

Notes to Chapter 1

[1]Paul Groth and Todd W. Bressi, eds., *Understanding Ordinary Landscapes* (New Haven and London, 1997).

[2]Paul Groth, "Frameworks for Cultural Landscape Study," in Groth and Bressi, *Understanding Ordinary Landscapes*, 1-2.

[3]Ibid., 3-16.

[4]Jay Appleton, "The Integrity of the Landscape Movement," in Groth and Bressi, *Understanding Ordinary Landscapes*, 189-90.

[5]Stephen Verderber and David J. Fine, *Healthcare Architecture in an Era of Radical Transformation* (New Haven and London, 2000), 280-82.

[6]John Allen, "Finsbury at 50: Caring and Causality," *Architectural Review* 183 (June 1988): 47-50; and Peter Coe, *Lubetkin and Tecton: Architecture and Social Commitment: A Critical Study* (London and Bristol, 1981).

[7]Ibid., 48.

[8]The criteria for architect selection were, in many instances, ad hoc.

[9]The Center for Health Design, based in Martinez, California, since its founding in 1985, has advocated for evidence-based design and research in architecture. The center has sponsored empirical research and is a clearinghouse for the presentation of new products. One early research project is Claire Cooper Marcus and Marni Barnes' *Gardens in Healthcare Facilities: Uses, Therapeutic Benefits, and Design Recommendations* (Martinez, CA, 1996). A current initiative is the Pebble Project, with twenty-five sponsoring clients assessing the performance and impact of evidence-based design in the private sector of the U.S. healthcare industry.

[10]The *American Journal of Public Health* devoted its September 2003 issue to the "Built Environment and Health." This issue contained articles on the unhealthful attributes of excessive communing distances, the deleterious health consequences of suburban sprawl, the health-promoting amenity of walkable communities, the history of public health and urban housing, the therapeutic value of nature engagement, and the illogic of current zoning laws in the United States. The *American Journal of Health Promotion* also devoted its September 2003 issue to this topic. Since, the CDC and the Robert Wood Johnson Foundation have sponsored research on this subject.

[11]Stephen Verderber and Ben Refuerzo, "Empowerment on Main Street: Implementing Research-Based Design," in R.M. Feldman, G. Hardie, and D.G. Saile, eds., *Power by Design: EDRA 24 Proceedings* (Oklahoma City, 1993), 281-84.

[12]Construction inactivity had reduced some to supporting cast roles as code analysts, in-house renovation project architects, and medical equipment planning coordinators.

[13]Appleton, "The Integrity of the Landscape Movement," 192-99.

[14]Peter Stringer, "The Myths of Architectural Creativity," *Architectural Digest* 10 (1975): 634-35.

[15]Sharon E. Sutton, "Power, Knowledge, and the Art of Leadership," *Progressive Architecture* 5 (May 1992), 65-68.

[16]Robert Gutman, *Architectural Practice, A Critical View* (New York, 1988).

[17]Ben Refuerzo and Stephen Verderber, "Beyond Static Conceptions of Research and Design in Architecture: An Integrative Paradigm," in Robert I. Selby, et al., eds., *Coming of Age, Proceedings of the Twenty-first Annual Conference of the Environmental Design Research Association* (Washington, D.C., 1990), 26-27.

[18]Steve Ritea and Ed Anderson, "Budget Gets $50 Million Trim; Health Agency Takes Biggest Hit," New Orleans *Times-Picayune*, December 12, 1999, A-4. On the same day on the editorial page, in a piece titled "It's Time for Fiscal Reform," Ritea and Anderson wrote

> Across the nation—including much of the South—state governments flush with money in a booming economy have slashed taxes. But here in Louisiana . . . lawmakers are slashing services and ogling tax hikes. The state's economy is anemic compared to the rest of the region. . . . Now apparently, state government is $104 million short of revenue for the current budget year. That, despite padding the budget last spring with $156 million from the first installment of the [state's share of a] tobacco industry legal settlement. It gets worse. Predictions are that revenues will come up $450 million short in 2000-2001. . . . The state's tax system is unstable and out of kilter. It relies too much on sales taxes, which are vulnerable to the whims of the economy and put an unfair burden on the poor. Plus, it gouges businesses. This is the only state that charges full sales tax on equipment and machinery purchases, and it also imposes a tax on money businesses borrow to set up shop or expand. . . . Combine that tax structure with the state's myriad social and education ills, and it's no surprise that Louisiana is lagging in economic development or that its population is shrinking. . . . Louisiana needs a tax system that will grow more and better jobs. Without that, it's going to lurch from one crisis to another.

Other newspaper articles included Steve Ritea, "Health Department Faces Millions in Cuts to Close Shortfall," *Times-Picayune,* January 19, 2000, A-3; Ed Anderson, "State Departments Will be Asked to Consider Program, Staff Cutbacks," *Times-Picayune*, January 21, 2000, A-2; and Christi Daugherty, "Cutting to the Bone," *Gambit Weekly*, February 15, 2000, 12-13. Federal auditors eventually detected numerous irregularities in the distribution of share funds, and Congress promptly reworked this federal program. The lion's share of the hundreds of millions of federal dollars flowing into Louisiana during this period was shifted to non-healthcare areas in the annual state budget. These and related problems were the subject of many subsequent articles in the popular press well into 2005.

[19]*Annual Report Card, Louisiana Office of Public Health*, 1997;. and Steve Ritea "Poverty Report Focuses on Kids to Raise Awareness in Louisiana," *Times-Picayune*, December 8, 1999, A-3.

[20]ReliaStar Forecasting Financial Report (Milwaukee, WI, 1996). The report was based on seventeen criteria, including disease rate, access to health care, occupational safety and disability, crime rate, and motor vehicle deaths data from 1995. In *Health Care State Rankings for 1997* (Lawrence, 1997) Louisiana ranked forty-eighth, among the worst in the nation, for health based on a set of commonly used population health status indicators. The state ranked first in persons with diabetes per 100,000 residents, first in the percentage of births by cesarean section and first for all types of cancer. The state's performance related to prenatal care was also dismal. The state was number two in the percentage of low birth weight babies and in the neonatal death rate. It had the twelfth highest infant mortality rate in the United States and Louisiana's rates of cancer and the cervical cancer morbidity rates for African-American women well exceeded the national average, whereas the rate for Caucasian women was below the national average. By 1997, 21 percent of Louisiana residents were uninsured and dependent on the public healthcare system for their care. By 2004, this number had grown to 27 percent. In 1995 Louisiana ranked fourteenth in the United States in the number of emergency outpatient visits to hospitals, and the number of such visits has since increased. Doug Simpson, "Louisiana Slips Back to Bottom Health Ranking," *Times-Picayune*, November 9, 2004, A-2.

[21]"Sister reports" for three DHH agencies were completed in the 1990s. See *An Architecture of Empowerment for Persons with Developmental Disabilities: Research-based Design*, Volumes 1-4 (New Orleans, 1993) and *Architecture for Community Health: Research-based Design*, Volumes 1-4, (New Orleans, 1996). In these sister reports the methodology generally mirrored the OPH report, and received two national awards from the American Institute of Architects. See *Health Facilities Research Review* (Washington, 1997), 5-19.

[22]In 2000, DHH had jurisdictional licensing oversight over a network of thirty-four small rural hospitals and eighty-six rural health clinics statewide. In 1998, Louisiana, through DHH and the LSU Medical Center, received a grant for the Rural Health Access Project, with additional funding from the Robert Wood Johnson Foundation. For many Louisianans access to primary or preventive health care is severely limited. Some rural areas are seriously underserved. Many of the state's almost 21 percent uninsured residents frequently must travel long distances to state public hospitals for non-emergency care. Pockets of persistent poverty and geographic isolation contribute to rural residents' problems of access. The unequal distribution of the state's health care resources between urban and rural communities accounted for the overall poorer health outcome status of rural residents, including higher mortality and morbidity rates. This program provided focus for Louisiana to renew its commitment to improving the health status of individuals and communities in the 72 percent of the state categorized as rural by the U.S. Census Bureau. Louisiana's Rural Health Access Project: A Part of the RWJ Southern Rural Access Program, Grant Proposal, November 12, 1998, 1. In 2003 the Louisiana State Legislature gave total administrative control of the Charity Hospital system to LSU.

[23]Frequently, architects were hired who lacked any prior experience with healthcare facilities. The bigger problem was that the designer typically dismissed the parish health unit staff during programming and design, opting to communicate only with the police jurors—those who paid the architect's invoices. A new facility, in the worst cases of negligence, would replicate the same problems that had plagued the clinic it replaced.

[24]In 1990-91 the people of Louisiana, the nation, and world, were subjected to ex-Ku Klux Klan grand wizard David Duke's rapid rise to power, and his candidacy for governor. Edwin W. Edwards narrowly beat Duke in a bitter, racially divisive runoff election. After Huey P. Long, Edwards was the dominant figure of twentieth-century Louisiana politics. Beginning in 1972, Edwards was elected to governor for four terms, the most in the state's history. In the 1990 runoff election Duke received 55 percent of the white vote. The election received international media attention because of Duke's candidacy. Edwards was responsible for the adoption of the new state constitution in 1974, and remained popular with the public. He was bedeviled by one self-inflicted legal controversy after another, and resulting in several federal indictments. At present, he is an inmate in federal prison, serving a ten-year sentence for interstate racketeering. In one of his trials, in the mid-1980s, he was accused of having an illegal role in the sale of Certificate of Need licenses. In 1995 the daily newspaper in New Orleans ran a series on how large amounts of federal Medicaid funds had been siphoned to more than twenty state legislators' private business interests. Edwards was directly implicated in these transactions. Meanwhile, between 1990 and 1995, healthcare spending doubled, and doubled again, to $4 billion. Chris Adams, "Health Care Bonanza for Those with Clout," *Times-Picayune*, March 22, 1995, A-1, A-11). In a signature event in Louisiana's quirky political history, in 1959 a federal judge committed Gov. Earl Long to a state psychiatric hospital. But the director of state hospitals (now DHH) was promptly fired the next morning and his replacement immediately released Long from incarceration. Earl Long's most memorable quote, among many, was "When I die—if I die—I want to be buried in Louisiana so I can remain active in politics."

[25]John Wilds, Charles L. Dufour and Walter G. Cowan, *Louisiana, Yesterday and Today: A Historical Guide to the State* (Baton Rouge and London, 1996). As a child I read about Huey P. Long, the infamous governor (1928-31) and senator (1932-35). Long thirsted for the U.S. presidency and his assassination by Dr. Carl Austin Weiss in the hallway of the Louisiana State Capitol in Baton Rouge in 1935 capped a bombastic career. His disdain for rules and established constitutional order was legendary and his rule was absolute. He constructed a virtual dictatorship and was cunning—his accumulated power permitted his heirs to maintain political control long after his assassination. Long's vocal opposition to Franklin Roosevelt's New Deal and his own competing Share Our Wealth program garnered national publicity. Long's legacy continues to influence Louisiana politics, such as the Homestead Exemption, which waives taxes on the first $75,000 of an owner-occupied home's assessed value.

[26]Visiting parish officials are often branded outsiders.

[27]The compendium of guidelines was formatted for ease of interpretation by architects as well as laypersons.

[28]Robert Sommer, *Social Design: Creating Buildings with People in Mind* (Englewood Cliffs, N.J., 1983). Some replacement facilities built in the early 1980s were in need of retrofitting by 2005. Sometimes new assignments appear out of the blue, such as when a new state highway displaced the parish health unit in Mansfield, DeSoto Parish.

[29]Janet R. Carpman and Myron A. Grant, *Design That Cares: Planning Health Facilities for Patients and Visitors*, 2d ed. (Chicago, 1993).

[30]Ben Refuerzo and Stephen Verderber, *Redefining the Place of Architecture in Community Public*

Healthcare: Research-Based Design/Implementation, volumes 1-5 (New Orleans and Los Angeles, 1991). Empirical work included a regression analysis of regional differences of user satisfaction in relation to site and facility attributes, i.e. size, site, age of facility, condition, parking, neighborhood context, and interior attributes such as the size of rooms by type, HVAC systems conditions and types, amenities and circulation patterns directly bearing on wayfinding behavior within the facility, lighting, furnishings, windows, sizes, views, and the amount of natural daylight in the main interior spaces. It was found that significant regional differences existed by geographic region. Facilities in the northernmost region of the state were found to be in significantly poorer condition than those in the southern half with respect to facility age, condition, user satisfaction levels, and dysfunctional HVAC systems.

[31]Franklin D. Becker, *The Total Workplace: Facilities Management in the Elastic Organization* (New York, 1990).

[32]Franklin D. Becker and Fred Steele, *Workplace by Design: Mapping the High Performance Workplace* (San Francisco, 1995).

[33]Jon Lang, *Creating Architectural Theory: The Role of the Behavioral Sciences in Environmental Design* (New York, 1987).

[34]Robert Grimshaw, "Space, Place and People: Facilities Management and Critical Theory," in Keith Alexander, Brian Atkin, Jan Brochner and Tore Haugen, eds., *Facilities Management: Innovation and Performance* (London, 2004), 15-32.

[35]T.M. Amabile, "Motivational Synergy: Toward New Conceptualizations of Intrinsic and Extrinsic Motivation in the Workplace," *Human Resource Management Review* 3 (1993): 185-201.

[36]Francis Duffy, "Design and Facilities Management in a Time of Change," *Facilities* 18 (1994), 371-75.

[37]Grimshaw, "Space, Place and People," 17.

[38]Bill Hillier, *Space Is the Machine: A Configurational Theory of Architecture* (Cambridge, 1996).

[39]Grimshaw, "Space, Place and People," 18.

[40]E. Casey, *The Fate of a Place: A Philosophical History* (Berkeley, 1997).

[41]H. Lefebvre, *The Production of Space* (Oxford, 1991).

[42]Z. Bauman, *Liquid Modernity* (Cambridge, 2000).

[43]Robert Grimshaw and D. Garnett, "Workplace Democracy," in P. McLennan and B. Nutt, eds., *Facility Management: Risks and Opportunities* (Oxford, 2000), 107-16.

[44]Grimshaw, "Space, Place and People," 22-28.

[45]Ben Refuerzo and Stephen Verderber, "Architecture for Community Public Healthcare," Thirty-ninth Annual *Progressive Architecture* (P/A) Awards Program, *Progressive Architecture*, January 1992, 94-95. Also Ben Refuerzo, Stephen Verderber, with Joan Burkhart, "Redefining the Place of Architecture in Community Public Healthcare," Paper 1 (Vol. 1-4) and Paper 2 (Vol. 5), *Proceedings of the 119th Annual Meeting of the American Public Health Association* (Atlanta, 1991); and Stephen Verderber, "Designing a Better Box," *Tulanian* 63 (1992): 24-29.

[46]Grassroots support for the SFI at the local community level has been a key factor in its longevity, fiscal sustainability, and efficacy.

[47]New Orleans is captivating, idiosyncratic, and unpredictable, offering a rich palette of Creole architecture, food, jazz and funk music, dancing, and cultural events such as Mardi Gras, the New Orleans Jazz and Heritage Festival, and neighborhood ethnic festivals. It is this enduring dialectic which intrigues tourists and locals alike.

[48]Sutton, "Power, Knowledge, and the Art of Leadership," 68.

[49]Stringer, "The Myths of Architectural Creativity," 635.

Notes to Chapter 2

[1]Federal grants through the Hill-Burton program were provided for construction of thirty-two health unit facilities in Louisiana. These parishes built new facilities in 1950, 1951, and 1952 as a result: East Baton Rouge, Winn, Natchitoches, Webster, Lafourche, Madison, St. Landry, Avoyelles, Terrebonne, Jefferson Davis, Tangipahoa, St. Tammany, Calcasieu, Evangeline, Rapides, Caldwell, LaSalle, Richland, Franklin, Grant, Union, Claiborne, East Carroll, St. Charles, St. Martin, Bienville, Bossier, Ascension, Iberville, Caddo, Morehouse, and Orleans. During the 1950 legislative session, the legislature passed an act that gave local police juries the authority to hold elections on imposing a millage tax of up to five mills to fund the construction and operation of new parish health units. The first parishes to do so were Calcasieu (1.5 mills), Jefferson (3 mills), Richland (1 mill), and Winn (1 mill). Barbara Cole, *Parish Health Units in Louisiana* (Baton Rouge, 2000), 12. Three facilities opened immediately after the end of World War II: one in Livingston Parish (1946), a second in East Feliciana Parish (1949) and one in West Feliciana Parish (1949). Records indicate that thirty-two Hill-Burton parish health units were built in Louisiana between 1950 and 1952 alone. However, for the entire decade of the 1950s this figure may have been as high as forty, although records of partial funding (less than a 50 percent match) are difficult to ascertain based on existing records, in some cases. The health unit in Vermilion Parish (Abbeville, 1952) was built entirely with funding from the Rockefeller Foundation.

[2]Ibid., 13. The last of the sixty-four parishes to open a health unit was Plaquemines Parish. Their facility opened in 1960 and in 1964 the parish broke away from the state system. This was due to its refusal to comply with Title VI of the 1964 Civil Rights Act, which prohibited discrimination on the basis of race or gender. This parish, a stronghold of racial segregation, defiantly set up its own health department, and this entity remains autonomous from the rest of the state to this day.

[3]Michel Foucault, *Madness and Civilization: A History of Insanity in the Age of Reason* (New York, 1965); Michael Foucault, *Discipline and Punish: The Birth of the Prison* (New York, 1979). Also see his *The Birth of the Clinic: An Archaeology of Medical Perception* (New York, 1975).

[4]John D. Thompson and Grace Goldin, *The Hospital: A Social and Architectural History* (New Haven, 1975).

[5]Heidi Johnson, *Angels in the Architecture: A Photographic Elegy to an American Asylum* (Detroit, 2001). These utopian designs for insane asylums sought to integrate nature and beauty as therapeutic treatment modalities. Nearly two hundred state mental hospitals were built in the United States between 1858 and 1885 based on the "Kirkbride System." Many of these campuses, so sturdily constructed and of such historic value now that the cost of tearing them down is often simply too great, live on as haunting reminders of a forgotten era in American psychiatry. Also see Carla Yanni, "The Linear Plan for Insane Asylums in the United States before 1866," *Journal of the Society of Architectural Historians* 62 (2003): 24-49. The Louisiana State Hospital in Jackson was built in 1843 and remains in use today. It is a classic example of the asylums in this period.

[6]Thompson and Goldin, *The Hospital*, 151.

[7]Ibid., 201.

[8]Grace Goldin, *Work of Mercy: A Picture History of Hospitals* (Ontario, 1994). Prior to the twentieth century, outpatient care was always dispensed in the hospital "Accident Room," later the "Emergency Room," and recently the Emergency Department.

[9]Stephen Verderber, "Exploring Person-Environment Transactions in Architecture through the Medium of Film," in Arthur E. Stamps III, ed., *Building Bridges Connecting People, Research and Design*, Proceedings of the 31st Annual Conference of the Environmental Design Research Association (San Francisco, 2000), 87-91. Films in this genre include *All's Quiet on the Western Front* (1924), *Gone With the Wind* (1939), *The Lost Weekend* (1945), *The Road to Wellsville* (1994), *A Clockwork Orange* (1971), *One Flew Over the Cuckoo's Nest* (1977), *Coming Home* (1980), *The Elephant Man* (1980), and *A/I* (2000). Also see Robert A. Clark, "Reel Oncology: How Hollywood Films Portray Cancer," available online, http://www.moffitt.usf.edu/pubs/ccj/v6n5/dept7.htm, accessed March 30, 2005.

[10]Martin S. Valins, *Primary Health Care Centres* (Essex, England, 1993). Primary healthcare care in the United Kingdom includes medical consultation, treatment and diagnostics, minor surgery, and health education. Some clinics include day care for physiotherapy and occupational therapy, outpatient emergency care, and inpatient short-stay beds for maternity and minor surgery patients. Staff consists of general medical practitioners, health visitors, nurse practitioners, district nurses, physicians, administrative and staff managers. Some clinics include midwives, chiropodists, therapists, dentists, physiotherapists, opticians, and radiologists. A primary care clinic serves a patient population of 10,000 to 30,000.

[11]Ibid., 7-8. A report issued by the Medical Planning Commission in 1942 was seen as further endorsement of the 1920 report and became an internationally acknowledged blueprint for the concept of community-based public healthcare. This document was built into the National Health Service Act of 1946 in England, which soon established a compulsory national health insurance plan for every citizen in the country. From that point on, according to Section 21 of the National Health Service Act, "It shall be the duty of every local authority to provide, equip and maintain to the satisfaction of the health minister premises which shall be called 'Health Centres.'"

[12]Stephen Verderber and David Fine, *Healthcare Architecture in an Era of Radical Transformation* (New Haven and London, 2000). Chapter Eight, "The Community Care Clinic," is an overview of the community-based health center as a building type in the period from 1965-2000. Chapters 5 and 9 define and discuss the phenomenon of functional deconstruction.

[13]Goldin, *Work of Mercy*, 264.

[14]Ben J. Refuerzo and Stephen Verderber, "Assessing Designers' Perceptions in the Provision of Shelter for the Homeless," in Ernesto G. Arias and Mark D. Gross, eds., *Equitable and Sustainable Habitat*, Proceedings of the 23rd Annual Conference of the Environmental Design Research Association (Oklahoma City, 1992), 200-10. Soon thereafter, in the wake of national media attention, including a piece on *60 Minutes*, its sponsors' underlying elitism was exposed. The homeless animals had been built a gleaming palace compared to the crude, unhealthy soup kitchen shelters only a few blocks away.

[15]Barbara Ehrenreich, *Fear of Falling: The Inner Life of the Middle Class* (New York, 1990).

[16]Ibid., 229-30.

[17]Ehrenreich cited the work of Deborah Silverman in *Fear of Falling*, 230.

[18]Editorial, "No Cure, Yet, for Health Care Blues," *Chicago Tribune*, December 19, 1999, C-14.

[19]Interview with the author, Luling, LA, December 9, 2000.

[20]"The Digital Divide," broadcast on National Public Radio, December 10, 1999. Few uninsured patients in 1999 had access to web-based healthcare. There is increasing concern among providers, public policy specialists, providers, and e-commerce entrepreneurs that this gap will persist and could become insurmountable.

[21]Web-MD, available online, http://www.web.MD.com.html, accessed December 12, 2004. This site is among a rapidly growing number of online medical sites related to personal wellness and health. The degree of interactivity will be largely determined by the ability to conduct synchronous consultative sessions between providers and care recipients in real time, anytime of the day or night, such as PlanetRX.com and Drugstore.com; Medem, in particular, signaled the decision on the part of the medical establishment to adopt a more aggressive stance with respect to the explosion in virtual healthcare. Medem was created in 1999 by the American Medical Association, and provides peer-reviewed medical information to the general public and broadens its global reach by establishing new forms of ties with the World Medical Association and the World Health Organization. Within community public health alone the possibilities are vast: teleconferencing with one's physician, scheduling appointments, consultation sessions, online medical encyclopedias, chat rooms on topics such as WIC, immunizations, post clinic follow-up treatment, family planning, discussions on sexually transmitted diseases, water quality inspection schedules, food quality, and early warning with respect to emergency preparedness.

[22]Erica Goode, "Social Status Might Affect Your Health, Scientists Find," *New York Times*, May 27, 1999, C-4. Goode added "What first compelled researchers' interest was the now-classic study, begun in the late 1960s, of men in the British civil service. *The Whitehall Study*, conducted by Dr. Michael Marmot, director of the International Center for Health and

Society at University College London, tracked mortality rates over 10 years for 17,530 male civil service employees. When the data were analyzed, the researchers were astonished to discover that mortality rates varied continuously and precisely with the men's civil services grade: the higher the classification, the lower the rates of death, regardless of cause. This finding was as perplexing as it was intriguing. The men all had jobs and equal access to health care under Britain's national health system. But mortality rates for men in the lowest civil service classification, the researchers found, were three times higher than those for men in the highest grade."

[23]Anonymous, "Many Ex-welfare Moms Lack Health Insurance" *Times-Picayune*, January 9, 2000, A-12. The problem stemmed largely from new eligibility rules enacted in 1999 for Medicaid benefits, and many caseworkers, public healthcare providers, and others remained unclear on the implications and logistics of the new rules.

[24]Megan O'Matz, "Residents Pushing to Save Clinic That Cares," *Chicago Tribune*, August 15, 1999, 4:1-2.

[25]Stephen A. Holmes, "Builders Ignore Law on Disabled Access," *Times-Picayune*, March 22, 1999, A-6. In suburban Chicago, for example, advocates for the disabled had found that out of fifty newly built multifamily developments, forty-nine had not followed federal law. In Baltimore, a similar survey found that 75 percent of fifty-nine new apartment and condominium complexes were not in compliance. Arizona advocates found that 75 percent of the new multifamily buildings in Tucson and 50 percent in Phoenix had not followed the law. The Justice Department and disability rights advocates in many cities and states have begun suing architects and developers to force them to conform to the law.

[26]Stephen Kaplan and Rachael Kaplan, *Cognition and Environment: Functioning in an Uncertain World* (New York, 1982). Functionalist-evolutionary theory is useful for architects to understand why the medically uninsured feel disempowered by a healthcare system and care setting which magnify uncertainty and alienation.

[27]Kirsten Day, "The Ethics of Care and Women's Experiences of Public Space," *Journal of Environmental Psychology* 20 (2000): 103-24.

Notes to Chapter 3

[1]Interview with the author, December 2, 1999. Disinterested in retirement, as of 2005, she had become the senior clerical staff person in the entire state OPH network of parish health units.

[2]Interview with the author, September 20, 2000.

[3]Interview with the author, August 25, 2000.

[4]The DHH-OPH Region V Environmental Health Program staff moved into their new Lake Charles quarters in September 2003 (see Chapter 5).

Notes to Chapter 4

[1]James Gleick, *Faster: The Acceleration of Just About Everything* (New York, 1999).

[2]James Bolner, ed., *Louisiana Politics: Festival in a Labyrinth* (Baton Rouge and London, 1982).

[3]See June Savoy Rowell, "Parish Government," in ibid., 143. In some parishes, the elected officials function, for the most part, as a closely-knit family. In other parishes, by contrast, "factional disputes and lack of cooperation are commonplace. Confronted with this pattern, the state acts as the benevolent parent, giving special benefits to favored children but refusing to mediate sibling rivalries," 145; and Roderick L. Carleton, *Local Government and Administration in Louisiana* (Baton Rouge, 1935), 1-31.

[4] Louisiana State Constitution as amended through the election of October 27, 1979, Section 8, Article XII, 95.

[5]Ibid., 43.

[6]Mary Jones, "The Shintech Controversy," *Gambit*, November 16, 2000, 26.

[7]Rowell, "Parish Government," 148. Data based on article by June Savoy, "New Police Juries Show Significant Changes," *Louisiana Parish Government* 12 (August 1976): 12-13.

[8]This pattern is most evident in the urban and suburban parishes.

[9]Rowell, "Parish Government," 150, 173.

[10]Interview with the author, December 17, 2000.

[11]This process begins with a form called an RL-2. On it, the space needs of the health unit are listed in relation to the building's occupants' job title classifications. This is very close to what is generally referred to in architecture as a functional space program. The RL-2 includes parking needs and special requirements. This form is submitted to the Legislative Capital Outlay Committee. The pool for a typical fiscal year might consist of requests for state funds for expansion of a major convention center (New Orleans), sports facilities and arenas, roads, bridges, regional parks, parish parks, or levee and related drainage improvements. Other projects could include schools and university facilities, facilities for annual use for parish-based festivals, historic preservation of noted buildings and places, or parish-based tourism attractions. The process for awarding funds is highly competitive, and any political advantage to be gained is gained. One parish recently sent every member of the legislature a fresh box of its local strawberries just before the final vote on the distribution of capital outlay funds for the next fiscal year. The parish received more than half of the $1.1 million needed for the total replacement of its obsolete facility.

[12]"A survey of Louisiana legislators serving in the period 1952-1974 showed that 48 percent had had previous experience in public service. Of those who held prior office, more had served at the parish level than at any other. This is especially noteworthy since there were more city-level elected positions available. The largest group of legislators who had been local officials were former police jurors." See Rowell, "Parish Government," 176. See also June Savoy, "Louisiana Lawmakers: A 25-year Profile," *Analysis* 3 (January 1975): 17-18.

[13]During this period the majority of health units built with capital outlay funds were in Office of Public Health's Region VII, centered in the Shreveport-Bossier City area. Elsewhere in the state, the picture was far different. In the period of 1988-98 only five health units were built, replacing obsolete facilities, entirely with capital outlay funds. These were in Vernon Parish (Leesville), Jefferson Davis Parish (Jennings), Allen Parish (Oberlin and Oakdale), Avoyelles (Marksville), with three facilities in the planning, design, or construction phase of development in 2000 for Iberville Parish (Plaquemine), Tensas Parish (St. Joseph), and Ouachita Parish (Monroe).

[14]Mary Swerczek, "Tax Urged to Build New Health Unit," *Times-Picayune*, December 23, 1999, B-1-2. The St. Charles Parish's health unit, despite limited resources, does a good job of serving the citizens, a parish council committee said. But the public health unit in Luling was too small and too old to adequately serve the parish's growing population, members of the council's Public Safety, Health and Environmental Committee rebutted. To solve the problem, the committee has recommended raising property taxes to pay for a new building. "In order to meet the parish needs for the new millennium, we need to update facilities," said Gail Hollins, the nursing supervisor. The health unit had been located in a rented 2,000 square-foot building at the corner of Post and Ellington streets in Luling. The new building should be at least twice that size, Hollins said. The safety committee recommended a tax increase for ten years to pay for a new facility. The $.75-mill tax would cost the owner of a house valued at $100,000 a mere $1.88 annually. The owner of a $150,000 house would pay $5.63. Health unit officials chose between two possible sites. One was a 5.3-acre tract offered at $800,000 and the other was four acres available for $327,000. A new building would cost $1.5 million. About $80,000 a year had been budgeted to maintain the health unit, said the parish's bond attorney. The millage would raise $442,500 per year. "It would relieve the general fund," Councilman Terry Authement said, adding that the millage could be renewed for a lesser amount in ten years to cover maintenance and operation of the health unit. The millage would pay for the purchasing of land, constructing the building, and maintaining it. "The state would continue to pay for staffing and programming. For the millage to be raised the parish council would have to vote to put the issue on the ballot and citizens would have to approve it." Hollins said they would be amenable to locating the health unit on the east bank (of the Mississippi River, because the parish is split by the river) but had "Not found a site. . . . At least one committee member was confident that residents would approve the millage: 'The public knows it's been long overdue.' . . . The council was going to vote on the millage at its meeting Monday but didn't because they didn't have a two-thirds majority."

[15]Rowell, "Parish Government," 176-78. Rural populism is being subjected to encroachment by the forces of urbanization. It no longer suffices to allow singular control of parish government by a "good 'ole boy network." Old, accepted ways of doing business within a parish are hard to let go. Cultural, social, and business ties are strong. Moreover, some influential

persons may be downright apathetic, persons for whom the health unit holds little meaning and instances of long-simmering racially motivated feuds persist.

[16]Ibid., 179. Also see Stephen K. Bailey, "Creative Leadership in Local Government," in Robert L. Moran, ed., *Capitol, Courthouse, and City Hall* (Boston, 1977), 340.

Notes to Chapter 5

[1]These visits occurred between October 1990 and March 1991.

[2]This typology was comprised of ten plan types: Axial Box; T plan, Courtyard/Partial Courtyard; Atrium; H plan; L plan; Linear Box; Cross plan; Adapted (derived) Box; and Designed Box. Second, a typology became discernable, generally based on urban, suburban, or rural contexts.

[3]Kenneth Frampton, "Prospects for a Critical Regionalism," *Perspecta: The Yale Architectural Journal* 20 (1983), 147-62; Kenneth Frampton, "Towards a Critical Regionalism: Six Points for an Architecture of Resistance," in Hal Foster, ed., *The Anti-Aesthetic: Essays on Postmodern Culture* (Port Townsend, CA, 1983); Kate Nesbitt, ed., *Theorizing a New Agenda for Architecture: An Anthology of Architectural Theory, 1965-1995* (New York, 1996), Chapter 11, 468-492.

[4]Carl D. Lane, *American Paddle Steamboats* (New York, 1943), 190; Adam I. Kane, *The Western River Steamboat* (College Station, 2004), 50-52; and Charles Preston Fishbaugh, *From Paddle Wheels to Propellers* (Indianapolis, 1970).

[5]Linda Treash, "Marksville Historical Site," *Times-Picayune*, June 16, 2000, Lagniappe Section, p. 4. Also see the Louisiana Department of Culture and Tourism pamphlet "Marksville Prehistoric Indian Park State Monument." This pamphlet is a useful background resource and is given to visitors to the site. Alan Toth, *Archaeology and Ceramics at the Marksville Site*, Anthropological Papers 56 (Ann Arbor, 1974).

[6]Charles Robert Goins and John Michael Caldwell, *Historical Atlas of Louisiana* (Norman and London, 1995), especially chapter three, for a description of Native American cultures in the region.

[7]Peter Nabokov and Robert Easton, *Native American Architecture* (New York, 1989), 56-58.

[8]Ibid., 306-8.

[9]Ibid., 68-71.

[10]Richard Sexton, *Vestiges of Grandeur* (San Francisco, 1999).

[11]Greg Lynn, *Animate Form* (New York, 1999).

[12]Ibid., 20.

[13]Jay Farbstein, "The Impact of the Client Organization on the Programming Process," in W.F.E. Preiser, ed., *Professional Practice in Facility Programming* (New York, 1993).

[14]The Commonwealth Fund, "Low Incomes Often Mean Poor Health and Poor Health Care," *The Commonwealth Fund Quarterly* 3 (Summer 1997): 1-2.

[15]American Anthropological Association, "Social and Cultural Aspects of Health," *Public Policy Briefing Sheet*, available online, http://www.ameranthassn.org/pphealth.htm, accessed February 14, 2002.

[16]D. Kirk Hamilton, "The Four Levels of Evidence-based Practice," *Healthcare Design* 3 (2003): 18-27.

[17]Robert M. Goodman, et al., "The Formation of a Complex Community Program for Diabetes Control: Lessons Learned from a Case Study of Project DIRECT," *Journal of Public Health Management and Practice* 7 (2001): 19-29.

[18]S.F. Verderber and B.J. Refuerzo, "Research-based Architecture and the Community Healthcare Consumer: A Statewide Initiative," *Journal of Architectural and Planning Research* 20 (2003): 57-67.

[19]R.M. Goodman, et al., "The Formation of a Complex Community Program."

[20]Michael Patton, *Utilization-Focused Evaluation*, 2d ed. (Beverly Hills, CA, 1986).

Notes to Chapter 6

[1]Fat, "Contaminating Contemplation," in Jonathan Hill, ed., *Occupying Architecture: Between the Architect and the User* (London and New York, 1998), 78-79. "Fat" is the name of an architectural co-op firm based in London. This "firm" is comprised of individuals who form teams on a project-by-project basis.

[2]Ibid., 80.

[3]Ibid., 81-82.

[4]Russell Ellis and Dana Cuff, eds., *Architects' People* (New York, 1989).

[5]Jon Lang, *Creating Architectural Theory: The Role of the Behavioral Sciences in Environmental Design* (New York, 1987).

[6]Le Corbusier, *Vers une architecture*, F. Etchells, trans. (New York, 1970). Corbusier wrote: "All men have the same organism, the same functions. All men have the same needs. The social contract which has evolved through the ages fixes standardized classes, functions and needs producing standardized products . . . I propose one single building for all nations and all climates."

[7]Lang, *Creating Architectural Theory*, 8.

[8]Claude Schnaidt, *Hannes Meyer: Buildings, Projects and Writings*, D.Q. Stephenson, trans. (Teufen, 1965).

[9]Owen B. Hardy and Lawrence P. Lammers, *Hospitals: The Planning and Design Process*, 2d ed. (Rockville, MD, 1986), 24-25.

[10]Christopher Alexander, et al., *A Pattern Language: Towns, Buildings, Construction* (New York, 1977). Alexander attacked healthcare architecture—and the hospital in particular as a building type—as having become disconnected from the patient. Alternatively, he called for numerous small-scale community-based neighborhood clinics in the place of highly concentrated urban megahospitals.

[11]Each pattern was a few pages in length, and the tone throughout was reformist.

[12]The individual was placed at the center of the pattern language, and this aspect of their work won praise from environmental psychologists, the staffs of grassroots community storefront design assistance centers, reform-minded urban planners, and landscape architects for its humanist perspective.

[13]Christopher Alexander, *The Timeless Way of Building* (New York, 1978).

[14]In 1983 the National Endowment of the Arts sponsored a national award program and publication titled *Exemplary Design Research 1983*.

[15]The American Institute of Architects' Academy of Architecture for Health is a 3,000-plus-member professional interest component of the AIA. This group, and the aforementioned Center for Health Design, are making inroads.

[16]Stephen Verderber and David J. Fine, *Healthcare Architecture in an Era of Radical Transformation* (New Haven and London, 2000), Chapters 5 and 9.

[17]Healthcare administrators have until recently remained, by and large, uncommitted to promoting the therapeutic value of architecture and interior design within their organizations.

[18]Stephen Verderber and Joseph Kimbrell, "The Role of the Architectural Environment in Community Health: An Evidence-Based Initiative," *Journal of Public Health Management and Practice* 11 (2005): 87.

[19]John R. Griffith, "A Step in the Right Direction: Revolutionizing Educational Outcomes," paper presentation, Association of University Programs in Health Administration/American College of Healthcare Executives Leadership Conference, Chicago, March 2000.

[20]Verderber and Fine, *Healthcare and Architecture in an Era of Radical Transformation*, Chapter 9.

[21]Verderber and Kimbrell, "The Role of the Architectural Environment," 88.

[22]Joan Harvey and Jacquelyn Vischer, "Environmental Design Research in Canada: Innovative Government Intervention," in Donna Duerk and Donald Campbell, eds., *The Challenge of Diversity: EDRA 15 Proceedings* (Washington, D.C., 1984), 278.

[23]Robert Sommer, *Social Design: Creating Buildings with People in Mind* (Englewood Cliffs, N.J., 1983).

[24]Sydney Arnstein, "A Ladder of Citizen Participation," *Journal of the American Institute of Planners* 35 (1969): 216-24.

[25]Donald Appleyard, "Elitists' versus the Public's Cry for Help," *Landscape Architecture* 61 (1970): 25-27.

[26]Peter Clavel, "The Evolution of Advocacy Planning," *APA Journal* 60 (1994): 146-49.

[27]Excessive scientific jargon and obfuscated prose have been frequent criticisms by architects of the work of social scientists and specialists in environmental psychology.

[28]M. Powell Lawton, "Therapeutic Environments for the Aged," in David Canter and Sandra Canter, eds., *Designing for Therapeutic Environments: A Review of the Literature* (London, 1979), 233-76.

[29]This replacement facility was built in Amite, Tangipahoa Parish.

[30]Warren G. Olsen, Thomas C. Wilson and Paul Flehmer, "Creating a Patient Friendly Environment," in *Developing Ambulatory Healthcare Facilities for Medical Groups, Hospitals, and Integrated Delivery Systems* (Madison, WI, 1996), 229-44.

[31]Sommer, *Social Design*, 16.

[32]Ibid.

[33]Charles Jencks, *Le Corbusier and the Tragic View of Architecture* (Cambridge, MA, 1973).

[34]Pedagogical approaches to the teaching and practice of architecture are needed where all steps in design, construction, and occupancy, from early stages of a project's conceptualization, to building completion and occupancy, are accorded equal weight.

[35]Fat, "Contaminating Contemplation," 83-86.

[36]Editorial, "Clean Up Mess at Health Unit," *Baton Rouge Sunday Advocate,* November 9, 2003, 12-B.

[37]Charles McConnell, *The Effective Health Care Supervisor* (Rockville, MD, 1993).

[38]U.S. Green Buildings Council, *Building Momentum: National Trends for High Performance Green Buildings*, available online, http://www.usgbc.org, accessed August 12, 2004.

[39]Barry Wasserman, et al., *Ethics and the Practice of Architecture* (New York, 2000).

[40]James McLarney and L.F. Chaff, eds., *Effective Health Care Facilities Management* (Chicago, IL, 1991).

[41]Franklin E. Becker, "Evaluation," in M. Beck and T. Meyer, eds., *Health Care Environments: The User's Viewpoint* (Boca Raton, FL, 1983). The SFI was modeled on Healthy Communities national program initiatives. With regard to the halo effect it is impossible to divorce the old from the new in one's consciousness, although after a period of a year following relocation, occupants are able to, by and large, be more objective.

[42]Robert K. Fullinwider, "Civil Society and Democratic Citizenship," *Report from the Institute for Philosophy and Public Policy* 18 (1998): 2-4.

[43]Jonathan Hill, *Occupying Architecture: Between the Architect and the User* (London, 1998).

[44]B. Kellerman, *Reinventing Leadership: Making the Connection Between Politics and Business* (Albany, NY, 1995).

[45]James L. Hargraves, et al., "Using Patient Reports to Measure Health Care System Performance," *Clinical Performance Quality Health Care* 1 (1993): 208-13.

[46]Kristin Day, "The Ethics of Care and Women's Experiences in Public Spaces," *Journal of Environmental Psychology* 20 (2000): 103-24.

[47]M.B. Heldring, "Collaborative Family Healthcare: Community and Compassion," *Families, Systems, and Health* 15 (1997): 333-36.

Notes to Chapter 7

[1]Delle Chatman, "Being Catholic in a Season of Trial and Love," *Chicago Tribune*, December 25, 2002, Section 1, p. 31.

[2]David Lordkipanidze, et al., "Anthropology: The Earliest Toothless Hominid Skull," *Nature* 434 (April 7, 2005), 717-18.

[3]Sir Norman Foster and Partners, *Architecture As Building* (London, 1993).

[4]Kurt W. Forster, *Frank O. Gehry: The Complete Works* (New York, 1998).

[5]Stephen Verderber. "Compassionism and the Design Studio in the Aftermath of 9/11," *Journal of Architectural Education* 56 (February 2003): 60-74.

[6]*Webster's New International Dictionary*, 2d ed. (Springfield, MA, 1946). Also see *The American Heritage Dictionary of the English Language*, 4th ed. (Boston, 2000).

[7]Ibid., 544.

[8]Lynn Brenner, "How Did You Do?" *Parade Magazine* (March 2, 2003): 4-5. Eight of the twelve biggest bankruptcies in U.S. history were filed within a thirteen-month period.

[9]Dolores Hayden, *The Power of Place: Urban Landscapes as Public History* (Cambridge, 1995).

[10]James T. Rojas, "The Enacted Environment of East Los Angeles," *Places* 8 (Spring 1993): 42-53.

[11]Bruce Allsopp, *Towards a Humane Architecture* (London, 1974).

[12]Stephen Verderber and Ben Refuerzo, "On the Construction of Research-Based Design: A Community Health Center," *Journal of Architectural and Planning Research* 16 (Autumn 1999): 225-41.

[13]Herbert J. Gans, "Towards a Human Architecture: A Sociologist's View of the Profession," *Journal of Architectural Education* 31 (1978): 26.

[14]Jay S. Garrott, "Interpreting Value System Milieus," in *The Role of the Architect in Society*, Peter G. Burgess, ed. (Pittsburgh, 1983), 21-29.

[15]Gans, "Towards a Human Architecture," 26.

[16]Robert G. Herschberger, "A Study of Meaning in Architecture," in Henry Sanoff and S. Cohen, eds., *Proceedings of the First Annual Environmental Design Research Association Conference* (Chapel Hill, 1968), 90-94. Also, Stephen Verderber and G.T. Moore, "Building Imagery: A Comparative Study of Environmental Cognition," *Man-Environment Systems* 7 (1977): 332-41. The everyday ordinary landscape was being seriously considered by "high" postmodern architects such as Robert Venturi and Charles Moore.

[17]Milton Rokeach, *The Nature of Human Values* (New York, 1979), 23-24.

[18]Ibid., 25.

[19]Garrott, "Interpreting Value System Milieus," 24.

[20]Peter Burgess, Elliott Littman, and James Mayo, "Political Knowledge and the Architectural Studio," *Journal of Architectural Education* 34 (1981): 24-28.

[21]Garrott, "Interpreting Value System Milieus," 25-26.

[22]Stephen A. Kurtz, *Wasteland: Building the American Dream* (New York, 1973). He writes "Renaissance architects attempted to incorporate in their buildings the esoteric concerns of the princes and bishops who employed them . . . by linking his efforts to those of philosophers and theologians and by connecting his art to the exactitude and spirituality of music and mathematics, the architect hoped to place himself within their charmed and elevated circles. . . . They succeeded so well that aristocrats became passionate (though non-professional) architects by the eighteenth century and professional ones by the end of the nineteenth. As the power of the professional grew . . . vernacular structures (homes built by the home-owner, public buildings constructed by local builders) declined. . . . How can we give architecture back to the people without taking it away from the architects?," 44.

[23]Joel Brinkley, "Deregulation Leaves Lobby with Free Time," *Times-Picayune*, October 23, 1999, C-3.

[24]However, there were notable exceptions.

[25]Research conducted by the author in 2000. Of these, 1,530 (74.7 percent) were buildings already built. The submissions were categorized into twelve building types: acute care hospitals, medical office buildings, outpatient hospital-based oncology centers, long-term care facilities, pediatric facilities, women's hospitals and health centers, rehabilitation hospitals and centers, outpatient community care clinics, outpatient surgery centers, psychiatric hospitals and clinics, and hospice. "Miscellaneous" facilities included outdoor gardens, dialysis centers, blood donor centers, fitness-wellness centers, and campus master plan reports. The main finding, not surprisingly, was a dramatic rise in the number of outpatient care buildings submitted to the awards program over this ten-year period. By the same measure, the number of hospital submissions fell precipitously across this period. As for the small number of outpatient clinic submittals, possible explanations for this include the low construction budgets for such projects, thereby allowing little room for "Design." Also, these clients tend to

not hire signature, high-end design firms for such commissions, instead often awarding the work to a local firm. In the 1990s the for-profit corporate sector of the healthcare industry clearly was where the action was from the standpoint of profits for architects.

[26]Robert K. Fullinwider, "Civil Society and Democratic Citizenship," *Report from the Institute for Philosophy and Public Policy* 18 (1998): 2.

[27]Benjamin R. Barber, "The Search for Civil Society: Can We Restore the Middle Ground Between Government and Markets?" *The New Democrat* 7 (1995): 21-33.

[28]Robert D. Putnam, *Bowling Alone: The Collapse and Revival of American Community* (New York, 2000).

[29]National Commission on Civic Renewal, *A Nation of Spectators: How Civic Disengagement Weakens America and What We Can Do About It* (College Park, MD, 1999), 5-6.

[30]Alan Wolfe, *One Nation, After All* (New York, 1998). Also see Peter L. Berger and Richard J. Neuhaus, *To Empower People: From State to Civil Society*, twentieth anniversary edition, Michael Novak, ed. (Washington, D.C., 1996); and Marvin Olasky, *The Tragedy of American Compassion* (Lanham, MD, 1992).

[31]National Commission on Civic Renewal, *A Nation of Spectators*, 6.

[32]David Osborne and Ted Gaebler, *Reinventing Government: How the Entrepreneurial Spirit is Transforming the Public Sector* (Reading, MA, 1992), 324.

[33]Mark Schneider, Paul Teske, with Michael Mintrom, *Public Entrepreneurs: Agents for Change in American Government* (Princeton, 1995), 1.

[34]Barbara Kellerman, *Reinventing Leadership: Making the Connection Between Politics and Business* (Albany, 1999), 10.

[35]Ibid., 215-31.

[36]Steve Ritea, "Edwards Will Appeal His 10-Year Sentence," *Times-Picayune*, Tuesday, January 9, 2001, A-1.

[37]Chris Adams, "Health Care Bonanza for those with Clout," *Times-Picayune*, March 22, 1995, A-1, A-11.

[38]Richard Wolf, "States Bracing for Leaner Times," *USA Today*, July 10, 2000, 1-A. See Richard Wolf, "Mississippi Uses Prosperity to Fix Itself Up," *USA Today* (July 10, 2000): 2-A.

[39]Laurie Garrett, *Betrayal of Trust: The Collapse of Global Public Health* (New York, 2001).

[40]James M. Mayo, "Critical Reasoning for an Enlightened Architectural Practice," *Journal of Architectural Education* 3 (Summer 1988): 46-57.

[41]Susan Popkin, "No Simple Solutions for Housing the Poor," *Chicago Tribune*, May 30, 1999, 1:22. These policies were rooted in the massive federal urban renewal programs conceived from visionary plans of the early 1920s, influenced by architects such as Le Corbusier. Despite compassionate aims, the projects were executed without genuine regard for the human condition, and therefore ultimately failed. These high-rise warehouses profoundly and

adversely affected the daily lives of their inhabitants. As is well known, fervent cries for abandonment and demolition arose among urban planners, politicians, and neighborhood activists alike. By 2010 all Chicago Housing Authority (CHA) high-rise developments will be demolished and the land redeveloped. This will displace more than 11,000 of the city's poorest families. CHA plans for these families to receive HUD Section 8 vouchers to transition into better housing.

[42]John R. Belcher and Frederick A. DiBlasio, *Helping the Homeless: Where Do We Go From Here?* (New York, 1990).

[43]Ibid., 90. Many liberal scholars, while lamenting the fact that many of the poor are inadequately housed, ignore structural aspects of the economy, such as tax favoritism for the middle and upper classes. Ironically, affluent individuals and families receive the major share of housing subsidies.

[44]Ibid., 100. Efforts to resolve the housing crisis require hard choices that challenge entrenched values. Home ownership is one such value. On the one hand, polices to increase the minimum wage are designed to allow more persons to enter the economic mainstream. On the other hand, such polices have not resulted in significantly more Americans being able to own their own home.

[45]Ibid., 16. To date, the *McKinney Homeless Assistance Act* (H.R. 286, 1987) remains the only major federal legislation developed to address the nation's chronic housing shortage. The competition for low income housing has become fierce. During the Reagan era there was a 75 percent cutback in funds for low income housing.

[46]Anthony Warnes and Maureen Crane, *Meeting Homeless Peoples' Needs* (London, 2000). It is the only shelter in the city specifically for elder persons and it targets those who have been abused, neglected, exploited or displaced. The residents stay, on average, three months, and the 24/7 staff works with them to restore independent living skills.

[47]Ibid., 99.

[48]Ibid., 101. Each resident has his or her own bedroom, toilet and verandah centered around a lounge room. All of the buildings are set in beautiful landscaped gardens, one feature being a fishpond. In addition, there is a centrally located facility called the 'shed,' with an adjacent barbecue area. Moving from night shelters or sleeping outside to private room apartments with fully equipped kitchens, stocked refrigerators, heating, carpets and in-suite showers can be jarring.

[49]Erin McClam, "NYC Looks at Retired Cruise Ships as Shelters," *Times-Picayune*, November 16, 2002, A-12.

[50]Chuck Mueller, "Housing Cure for Homeless?" *The Sun*, April 11, 2002, 14. They are expected to cost $1,000 per inhabitant. This would be the first project of its kind in Senegal. About 90 percent of the material, including clay, sand and lime for cement slurry, would be available at the new town's site. The technology of this "Superadobe System" is an offshoot of space technology that the architect developed and presented to NASA in the late 1980s for lunar and Martian habitation in the twenty-first century. This prototype is rooted in traditional African housing—the ubiquitous hut. The houses are expected to cost about 50 percent less

than the houses of similar standard built by other methods. Better housing is a pressing need in Senegal, especially after periodic floods, which devastate the country.

[51]Tom Boland, "Shelter Design: Homeless People Judge UCLA Student Architecture," *Los Angeles Times*, April 23, 1999, 22-23.

[52]Robert Kronenburg, *Houses in Motion: The Genesis, History and Development of the Portable Building* (London, 1995).

[53]Portable Building Research Unit, *Portable Architecture Conference and Symposium* (Liverpool, 1997).

[54]International Red Cross Report, *Response Preparedness in Bangladesh*, available online, http://www.ifrc.org.html, accessed December 12, 2002. Also see International Red Cross report, *Principles of Disaster Mitigation in Health Facilities: Preparedness and Relief Coordination* (New York, 2000).

[55]Cameron Sinclair, *Architecture for Humanity: Building a Better World: Mobile HIV/AIDS Health Clinic Design*, Architecture for Humanity, available online, http://www.architecturefor humanity.org, accessed December 12, 2002.

[56]Peter Duby, "Flood Adaptive Housing in Bangladesh," available online, http://www.archnet.org.html, accessed December 12, 2002.

[57]Mary C. Comerio, *Disaster Hits Home: New Policy for Urban Housing Recovery* (Berkeley, 1998).

[58]Andres Duany, Elizabeth Plater-Zyberk, and Jeff Speck, *Suburban Nation: The Rise of Sprawl and the Decline of the American Dream* (Boston, 2002). Duany, et al. argue that suburban sprawl, now the standard North American pattern of growth, ignores historical precedent and human experience.

[59]Ibid., 15.

[60]Ibid., 5. The authors list the five main components of sprawl. These are housing subdivisions, shopping centers, office parks, civic institutions, and roadways.

[61]Peter Calthorpe, *The Next American Metropolis: Ecology, Community, and the American Dream* (New York, 1993). Since the 1990s, sprawl has been linked with numerous deleterious public health outcomes. These include acts of road rage among weary, stressed commuters, the isolation and alienation of elderly persons, and the poor, who are stranded without access to public transit because they can't afford an auto.

[62]Dave Benjamin, "Hopefuls Cite Preservation of Open Space as Key Issue," *News Transcript*, available online, http://www.newstranscript.gmnews.com.html, accessed March 15, 2003.

[63]David Brooks, "For Democrats, Time to Meet the Exurban Voter," *New York Times*, November 10, 2002, WK-3. In reality, America has a long way to go if the results of the 2002 and 2004 elections are any indication. He writes: "Before 1980, only a quarter of all office space was in the suburbs. But about 70 percent of the office space created in the 1990s was in suburbia, and now 42 percent of all offices are located there. You have a tribe of people who don't live in cities, or commute to cities, or have any contact with urban life. Mesa,

Arizona, another quintessential exurb east of Phoenix, already has more people than St. Louis. Extrapolate out a few years, and some of these sprawling suburbs will have political clout equal to Chicago's . . . ex-urban voters are not, by and large, ideological conservatives. But many of them have recently left inner-ring suburbs they found too congested . . . you find a pretty consistent set of priorities, which can be summarized with the motto: More Highways, Less Growth."

[64]Jim Hopkins, "Wal-Mart's Influence Grows," *USA Today*, January 29, 2003, B-1-2. Wal-Mart alone accounted for as much as 25 percent of U.S. productivity gains from 1995-99. With 1.3 million workers, it is now the world's largest private employer, employing one of every 123 U.S. workers and nearly one of every twenty retail employees.

[65]Michael D. Kinerk and Dennis W. Wilhelm, *Popcorn Palaces: The Art Deco Movie Theatre Paintings of Davis Cone* (New York, 2001).

[66]Karen Stoner, "Lake Theatre an Oak Park Gem," *Chicago Tribune*, July 5, 2002, 7-A.

[67]Michael A. Tomlan, "Preservation Education: In Service to the Community," *Community Resource Management* 3 (1998): 3-4.

[68]Anthony M. Tung, *Preserving the World's Great Cities: The Destruction and Renewal of the Historic Metropolis* (New York, 2001).

[69]Ben Tuxworth, "Sit Still while I Empower You . . . ," *Green Futures*, 35 (July/August 2002): 14. Community development professionals have known for many years that in order to compassionately engage with disadvantaged groups one must first address the preexistent power imbalances and status hierarchies.

[70]Douglas Jehl, "Parched Santa Fe Makes Rare Demand on Builders," *New York Times*, November 3, 2002; National Report, 14. In every new home a contractor builds, they must first install, without charge, eight to twelve new high-efficiency toilets in existing homes, hotels, and shops.

[71]Martha Carr, "Developers Float Water Park Idea to Jefferson Officials," *Times-Picayune*, January 30, 2003, B-2.

[72]Andrea Oppenheimer Dean and Timothy Hursley, *Rural Studio: Samuel Mockbee and Architecture of Decency* (New York, 2002). Also see Brian Bell, ed., *Good Deeds, Good Design: Community Service Through Architecture* (New York, 2004).

[73]Ibid., 1.

[74]Ibid., 3.

[75]Ibid., 126.

[76]Stephen Verderber, "Compassionism and the Design Studio in the Aftermath of 9/11," *Journal of Architectural Education*, 56 (February 2003): 48-62. This author initiated a rapid response design studio at Tulane University in 2001, in direct response to the events of 9/11. Studio projects completed to date include prototypes for transportable medical facilities for rapid deployment globally in the aftermath of natural or man made disasters, i.e. hurricanes, earth-

quakes, and bioterrorism. Also see Stephen Verderber, "Architecture for Health—2050: An International Perspective," *Journal of Architecture* 8 (Autumn 2003): 281-304.

[77]Sarah Williams Goldhagen, "Our Degraded Public Realm: The Multiple Failures of Architecture Education," *Chronicle of Higher Education* (January 10, 2003): 5.

[78]Ibid., 6.

[79]Ibid., 9.

[80]Benjamin R. Barber, *A Place for Us: How to Make Society Civil and Democracy Strong* (New York, 1998).

[81]Morris Berman, *The Twilight of American Culture* (New York, 2000).

[82]George Will, "Greenspan Oversees Changed Economy," *Washington Post*, January 10, 2000, C-8.

[83]Harry S. Dent, Jr., *The Roaring 2000s Investor: Strategies for the Life You Want* (New York, 1999), 135.

[84]Ibid., 136.

[85]Larry Dossey, *Beyond Mind-Body to a New Era of Healing* (San Francisco, 1999), 18-27, 196-98.

[86]Gerard F. Anderson, Uwe E. Reinhardt, Peter S. Hussey, and Varduhi Petrosyan, "It's the Prices, Stupid: Why the United States is so Different from Other Countries," *Health Affairs* 22 (2003): 89-105.

[87]Sara Carmel and Seymore M. Glick, "Compassionate-Empathic Physicians: Personality Traits and Social Organizational Factors that Balance or Inhibit This Behavior Pattern," *Social Science and Medicine* 43 (1996): 1253-61.

[88]Margaret B. Heldring, "Collaborative Family Healthcare: Community and Compassion," *Families, Systems, and Health* 15 (1997): 333-36.

[89]Betty K. Cheng, "Cultural Clash Between Providers of Majority Culture and Patients of Chinese Culture," *Journal of Long Term Home Health Care* 16 (1997): 39-43.

[90]Robert Wuthnow, *Acts of Compassion: Caring for Others and Helping Ourselves* (Princeton, N.J., 1991). Also Gregory L. Fricchione, "Illness and the Origin of Caring," *Journal of Medical Humanities* 14 (1993): 15-21.

[91]Philip Cushman, *Constructing the Self, Constructing America* (New York, 1995). Also Lindsay Prior, "Cruel Compassion: Psychiatric Control of Society's Unwanted," *Science, Technology and Human Values* 20 (1995): 269-70.

[92]Stefani Ledewitz, "Community Design: Creating a Public Architecture," in Robert Burgess, ed., *Community Design* (New York, 1998), 49-60.

[93]Jim Murphy, "Health and Packaging," *Progressive Architecture* (July 1976): 46-50.

[94]Stanford Anderson, "Postscript: Regrounding Architecture," in Malcolm Quantrill and Bruce Webb, eds., *Constancy and Change in Architecture* (College Station, 1991).

[95]Ben J. Refuerzo and Stephen Verderber, "Effects of Personal Status and Patterns of Use on Residential Satisfaction in Shelters for Victims of Domestic Violence," *Environment and Behavior* 21 (1990): 413-34; Refuerzo and Verderber, "Dimensions of Person-Environment Relationships in Shelters for Victims of Domestic Violence," *Journal of Architectural and Planning Research* 7 (1990): 33-52. Also, Refuerzo and Verderber, "In Support of a New Life: A Shelter for Victims of Domestic Violence," *Journal of Architectural and Planning Research* 10 (1993): 40-58; and Stephen Verderber, "Recent Trends in the Design of Shelters for Victims of Domestic Violence," *Loyola Law Review* 47 (2001): 457-70.

[96]C. Richard Hatch, ed., *The Scope of Social Architecture* (New York, 1984).

[97] Robert Ivy, "It's in the Air," *Architectural Record* 96 (May 2005), 2. This article was posted on the ArchVoices web site along with additional background information, available online, http://www.archvoices.org, accessed May 15, 2005. These organizations include Architects/ Designers/Planners for Social Responsibility, Architects Without Borders, Architecture for Humanity, Association for Community Design, Design Coprs, Habitat for Humanity International, Public Architecture, and Rebuilding Together. Post-graduate service fellowships are available through Americorps, Blue Moon Urban Fellowship, Peace Corps, and Rose Architectural Fellowship program. The web site addresses for these organizations are provided in this same issue of *ArchVoices*. This is precisely the type of activity Ernest Boyer and Lee Mitgang called for in their seminal report on the status of architectural education and practice in the 1990s, entitled *Building Community: A New Future for Architecture Education and Practice* (Princeton, 1996).

[98]Thomas A. Markus, *Buildings and Power: Freedom and Control in the Origin of Modern Building Types* (London and New York, 1993).

Notes to Appendix A

[1]John Wilds, Charles L. Dufour and Walter G. Cowan, *Louisiana, Yesterday and Today: A Historical Guide to the State* (Baton Rouge and London, 1996), 84.

[2]Ibid., 85-87.

[3]Barbara Cole, *Parish Health Units in Louisiana*, unpublished report, March 2000. Much of the information incorporated in this report was culled from the Biennial Reports of the Louisiana State Board of Health, housed in the State Archives in Baton Rouge. Also see Gordon E. Gillson, *Louisiana State Board of Health—The Progressive Years* (Baton Rouge, 1993), and Virgil L. Mitchell, *The Civil Works Administration in Louisiana: A Study in New Deal Relief, 1933-1934*, USL History Series 7 (Lafayette, LA, 1976).

[4]Cole, *Parish Health Units in Louisiana*, 2. These five parishes were Natchitoches, on June 1, 1921, DeSoto, on July 1, 1921, Beauregard, on August 15, 1921, Caddo, on September 1, 1921, and Ouachita, on September 15, 1921. Each of these parish health units was provided in 1921 with an operating budget of $10,000. The money was from the following sources: $5,000

from the police jury, $2,500 from the State Board of Health, and $2,500 from the Rockefeller Foundation. Each health unit had the authority to employ four full-time staff members: the director ($3,000 annual salary), one public health nurse ($1,800 annual salary), one sanitary inspector ($1,800 annual salary), and one clerical assistant ($600 annual salary). Later in 1921 a health unit in Washington Parish (Bogalusa) began full-time operation.

[5]Ibid., 5. These new clinics were in the following parishes: Calcasieu (1915), Rapides (1918), Tangipahoa (1923), Claiborne (1924), Lafourche, St. Mary, Webster, Plaquemines (1925).

[6]Ibid., 4.

[7]Ibid., 5.

[8]Ibid., 6. In the seven states where the worst flooding occurred, seventy-four full-time parish-county health units were established within a year.

[9]Ibid., 6.

[10]This group of personnel consisted of forty-four non-medical persons, fourteen physicians, eight nurses, and twenty-two sanitary inspectors. The first of the new health units to open under this cooperative agreement was in Morehouse Parish (August 27, 1927). Before the end of the year eleven new ones would open, with two others (Lafourche and St. Mary) reorganized to conform to the new model of care. These parishes were: Morehouse, St. Martin, Richland, Lafayette, Assumption, Caldwell, Concordia, LaSalle, Madison, Lafourche, St. Mary, Tensas, and Avoyelles. The combined first year annual fiscal budget for these thirteen facilities was $121,400 (Cole, *Parish Health Units in Louisiana*, 6). An excellent account of the flood and its aftermath is provided in John M. Barry's book *Rising Tide: The Great Mississippi Flood of 1927 and How it Changed America* (New York, 1997).

[11]In 1928 alone nine new health units opened. These were in the following parishes: Catahoula, East Carroll, Franklin, Iberia, St. Landry, West Carroll, Iberville, Terrebonne, and Pointe Coupée. Cole, *Parish Health Units in Louisiana*, 8.

[12]These twelve new facilities were opened in the following parishes: Evangeline (1931), Red River (1934), Acadia (1935), Jefferson Davis (1935), Bienville (1936), Union (1936), Bossier (1937), Vermilion (1937), St. Charles (1938), Vernon (1938), St. Tammany (1939), and Allen (1939). Ibid., 10.

[13]These eight new facilities were opened in the following parishes: Evangeline (number 2, 1940), Grant (1940), Jackson (1940), Vernon (1940), Winn (1940), Ascension (1941), Beauregard (1941), and East Baton Rouge (1941). Ibid., 11.

[14]Construction funds for new facilities in nineteen towns were obtained. Cities received as much as $100,000, smaller towns which also served as parish seats received on average $30,000 in construction funds, and small towns received on average $5,000. Ibid., 12.

[15]These five parishes were Sabine, St. James, Calcasieu, Cameron, and Jefferson. Ibid., 9.

Illustration Credits

Stephen Verderber (photos)—Figs. 1.1, 1.3, 1.4, 1.10. 1.14, 2.1, 2.13, 3.2, 3.7, 3.13-3.15, 4.1, 4.5-4.8, 5.1, 5.2, 5.5-5.14, 5.17-5.20, 5.22, 5.27, 5.32, 5.33, 5.52, 5.55, 5.60, 5.61, 5.63, 7.8

Francisco J. Arens/Ott Gira/Christopher Roth (drawings)—Figs. 1.5-1.8, 1.11-1.13, 2.2, 2.14, 3.1, 3.3, 3.6, 3.8, 3.11, 3.12, 4.2-4.4, 6.2, 6.7

Courtesy of the Morehouse Parish Health Unit (photo archive)—Figs. 1.9, 2.3 2.4, 3.9, 3.10

Jessica Gramcko (photos)—Figs. 1.2, 2.15, 5.28, 5.29, 5.34, 5.51, 5.53, 5.54, 5.58, 5.59, 5.64, 7.2, 7.3, 7.5, 7.6

Courtesy of the Beauregard Parish Health Unit (photo archive)—Figs. 2.5, 2.6, 2.12

Courtesy, E.T. Archive, London—Figs. 2.7, 2.9, 2.10

Courtesy of the Wellcome Institute Library, London—Fig. 2.8

Courtesy, Bridgeman Art Library, London—Fig. 2.11

Courtesy, Estate of M.C. Escher (engraving)—Fig. 2.16

Stephen Verderber/Victoria Yee/Jessica Gramcko (drawings)—Figs. 5.3, 5.4, 5.15, 5.16, 5.30, 5.31, 5.35-5.36

Ava Brucato/Jessica Gramcko (drawings)—Fig. 5.25, 5.26

Courtesy of Tensas Parish Historical Society (archive illustration)—Fig. 5.21

Courtesy, The Mariners' Museum Archive (illustration)—Fig. 5.23

Courtesy Library of Congress (illustration)—Fig. 5.24

Julia Ford/Claudia Foronda (graphics)—Figs. 5.37-5.44

L.H. Morgan (illustration, 1881)—Fig. 5.45

Courtesy, Santa Barbara Museum of Natural History (E.S. Curtis: photo)—Fig. 5.46

Courtesy, Peabody Museum, Harvard University (H. Burger: photo)—Fig. 5.47

Courtesy of the Smithsonian Institution, National Anthropological Archives (photo)—Fig. 5.48

Courtesy of Louisiana State University Special Collections, Hill Memorial Library (map illustration)—Fig. 5.62

Stephen Verderber (Romy Diaz/Jessica Gramcko: graphics)—Figs. 5.65-5.73

Stephen Verderber (Jessica Gramcko: graphics)—Figs. 5.74-5.76

Ian Lambot (photo)—Fig. 7.1

Courtesy, Progressive Architecture magazine (photo)—Fig. 7.4

Timothy Hursley (photo)—Fig. 7.7

INDEX